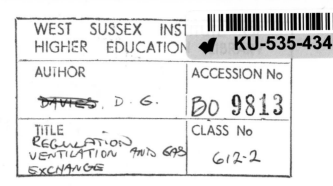
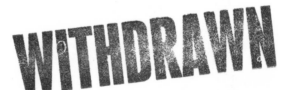

Regulation of Ventilation and Gas Exchange

Research Topics in Physiology

Charles D. Barnes, *Editor*
Department of Physiology
Texas Tech University School of Medicine
Lubbock, Texas

1. Donald G. Davies and Charles D. Barnes (Editors). Regulation
   of Ventilation and Gas Exchange, 1978

Regulation of Ventilation and Gas Exchange

Edited by

DONALD G. DAVIES
CHARLES D. BARNES

Department of Physiology
Texas Tech University School of Medicine
Lubbock, Texas

ACADEMIC PRESS
New York   San Francisco   London   1978
A Subsidiary of Harcourt Brace Jovanovich, Publishers

ACADEMIC PRESS, INC.
111 Fifth Avenue, New York, New York 10003

United Kingdom Edition published by
ACADEMIC PRESS, INC. (LONDON) LTD.
24/28 Oval Road, London NW1   7DX

Library of Congress Cataloging in Publication Data

Main entry under title:

Regulation of ventilation and gas exchange.

    (Research topics in physiology ; 1   )
    Includes bibliographies.
    1.   Respiration––Regulation.   2.   Blood gases.
3.   Ventilation–perfusion ratio.   I.   Davies, Donald G.
II.   Barnes, Charles D.   III.   Series.
QP121.R4   596'.01'2   78–3332
ISBN   0–12–204650–1

CONTENTS

LIST OF CONTRIBUTORS

Numbers in parentheses indicate the pages on which the authors' contributions begin.

ROBERT A. BERKMAN (69), Departments of Physiology and Medicine, Albany Medical College, Albany, New York 12208

B. BURNS (197), Departments of Medicine (Respiratory Division) and Environmental Health Sciences, The Johns Hopkins Medical Institutions, Baltimore, Maryland 21205

DONALD G. DAVIES (167), Department of Physiology, Texas Tech University School of Medicine, Lubbock, Texas 79409

ROBERT E. DUTTON (69), Departments of Physiology and Medicine, Albany Medical College, Albany, New York 12208

G. H. GURTNER (197), Departments of Medicine (Respiratory Division) and Environmental Health Sciences, The Johns Hopkins Medical Institutions, Baltimore, Maryland 21205

J. HILDEBRANDT (261), Virginia Mason Research Center, Seattle, Washington 98101

DONALD C. JACKSON (93), Division of Biology and Medicine, Brown University, Providence, Rhode Island 02912

SANFORD LEVINE (31), Cardiovascular-Pulmonary Division, Department of Medicine, University of Pennsylvania, Veterans Administration Hospital, Philadelphia, Pennsylvania 19104

C. J. MENDOZA (197), Departments of Medicine (Respiratory Division) and Environmental Health Sciences, The Johns Hopkins Medical Institutions, Baltimore, Maryland 21205

JOHN OREM (131), Department of Physiology, Texas Tech University School of Medicine, Lubbock, Texas 79409

H. H. PEAVY (197), Departments of Medicine (Respiratory Division) and Environmental Health Sciences, The Johns Hopkins Medical Institutions, Baltimore, Maryland 21205

WALTER M. ST. JOHN (1), Department of Physiology, Dartmouth Medical School, Hanover, New Hampshire 03744

A. M. SCIUTO (197), Departments of Medicine (Respiratory Division) and Environmental Health Sciences, The Johns Hopkins Medical Institutions, Baltimore, Maryland 21205

W. SUMMER (197), Departments of Medicine (Respiratory Division) and Environmental Health Sciences, The Johns Hopkins Medical Institutions, Baltimore, Maryland 21205

R. J. TRAYSTMAN (197), Departments of Medicine (Respiratory Division) and Environmental Health Sciences, The Johns Hopkins Medical Institutions, Baltimore, Maryland 21205

PETER D. WAGNER (217), Department of Medicine, University of California–San Diego, San Diego, California 92117

PREFACE

For a number of years the Department of Physiology at Texas Tech University School of Medicine has conducted an annual seminar series designed around a specific topic with invited lectures from leading researchers in the area. The criteria for selecting the topic is that the subject be in a research area which is undergoing rapid development and from which further development can be expected, with the further proviso that a recent review at an advanced comprehensive level is not available in the topic area at the present time.

The overwhelming success of the seminar has generated the idea of formalizing each topic into a published volume. "Regulation of Ventilation and Gas Exchange," the first volume in the series, presents an in-depth view of several specialized areas of research in respiratory physiology that are currently in a state of expansion. Eminent investigators in discrete areas of respiratory physiology were asked to review their own work and place it in perspective. They were charged with presenting the historical basis and theory from which their particular research interest originated, the current status of the field, and directions for future research. Special emphasis was placed on critical evaluation of the experimental data in each scientist's research area.

The regulation of ventilation and gas exchange have been covered in a comprehensive manner; at the same time, however, due to the plenitude of information in this area, specific subtopics are treated in depth as individual chapters. The first five chapters are devoted to the regulation of ventilation. The presentation begins with a unique view of the neural elements which modify and/or are intrinsic to the respiratory rhythm. The next two chapters deal with the contribution of metabolic factors in the control of ventilation: the importance of metabolic factors during muscular exercise and the specific role of ammonia in respiratory regulation are evaluated. A view of ventilatory control from a comparative standpoint, stressing both adaptive and mechanistic phenomena, is presented in the following chapter. The remaining chapter describes the newly emerging and important area of the regulation of breathing during sleep.

Chapter 6 bridges the subjects of ventilatory regulation and gas exchange, discussing the current hypotheses for the regulation of cerebral extracellular fluid acid–base composition and its role in the control of ventilation and cerebral blood flow.

The next two chapters deal specifically with gas exchange. The evidence for carrier-mediated transport of respiratory gases is updated, and an in-depth presentation of the current theoretical and experimental aspects of the multiple inert gas technique for the measurement of ventilation–perfusion ratios is presented. The last chapter addresses both the historical development of the current concepts of the function and properties of surfactant and current research activity in the area.

This volume is designed not only for respiratory physiologists but for students and researchers in other areas with an inclination toward respiratory physiology. It is the hope of the Editors that this book will be provocative and stimulate future research in respiratory physiology.

Donald G. Davies
Charles D. Barnes

CHAPTER 1

Central Nervous System
Regulation of Ventilation

WALTER M. ST. JOHN

I. INTRODUCTION

Two interrelated phenomena are intrinsic to any discussion of the neural mechanisms controlling ventilation: the neurogenesis of respiratory rhythmicity per se, and the neural modulation of this basic respiratory rhythm. In this context, a large quantity of information is available concerning both the role of various neural elements in potentially modifying the respiratory rhythm and the manner in which various neural elements are integrated into the respiratory rhythm. However, those

1

Regulation of Ventilation and Gas Exchange
Copyright © 1978 by Academic Press, Inc.
All rights of reproduction in any form reserved.
ISBN 0-12-204650-1

neurophysiological processes responsible for the genesis of the respiratory rhythm are, at present, largely undefined. Therefore, the main focus of the present discussion will be a consideration of those neural elements which modify and/or are intrinsic to the respiratory rhythm.* The reader is referred to several recent reviews (Cohen, 1970; Mitchell and Berger, 1975) which deal both theoretically and experimentally with those processes which may be responsible for the neurogenesis of respiration.

II. BRAINSTEM RESPIRATORY CENTERS

A. General Categorization

It has long been recognized that, if, in an anesthetized animal, the entire neocortex, cerebellum, and precollicular brainstem are removed, the pattern of ventilation is not markedly altered (see, e.g., Lumsden, 1923; Tenney and Ou, 1977). The fact that an eupneic respiratory pattern can be maintained in an animal having only the caudal midbrain, pons, and medulla of the brain remaining intact does not mean that the other components of the brain do not exert a role in respiratory regulation. It is quite apparent that voluntary ventilation and changes in ventilation in animals exposed to warm environments, respectively, are dependent on neocortical and hypothalmic influences. Moreover, Tenney and Ou (1977) reported that both the diencephalon and the cerebrum exert important functions in the regulation of hypoxia-induced ventilatory alterations. Thus, it might be concluded that although the portion of the central nervous system caudal to the midbrain level is capable of supporting eupnea and may represent the site of primary importance for the control of "automatic" ventilation, the contribution of the telencephalon and diencephalon to overall ventilatory control may be appreciable.

If, in the experimental preparation with the midbrain transection, additional sequential transections of the brainstem are begun (see Lumsden, 1923; Wang *et al.*, 1957) (Fig. 1), it is found that subsequent to removal of the caudal midbrain and rostral pons, the respiratory pattern is changed in that the frequency of ventilation diminishes and the tidal volume augments slightly. The next major change in ventilation occurs when the brainstem is transected at the pontomedullary junction. Respiration is

---

* Symbols used in this chapter: Alveolar partial pressures of carbon dioxide ($P_{A_{CO_2}}$) and oxygen ($P_{A_{O_2}}$), arterial partial pressures of carbon dioxide (Pa_{CO_2}), and oxygen (Pa_{O_2}), arterial pH pHa), dorsal medullary respiratory nucleus (DRN), duration of expiratory phase (T_E), duration of inspiratory phase (T_I), frequency (f), tidal volume (V_T), and ventral medullary respiratory nucleus (VRN).

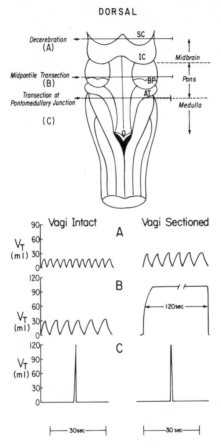

Figure 1. Ventilatory patterns obtained subsequent to (A) intercollicular decerebration, (B) transection of the brainstem at a midpontile level, and (C) transection at the pontomedullary junction in cats having intact vagal nerves (left-hand side) or bilateral vagal section (right-hand side). See Section II,A of text for full discussion.

now usually characterized by infrequent excursions which, when they occur, are of great magnitude and very minimal durations (see pages 12–15). This latter ventilatory pattern is termed *gasping*. Finally, if a transection is performed at the first cervical level of the spinal cord, expiratory apnea is obtained.

If the above sequence of brainstem transections is repeated in an experimental animal having bilateral vagal section (see Fig. 1), some strikingly different results are obtained (see e.g., Lumsden, 1923; Wang *et al.*, 1957). Thus, subsequent to the midpontile transection in the vagotomized animal, respiration changes to a pattern marked by very large increases both in tidal volume and in the duration of the inspiratory phase. This pattern of respiration is termed *inspiratory apnea* or *apneusis*. During apneusis, the tidal volume of the cat typically exceeds 100 ml and the inspiratory duration is often in excess of 120 seconds (see e.g., St. John and Wang, 1977b). These values of tidal volume and inspiratory duration are in contrast to those of the vagotomized cat having a midcollicular transection. In the latter preparation, V_T is typically about 25 ml and T_I is approximately 1.0–2.5 seconds (W. M. St. John, unpublished observations). Continuing the brainstem transections, it is found that the depth and duration of apneusis decreases in direct proportion to the quantity of caudal pons ablated until, subsequent to a transection at the pontomedullary junction, gasping is again usually obtained.

As the result of these transection experiments, three major respiratory centers were designated by Lumsden (1923) within the brainstem. The area of the caudal pons responsible for apneusis generation in the vagotomized animal having a midpontile transection is termed the *apneustic center*. In the rostral pons, the structure preventing apneusis in the vagotomized animal is termed the *pneumotaxic center*. Finally, the area of the medulla responsible for gasping has been designated as the *medullary respiratory center*. It was noted above that, subsequent to the brainstem transections, the patterns of ventilation differ depending upon whether the vagi are intact or sectioned. Therefore, there must be feedback connections from the vagal system to the brainstem. At present, such vagal afferent input has been experimentally demonstrated only upon medullary sites (see Section II,C,3 below). However, indirect evidence suggests that vagal afferent influences are also distributed to the apneustic center (Wang *et al.*, 1957) and possibly also to the pneumotaxic center (Feldman *et al.*, 1976) (see Fig. 1).

B.   Respiratory-Modulated Units within the Brainstem

Single units, whose pattern of activity is linked to some portion of the respiratory cycle, can be localized throughout the pons and medulla of cats (Batsel, 1964, 1965; Bertrand and Hugelin, 1971; Bertrand *et al.*, 1973, 1974; Bianchi, 1971; Bianchi and Barillot, 1975; Burns and Salmoiraghi, 1960; Cohen, 1968, 1969, 1970, 1971, 1974; Cohen and Wang, 1959; Feldman *et al.*, 1976; Haber *et al.*, 1957; Hassen *et al.*, 1976; Hilaire and Monteau, 1975, 1976; Hildebrandt, 1974; Hugelin and Bertrand, 1973; Hukuhara, 1973; Kahn and Wang, 1967; Merrill, 1974; Mitchell and Berger, 1975; Mitchell and Herbert, 1974; Nesland *et al.*, 1966; Richter *et al.*, 1975; St. John and Wang, 1977a; Salmoiraghi and Burns, 1960a,b;

Vibert *et al.*, 1976a,b; von Baumgarten and Kanzow, 1958; von Baumgarten *et al.*, 1957; von Euler *et al.*, 1973a,b; Wyman, 1977). These respiratory-modulated units have been classified (Fig. 2) as (a) inspiratory, having a phasic discharge pattern linked to the inspiratory phase; (b) expiratory, in which the phasic discharge occurs during expiration; and (c) phase-spanning, whose activity is not exclusively limited to either the inspiratory or expiratory phases but rather "spans" a portion of both respiratory phases. These latter phase-spanning units, in contrast to inspiratory or expiratory neurons, may exhibit either phasic or tonic patterns of activity. The activity of tonic phase-spanning units is characterized by an increase in discharge frequency during one portion of the respiratory cycle. This categorization of brainstem respiratory neuronal types may be further amplified by definition of that portion of the respiratory cycle during which the phasic units discharge. Thus, for example, expiratory units have been designated as "early," "late," or "all" depending on whether their discharge occurs during the beginning, end, or throughout the expiratory phase (see Fig. 2). In a similar fashion, the discharge pattern of phase-spanning units have been designated as inspiratory–expiratory (I–E) or expiratory–inspiratory (E–I) depending on those portions of the respiratory cycle during which their discharge commences and ceases.

Although phasic inspiratory and expiratory units and phase-spanning units can be localized throughout the pons and medulla, most inves-

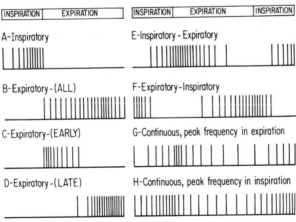

Figure 2. Schematic representation of the major discharge patterns of respiratory units. Phasic inspiratory (A) and expiratory (B–D) unit discharges are illustrated in the left-hand side, whereas the right-hand side illustrates phasic phase-spanning units (E–F) and tonic phase-spanning units (G–H). (Redrawn from Cohen, 1968, by permission of the author and publisher.)

tigators have noted that inspiratory and expiratory units are predominant in the medulla, whereas phase-spanning units represent the predominant population of respiratory units in pons (see, e.g., Cohen and Wang, 1959; Kahn and Wang, 1967; Hassen *et al.*, 1976). In this latter context, however, Vibert *et al.* (1976a,b), on the basis of a computer analysis of the temporal discharge pattern of a very large number of pontile units, have reported that, exclusive of the pneumotaxic center, the probability of observing phase-spanning units in pons is quite low. These authors have further concluded that "no evidence can be provided to support the existence of definite phase-spanning populations in the brainstem caudal to the pneumotaxic center." This conclusion of Vibert *et al.* should not be taken as evidence that phase-spanning units do not exist. Rather, these results may imply that, statistically, phase-spanning respiratory units can be envisaged as a continuum of the inspiratory or expiratory neuronal populations.

It is well documented (see, e.g., Karczewski, 1973; Severinghaus and Larson, 1965) that the presence of anesthesia may profoundly alter the behavior of the respiratory control system. This statement critically applies to studies concerned with brainstem respiratory neuronal activity. Thus, while respiratory-modulated units can be localized in both the pons and the medulla of "unanesthetized" (i.e., decerebrate, encephale isolé) cats, respiratory units can only be found in the medulla of animals anesthetized with barbiturates. The profound effects of barbiturates on pontile respiratory unit activities has been demonstrated by Hukuhara (1973). This investigator recorded simultaneously from a pontile and a medullary respiratory unit in an unanesthetized cat and noted that, subsequent to administration of only 1–5 mg of pentobarbitone, the pontile unit lost its respiratory periodicity while the medullary unit continued periodic respiratory-linked discharges. Similar differential changes in pontile and medullary unit activities have been noted subsequent to morphine administration (Hassen *et al.*, 1976). Whether other anesthetic types similarly alter the activity of pontile respiratory units has not been defined at present.

C. Functions of the Brainstem Respiratory Centers in Ventilatory Control

1. Caudal Midbrain, Rostral Pons, and the Pneumotaxic Center

For a considerable period, investigators attempted to localize the pneumotaxic center to a specific rostral pontile or midbrain locus (Fig. 3).

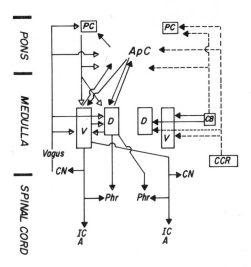

Figure 3. Interconnections between the brainstem respiratory centers and the major afferent and efferent projections to and from these centers. At the left, solid lines indicate pathways which have been established or proposed based on experimental observations, interconnecting the pneumotaxic center (PC), apneustic center (ApC), and the dorsal (D) and ventral (V) medullary respiratory nuclei. Proposed vagal afferent inputs to these brainstem centers are also shown. The efferent projections, both ipsilateral and contralateral, from D and V to cranial (CN), abdominal (A), intercostal (IC) and phrenic (Phr) respiratory motoneurons are illustrated on the left-hand side. At the right, possible afferent inputs from the central chemoreceptors (CCR) and carotid body (CB) peripheral chemoreceptors are illustrated. Solid lines indicate pathways defined from experimental observations; dashed lines indicate possible pathways for which no experimental support is yet available. Terminations which are primarily excitatory to respiratory unit activity are shown by solid arrows, open arrows designate inhibitory terminations, and half-solid arrows are for terminations which may be excitatory or inhibitory. Note that no assumption as to the number of synapses between various sites is implied in the figure.

At various times, such structures as the red nucleus (Henderson and Sweet, 1929), the inferior colliculus (Marckwald, 1888), and the locus coeruleus (Johnson and Russell, 1952) were considered the site of the pneumotaxic center. One important method by which the pneumotaxic center was definitively localized at a site in the rostral pontile tegmentum and by which more information was obtained concerning the function of this structure in ventilatory control was through the use of electrical stimulation. These studies (see, e.g., Bertrand and Hugelin, 1971; Cohen, 1971) led to the interesting and important observation that stimuli delivered at appropriate sites in the rostral pons provoke a "phase-switch" of the respiratory cycle (Fig. 4). Thus, stimuli delivered at dorsal sites in the rostral pontile tegmentum caused a premature inspiration, whereas

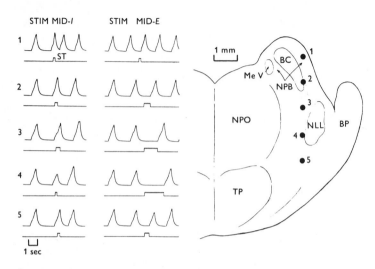

Figure 4. Phase-switching of the respiratory cycle resulting from electrical stimulation of the region of the pneumotaxic center. The effects on the respiratory cycle and integrated phrenic discharge of stimulus trains (ST) delivered during midinspiration and midexpiration to each of five points in the rostral pons (right-hand side) are illustrated. Abbreviations: BC, brachium conjunctivum; BP, brachium pontis; MeV, mesencephalic root of Vth nerve; NLL, nucleus of lateral lemniscus; NPB, nucleus parabrachialis; NPO, nucleus pontis oralis; and TP, pyramidal tract. (From Cohen, 1971, p. 138, by permission of the author and the publisher. See this original article for description of stimulus parameters.)

stimuli delivered at ventral sites resulted in a premature expiration. Also, it has been found that the placement of extremely small lesions within the area of stimulation, most critically within the dorsal region, results in apneusis in vagotomized cats. As the result of all these studies, the pneumotaxic center is presently considered as synonymous with the nucleus parabrachialis medialis complex of the rostral pontile tegmentum. According to Bertrand *et al.* (1973), this nucleus parabrachialis medialis complex includes the nucleus parabrachialis as well as the adjacent region of the anterior part of the brachium conjunctivum and the Kölliker–Fuse nucleus.

On the basis of ablation studies, Pitts *et al.* (1939) have concluded that those pathways interconnecting the pneumotaxic center with more caudal respiratory areas lie in the ventral part of the lateral tegmentum, ventral and slightly lateral to the descending root of the trigeminal nerve. In seeming confirmation of this early work of Pitts, Hugelin and his colleagues have found that the placement of small unilateral lesions in that lateral tegmentum of the rostral pons, in the ventrolateral portion of the rostral medulla, or in various sites in the caudal medulla results in an immediate but not persistent apneusis in unanesthetized cats (A. Hugelin, personal communication). Other studies (Cohen, 1971) based on recordings of respiratory unit activities within the brainstem have demonstrated that efferents from the pneumotaxic center are connected by a pathway having few synapses with the apneustic and medullary respiratory complexes.

Within the caudal midbrain and rostral pons, the greatest concentration of respiratory-modulated units are found within the nucleus parabrachialis medialis complex (Bertrand et al., 1973). Exclusive of this pneumotaxic center, respiratory-modulated units were located in the greatest concentration in the trigeminal nuclear complex and in the rostral pontile reticular formation. Three major types of respiratory units have been recorded within the pneumotaxic center: inspiratory (I), inspiratory–expiratory phase-spanning (I–E) and expiratory (E) (Bertrand et al., 1973, 1974). Through an elaborate and elegant analysis of the discharge pattern of these units and their anatomical location Bertrand and her colleagues have concluded that there is a wave of excitation which proceeds from I to I–E to E and back to I from E, at which point an inhibition of the I unit activity occurs. Thus, according to this model system, there is a recycling of activity within the pneumotaxic system. Activation of the pneumotaxic system is envisaged to occur either by extrinsic stimuli from other sites in the central and/or peripheral nervous system or, as Bertrand et al. hypothesize, by an intrinsic pacemaker generator within the pneumotaxic center.

As noted above, apneustic respiration is characteristic of anesthetized, decerebrate, or encéphale isolé animals in which bilateral pneumotaxic center ablation and vagal section have been performed acutely. However, if a temporal period of several weeks is allowed between the pneumotaxic center lesioning and vagal sections, rhythmic respiration, and not apneusis, characterizes the ventilatory pattern of the unanesthetized animal (Gautier and Bertrand, 1975; St. John et al., 1972). Reinstatement of general anesthesia in the chronic animal results in a reestablishment of apneusis (St. John et al., 1971, 1972). The implications of these studies are twofold: that other portions of the central nervous system may compensate for removal of the pneumotaxic mechanism, and that these compensatory mechanisms are suppressed by general anesthesia. In this same context, Webber and Peiss (1972; Webber, 1974) have demonstrated that in intact cats anesthetized with an intraperitoneal dose of 30 mg/kg of pentobarbital, administration of an additional intravenous dose of approximately 22 mg/kg of pentobarbital or 11 mg/kg of thiopental results in an alteration of ventilation from an eupneic to an apneustic pattern. In similarly prepared animals having bilateral vagal section, the intravenous dose of these barbiturates required to produce apneusis was significantly reduced (pentobarbital 7 mg/kg i.v., thiopental 3 mg/kg i.v.). Qualitatively similar results have been obtained by other investigators (St. John *et al.*, 1971). As a result of these studies, Webber and Peiss have concluded that, with respect to respiratory control, inhibitory mechanisms are more susceptible to barbiturate depression than are facilitatory ones. These results further reinforce the concept that the presence of general anesthesia may profoundly alter the functions of the brainstem respiratory controller.

2. Caudal Pons and the Apneustic Center

In contrast to the pneumotaxic center, an apneustic center has not been localized to a specific anatomical entity within the caudal pons. Indeed, in recent reports, Vibert *et al.* (1976a,b) were unable to demonstrate either a difference in the distribution of firing patterns between caudal pontile and medullary respiratory units or a clear anatomical separation between respiratory units of the pons and medulla. These results have led Vibert *et al.* to conclude that the designation of an apneustic center within the caudal pons may be inappropriate. These results of Vibert *et al.* stand in some contrast to those obtained with sequential brainstem transections, as noted above, or results obtained in studies involving electrical stimulation of the caudal pons. In these latter stimulation experiments, Ngai and Wang (1957) found that inspiratory spasms might be obtained by stimulation of structures extending from the rostral pons to the area of the trapezoid body. The effective sites for eliciting inspiratory spasms proceeded from lateral to medial as more rostral pontile sites were stimulated. The net result of all these studies might be a consideration of the apneustic center as a functional and not an anatomical entity within the caudal pons.

3. Medullary Respiratory Centers

Although in the decerebrate, encéphale isolé, or even anesthetized animal, respiratory-modulated units can be localized at diverse sites throughout the medulla, it is generally agreed (see Mitchell and Berger, 1975, for review) that these respiratory units are primarily concentrated into two major aggregates: an area, termed the *dorsal respiratory nucleus* (DRN), localized in approximation to the nucleus of the tractus solitarius and a site in approximation to the nucleus ambiguus and retroambiguus, termed the *ventral respiratory nucleus* (VRN). These two respiratory nuclei are of considerable interest in view of their position as the final integrative site within the brainstem respiratory controller. Within the ventral nucleus, both inspiratory and expiratory units can be located (see, e.g., Bianchi, 1971; Merrill, 1974; Mitchell and Berger, 1975). Studies, using antidromic activation of proposed efferents from the brainstem and/or cross-correlation analyses between medullary respiratory unit activities and activities in efferent nerves to respiratory muscles, have attempted to define the output connections of VRN units (Bianchi, 1971; Bianchi and Barillot, 1975; Hilaire and Monteau, 1976; Merrill, 1974). Efferent activity from the VRN is concluded to be distributed to abdominal, intercostal, and cranial respiratory motoneurons and also, to a considerable extent, to phrenic motoneurons. Additionally, a number of VRN units appear to have efferent connections which remain entirely within the brainstem (propriobulbar units). In this context, Merrill (1974) has presented evidence that the efferent fibers of a considerable number of inspiratory units within the nucleus retroambiguus, which ultimately terminate at thoracic levels, have collaterals which arborize to the phrenic nucleus. Merrill has concluded that these collaterals account for the entire distribution of ventral nucleus unit efferents to phrenic motoneurons; hence, there are no exclusive efferent connections from the VRN to phrenic motoneurons. These results of Merrill are in agreement with those of Hilaire and Monteau (1976), who further conclude that these connections between VRN units and phrenic or intercostal motoneurons are monosynaptic.

Since Breuer's description of the Hering–Breuer vagal reflex in 1868 (see Widdicombe, 1964), it has been recognized that overinflation of the lungs results in a marked prolongation of succeeding expiratory phase whereas, conversely, if the lungs are overdeflated, the succeeding inspiratory effort is temporally advanced and augmented in amplitude. In view of this Hering–Breuer reflex, it might be expected that lung inflation would result in an inhibition of inspiratory neuronal activity; indeed, such an inhibition has been observed for inspiratory bulbospinal units of the VRN (Bianchi and Barillot, 1975). Bulbospinal expiratory units within the VRN typically exhibited an augmentation of activity concomitant with lung inflations. In contrast to these results with bulbospinal units, most VRN inspiratory units, having efferent connections to the larynx, exhibited an increase in discharge concomitant with lung inflation, whereas most VRN expiratory laryngeal motoneurons were depressed by these inflations. A third group of VRN units are, as noted above, the so-called *propriobulbar* units. Approximately half of these propriobulbar units behaved as bulbospinal units in response to lung inflations; the remaining propriobulbar units responded as did the laryngeal units (Bianchi and Barillot, 1975).

Within the dorsal respiratory nucleus, inspiratory units have been grouped into two classes, depending on their response to lung inflation or vagal stimulation (von Baumgarten *et al.*, 1957; von Baumgarten and Kanzow, 1958). One group of inspiratory units, termed Rα, exhibited an inhibition of discharge concomitant with lung inflation, whereas the second group of inspiratory units, termed Rβ, showed an increase in discharge in response to lung inflations. Von Baumgarten and Kanzow (1958) have hypothesized that the Rα units might serve as efferents to spinal inspiratory motoneurons, whereas the Rβ units would be reflexly connected to the Hering–Breuer vagal mechanisms and would serve to inhibit the Rα unit activity. Support for this hypothesis has been derived from the work of von Euler *et al.* (1973a,b). These investigators found two groups of inspiratory units within the DRN: a group which responded to vagal stimulation but did not appear to have spinal efferents, and a group which did not respond to vagal stimulation but did have efferent connections in the contralateral spinal cord. Furthermore, Cohen *et al.* (1974) and Hilaire and Monteau (1976) have concluded that DRN units are connected monosynaptically with the contralateral phrenic motoneurons and disynaptically with the ipsilateral phrenic motoneurons. However, Hilaire and Monteau (1976) were unable to find any propriobulbar units within the dorsal nucleus. Such propriobulbar units, having their axons entirely within the medulla, would seemingly be required for the Rβ units described by von Baumgarten *et al.* (1957; von Baumgarten and Kanzow, 1958) and Euler *et al.* (1973a,b). The reason for this discrepancy in results is unclear. It must be noted, for completeness, that several authors have noted that the DRN consists entirely of inspiratory units (see, e.g., von Baumgarten *et al.*, 1957; von Baumgarten and Kanzow, 1958; von Euler *et al.*, 1973a,b). However, expiratory units have been demonstrated in the region of the nucleus tractus solitarius in the recent study of Vibert *et al.* (1976b). This difference in results may reflect the relatively greater number of respiratory units that Vibert *et al.* are capable of examining with their computer recognition technique.

   a.   Patterns of Respiration in the Medullary Preparation.   In his now classic paper in 1923, "Observations on the Respiratory Centres in the Cat," Lumsden noted that following section of the brainstem immediately caudal to the level of the striae acousticae, "rhythmic respirations continue, but both inspirations and expirations are more sudden in beginning and ending. They are a series of brief gasps. . . ." Despite this seemingly clear description of gasping and Fig. 2 of Lumsden's article, in which gasping is visually contrasted with the eupneic respiratory pattern of the decerebrate cat, there is still considerable confusion concerning the pattern of ventilation in the medullary animal. Part of this confusion may have arisen from interpretation of studies performed in the laboratories of Pitts *et al.* (1939; Pitts, 1946), Hoff and Breckenridge (1949; Breckenridge and Hoff, 1950), and Wang *et al.* (1957) from 1939 to 1957 which mainly emphasized the phenomenon of apneusis. In these studies, considerable discussion was devoted to the brainstem site (i.e., pontile or medullary) responsible for apneusis generation and to those procedures which would alter apneusis and restore a "normal" respiratory pattern. Hence, the observations that the respiratory pattern of the vagotomized animal having brainstem transections at the pontomedullary junction more closely approximated a normal ventilatory pattern than did the animal having a midpontile brainstem transection was emphasized. A further complicating factor in these studies may have arisen from the use of various species of experimental animals. Thus, in a 1949 report, Hoff and Breckenridge note that, in dogs having the brainstem transected at the pontomedullary junction, respiration was characterized by one of three patterns: (a) "regular, slow" (i.e., infrequent) "and complete inspirations and expirations, suggesting an all or nothing discharge with each inspiration" (i.e., gasping); (b) "respirations of lesser amplitude which vary in depth and interval" (an "ataxic" pattern, the most common type observed in the dog); and (c) Biot's breathing. In a 1950 report concerning the ventilatory pattern of the cat having the brainstem transected at the pontomedullary junction, Breckenridge and Hoff note that, although the ataxic pattern of respiration mentioned above was observed for some animals, "in almost all preparations, a type of respiration which Lumsden described as gasping" was obtained. Unfortunately, Hoff and Breckenridge do not consider the differences between the results obtained in dog and cat in their discussion of this work; rather, they emphasize the "rhythmic" character of the respiration in the medullary preparation.

In essential agreement with the work of Hoff and Breckenridge, Wang *et al.* (1957) note that when transections were made caudal to the trapezoid body in cats, "in a few animals, the respiratory movements appeared entirely normal but, in most instances, they were gasping." Similar results have been reported by Ngai (1957). Other investigators report only gasping following isolation of the medulla from the pons in cats (Brodie and Borison, 1956; Hukuhara *et al.*, 1951; Tang, 1967). However, in the 1967 study by Tang, it would appear that in his illustrations of ventilation in the medullary preparation, one ventilatory pattern resembles the ataxic pattern noted by Hoff and Breckenridge and the other pattern that of gasping respiration. Furthermore, in the doctoral dissertation which served as the basis for his 1957 report, Brodie notes that the ataxic pattern was obtained in some cats following transections at the pontomedullary junction.

The sum of the experimental evidence leads to the conclusion that, in the cat or dog having the brainstem transected at the pontomedullary junction, the respiratory pattern is usually not eupneic or normal in character but is, in the very great majority of instances "gasping" or, in fewer instances, "ataxic." This conclusion is contrary to that which Wyman (1977) has drawn in his recent review. Wyman notes that "although the pons and higher centers have great influence on breathing, they are not necessary for the generation of periodic breathing." In support of this thesis, Wyman states (p. 419) that "Wang, Ngai and Frumin confirmed that, in the best cases, after vagotomy and section in the rostral medulla 'respiratory movements appeared entirely normal.' " I believe the full quotation from Wang *et al.* (1957, p. 336) more accurately reflects the net evidence of most investigators concerning the respiration of the medullary preparation: "In a few animals the respiratory movements appeared entirely normal, but in most instances, they were gasping."

Despite the confusion considered above, it is important to note that, in the hands of very skilled investigators, gasping, ataxic, and eupneic-like respiratory patterns have been obtained in the medullary preparation. There are several factors which might account for these differing ventilatory patterns. It has recently been demonstrated that, in the decerebrate cat having bilateral pneumotaxic center lesions and sectioned vagi, a wide variety of punctate lesions within the pons and medulla caused an alteration of ventilation, from apneusis to a more rhythmic respiratory pattern (St. John and Wang, 1977b). These results, taken together with the well-established experimental observation (Breckenridge and Hoff, 1950; Wang *et al.*, 1957) that both the tidal volume and inspiratory duration of apneusis diminishes as the caudal pons is transected, might imply that in some of the studies noted above a remnant of caudal pons remained in the "medullary preparation." However, the established skill of these investigators and the similarity of results between different laboratories lead to the conclusion that this possibility is quite improbable. A second possibility is that gasping and ataxic respiration may be a continuum of the same phenomenon. Because, in all the studies noted above, spontaneously breathing animals were evaluated, and, in all but the study of Ngai (1957), no measurements of alveolar gas concentrations or blood gas and acid–base status were undertaken, it is possible that the different ventilatory patterns of the medullary preparation might be reflective of differences in Pa_{CO_2}, Pa_{O_2}, and pHa. Indeed, in the Ngai report, it is noted that the medullary preparation exhibiting gasping was extremely acidotic (Pa_{CO_2} = 71–74 mm Hg, pHa = 6.91–6.89), whereas in the medullary animal exhibiting quasi-normal respiration, values of Pa_{CO_2} were much lower (34–35 mm Hg) and pHa much higher (7.21–7.41). Also, in only a few studies was arterial blood pressure monitored and, in some of these, sympathomimetic agents were administered to maintain arterial blood pressure at relatively normal levels. This elevation of blood pressure by pharmacological agents was necessary, for a profound hypotension develops following transections at the pontomedullary junction. Thus, in many studies of gasping, the absence of alveolar or arterial blood gas measurements and the absence of arterial blood pressure measurements lead to the conclusion that the effective tissue oxygen pressure might have been quite different in various medullary preparations.

Despite these considerations, however, I must conclude, in agreement with Wang *et al.* (1957) that there is no firm information as to why in some medullary animals gasping was obtained whereas, in others, a quasi-normal respiratory pattern was observed. It is entirely possible that, as Wang *et al.* suggest, there may be separate neural mechanisms responsible for the different respiratory patterns seen in the medullary animal.

III. NERVOUS SYSTEM INTEGRATION OF CHEMORECEPTOR AFFERENT STIMULI

The above discussion of nervous system control of ventilation has focused on a description of the location and organization of the various brainstem respiratory centers. The manner in which various neural elements might serve to define the ventilatory output of the organism has been only superficially considered. It would seem most appropriate to consider these mechanisms by which the various neural components serve to define the tidal volume and frequency of the organism in the context of the response of the animal to changes in respiratory drive arising from peripheral and central chemoreceptor stimuli.

It is, of course, well recognized that ventilation is increased subsequent to exposure of experimental animals to hypercapnia or hypoxia. Diminutions in the arterial partial pressure of oxygen are sensed by the so-called *peripheral chemoreceptors*, localized in the carotid and aortic bodies (Duffin, 1971; Sørensen, 1971). Although these peripheral chemoreceptors are also responsive to elevations in Pa_{CO_2}, the primary detectors for Pa_{CO_2} changes are the central chemoreceptors which Mitchell *et al.* (1963a,b), Loeschcke *et al.* (1963; Loeschke, 1973), and Schlaefke *et al.* (1970, 1973, 1975; Schlaefke, 1973) have localized on the ventrolateral surface of the medulla. Typically, both the tidal volume and the frequency of ventilation are increased subsequent to exposure to hypercapnia or hypoxia.

A. Vagal Mechanisms

Many investigators (e.g., von Euler *et al.*, 1970; Clark and von Euler, 1972; Florez and Borison, 1967; Rosenstein *et al.*, 1974) have noted that, in the anesthetized or decerebrate animal, frequency alterations in response to either hypercapnia or hypoxia are almost entirely eliminated following bilateral vagotomy. The "baseline" or "minimal" respiratory frequency which remains relatively constant following vagotomy is taken to be that frequency which is defined by the "bulbopontile pacemaker." In contrast to these results obtained in the anesthetized or decerebrate animal, unanesthetized animals do show some frequency changes following vagotomy (Gautier, 1975). In addition to slight elevations of frequency, these animals may exhibit a diminution of frequency as tidal volume increases in response to increased ventilatory drive. From what has been discussed above, it might also be concluded that the pneumotaxic center may exert a function in the definition of respiratory frequency.

B. Pneumotaxic Center

In the ketamine-anesthetized or decerebrate animal (St. John, 1973a, 1975; St. John *et al.*, 1975), the placement of lesions in the rostral pontile tegementum, which ablated the pneumotaxic center and adjacent structures, or midpontile transection, resulted in a significant suppression of the frequency response to hypercapnia, whereas the tidal volume response was mainly unaltered. The net effect of these changes was that, following these rostral pontile lesions, the minute volume response to hypercapnia was significantly suppressed. Upon vagal section in these animals, apneusis was obtained.

In recent studies using pentobarbital-anesthetized animals, von Euler *et al.* (1976) found that very small lesions which affected only the nucleus parabrachialis medialis resulted only in a diminution of hypercapnia-induced frequency responses and that the cumulative inspiratory activity (i.e., peak-integrated phrenic height $\times$ frequency) in response to hypercapnia remained unaltered. These investigators did note a suppression of hypercapnia-induced cumulative inspiratory activity in some experimental animals in which the rostral pontile lesions encroached upon structures adjacent to the pneumotaxic center. Apneusis was obtained in those animals having the small lesions within the nucleus parabrachialis medialis upon vagal section. As a result of these studies, von Euler *et al.* have concluded that the phase-switching capabilities of the pneumotaxic center are separable from the proposed role of this area in the integration of central chemoreceptor afferent stimuli. However, these results and the conclusion of von Euler *et al.* are also complicated by the use of pentobarbital-anesthetized animals for their evaluations. Thus, it is well demonstrated that pentobarbital anesthesia suppresses ventilatory responses to hypercapnia to a much greater degree than does either ketamine anesthesia (St. John, 1973b) or decerebration (Wang and Nims,

1948). Moreover, in contrast to the ketamine-anesthetized or decerebrate cat in which no change in tidal volume response to hypercapnia is obtained following pneumotaxic center ablation, pentobarbital-anesthetized animals exhibit a pronounced increase in hypercapnia-induced tidal volumes following similar ablations (St. John, 1973a). Wyman (1977) recently concluded, however, that the phase-switching functions of the nucleus parabrachialis medialis and the functions of this locus in the integration of central chemoreceptor afferent stimuli are "clearly separable." Additional experimentation, involving the placement of discrete lesions only within the nucleus parabrachialis medialis of decerebrate and nonpentobarbital-anesthetized animals, is obviously needed. In spite of the difference in results concerning hypercapnia-induced minute volume changes, however, all studies agree that hypercapnia-induced frequency increases are diminished following pneumotaxic center ablations.

In similar fashion to hypercapnia-induced responses, hypoxia-induced respiratory frequency responses are significantly suppressed following pneumotaxic center ablations in ketamine-anesthetized or decerebrate cats (St. John, 1973a, 1975; St. John *et al.*, 1975). However, in contrast to the hypercapnia-induced changes in these animals, hypoxia-induced minute volumes might remain unaltered following pneumotaxic center ablations. Because the hypoxia-induced frequency responses were significantly suppressed, this maintenance of hypoxia-induced minute volumes was due to significant tidal volume elevations.

These results, i.e., a significant suppression of minute volume response to hypercapnia but not to hypoxia following pneumotaxic center ablation, might imply that there is a difference in the brainstem processing of peripheral and central chemoreceptor afferent stimuli. This conclusion is supported by other investigations which have demonstrated that the pattern of ventilatory response to hypercapnia may differ from that resulting from exposure to hypoxia (see, e.g., Fitzgerald, 1973; Gautier, 1976; Haldane *et al.*, 1919). It might be concluded that respiratory frequency alterations are defined both by vagal mechanisms and by mechanisms of the bulbopontile pacemaker of which the pneumotaxic center constitutes an integral element.

C. Apneustic Center

It was noted above that, during apneusis, the respiratory tidal volume is maximal. Therefore, it might be hypothesized that caudal pontile sites may exert a fundamental role in the determination of ventilatory tidal volume in response to either hypercapnia or hypoxia. In studies (St. John *et al.*, 1975) involving sequential brainstem transections, it was found that, as noted above, there was no significant depression of the tidal volume response to either hypercapnia or hypoxia in decerebrate animals subsequent to a midpontile brainstem transection. However, if a further transection was made through the caudal pons (St. John and Wang, 1976), the tidal volume responses to both hypercapnia and hypoxia were significantly suppressed, whereas the comparable frequency responses were significantly elevated. The net effect of these changes in tidal volume and frequency was to maintain hypercapnia- and hypoxia-induced minute volumes at those same levels as were observed subsequent to the midpontile transections. Comparable changes to those occurring following the caudal pontile transections could be obtained by the placement of punctate lesions on the midline at the pontomedullary junction. It has been concluded (St. John and Wang, 1976) that these lesions produce ventilatory change by ablating a functional pathway interconnecting the caudal pontile apneustic center with the medullary respiratory complex.

The most obvious conclusion to be drawn from the above studies is that the pontile apneustic center is intimately involved in the brainstem definition of tidal volume. It must be stated, however, that tidal volume cannot be a direct output parameter exclusively defined by the apneustic center for, as noted previously, both pneumotaxic center ablation and/or vagal section may alter the ventilatory tidal volume. Moreover, the final integrative area of the brainstem respiratory controller is within the medullary respiratory complex and not within the apneustic center. Thus, while it might be concluded that the apneustic center exercises a primary role in the definition of tidal volume, tidal volume definition per se is nevertheless a complex process involving the interaction among and between the brainstem respiratory centers and the afferent activity impinging upon these centers.

D. Medullary Centers

As noted above, the medullary respiratory complex represents the final integrative area within the brainstem respiratory controller; therefore, it would seem probable that significant information concerning the brainstem integration of chemoreceptor afferent stimuli could be obtained from examination of the medullary preparation. Unfortunately, results concerning the effects of hypercapnia and hypoxia upon the ventilatory pattern of animals having the brainstem transected at the pontomedullary junction are as confused and conflicting as those results conerning the ventilatory pattern of these animals per se. Thus, Ngai (1957) reports that in the medullary preparation, elevation of the inspired carbon dioxide concentration "caused an increase in the rate and depth of the periodic respiration, whether eupneic or gasping.'' In contrast, Tang (1967) reports that "changing from breathing air to breathing 7% CO_2 did not alter the rate or depth of gasping.'' Likewise, Ngai (1957) found that the depth and rate of respiration increased in response to peripheral chemoreceptor stimulation arising from intracarotid injections of sodium cyanide or lobaline. Again, in contrast to Ngai's results, Tang observed that in animals having intact carotid chemoreceptors and in those with carotid chemoreceptor denervation, the rate but not the depth of gasping decreased when 100% oxygen rather than air was breathed. Thus, according to Tang's study, the peripheral chemoreceptor afferents would not appear to influence the pattern of gasping. Obviously, much work remains to be done to characterize the ventilatory pattern of the medullary animal and the ability of peripheral and central chemoreceptor afferent stimuli to alter this pattern.

E. Hypercapnia- and Hypoxia-Induced Alterations in Brainstem Respiratory Neuronal Activity

Changes in ventilation resulting from exposure to hypercapnia or hypoxia are, of necessity, reflective of changes in the activity of brainstem respiratory units. The most detailed study of alterations in brainstem neuronal activity resulting from changes in $P_{A_{CO_2}}$ was that of Cohen (1968). Cohen found that as $P_{A_{CO_2}}$ was lowered, respiratory units exhibited one of three altered patterns of activity: type 1, in which the discharge frequency of the unit declined as $P_{A_{CO_2}}$ was lowered until, at some hypocapnic level, all discharge of the unit ceased; type 2, wherein, as the $P_{A_{CO_2}}$ was lowered the discharge frequency increased during some portions of the respiratory cycle and decreased during other portions such that, at sufficiently low $P_{A_{CO_2}}$ levels, the neuron fired continuously and without respiratory periodicity; and type 3, observed for continuously firing respiratory-modulated units, in which a reduction in discharge frequency was observed during all portions of the respiratory cycle as $P_{A_{CO_2}}$ was lowered and, at low $P_{A_{CO_2}}$ levels, the unit fired tonically and without respiratory periodicity. Cohen found that most phasic inspiratory and expiratory units exhibited type 1 responses. Likewise, most inspiratory–expiratory phase-spanning units exhibited a type 1 response, whereas expiratory–inspiratory phase-spanning units predominantly showed a type 2 response. As noted above, continuously firing phase-spanning units had predominantly type 3 responses. As a corollary to Cohen's observations, most respiratory-modulated units exhibited a synchronization of discharge and an augmented discharge frequency as $P_{A_{CO_2}}$ was elevated. This increase in respiratory neuronal activity concomitant with an increase in $P_{A_{CO_2}}$ is in agreement with work of other authors (Batsel, 1965; Nesland et al., 1966; St. John and Wang, 1977a).

In contrast to these rather well-documented changes in respiratory neuronal activity in response to hypercapnia, relatively few similar studies of hypoxia-induced changes have been attempted. Thus, Batsel (1965) has reported that the discharge of medullary respiratory units increased upon presentation of hypoxic gases. In partial agreement with Batsel's results, Nesland et al. (1966) noted that, although medullary inspiratory unit discharge increased in response to hypoxia, there was considerably more variability in the neuronal responses to hypoxia than to hypercapnia, and that hypoxia depressed medullary expiratory unit activity. Nesland et al. have concluded that the lack of maintenance of isocapnia in their studies might be the major cause of this variability in hyposia-induced responses. Recently, St. John and Wang (1977a) have examined the response of respiratory units within the DRN and VRN to hypercapnia and isocapnic hypoxia. We found that, as noted above, hypercapnia consistently resulted in an increased discharge frequency of respiratory units. Although isocapnic hypoxia usually resulted in comparable changes in medullary respiratory neuronal activity, the discharge frequency of some units was depressed. Moreover, this hypoxia-induced depression was frequently observed simultaneously with an overall increase in ventilatory activity, as evidenced by an increase in the peak-integrated phrenic nerve discharge. As a result of these studies, St. John and Wang (1977a) have concluded that central chemoreceptor afferent influences are ubiquitously distributed to the medullary respiratory complex, whereas peripheral chemoreceptor afferents produce only a discrete and unequal excitation of respiratory units. These results also further support the concept that hypoxia-induced ventilatory changes are the net result of peripheral chemoreceptor excitation of respiratory units and a direct depression of the brainstem respiratory complex by hypoxia (Bjurstedt, 1946; Lee and Milhorn, 1975).

F. Afferent Pathways Interconnecting the Central and Peripheral Chemoreceptors with the Brainstem Respiratory Complex

An obviously important element for the consideration of the brainstem integration of chemoreceptor afferent stimuli is the pathway interconnecting the central and peripheral chemoreceptors with the brainstem respiratory controller. As has been detailed above, Mitchell, Loeschcke, Schlaefke, and their colleagues have localized the central chemoreceptor mechanism to the ventrolateral medullary surface. However, despite the evidence in support of this site, there is still controversy concerning the precise location and mechanism of action of these central chemoreceptors (see, e.g., Fukuda and Honda, 1976; Lipscomb and Boyarsky, 1972; Pappenheimer *et al.*, 1965; Pokorski, 1976; Schlaefke *et al.*, 1975). Moreover, there is essentially no information as to the pathways interconnecting the central chemoreceptors, as described by Mitchell *et al.* (1965a,b), with the brainstem respiratory controller.

In contrast to the central chemoreceptors, there is, of course, rather complete agreement that afferent impulses from the carotid and aortic chemoreceptors are conveyed to the brainstem via the IX and X cranial nerves, respectively. To my knowledge, only the connections between the carotid body afferents and specific brainstem sites have been examined in detail. In this context, Davies and Edwards (1973, 1975) have reported that carotid chemoreceptor afferents are connected monosynaptically with units of the DRN and VRN. Lipski *et al.* (1976) have located nonrespiratory-modulated units in approximation to the DRN and VRN which appear in close physiological proximity to carotid chemoreceptor afferents. In contrast to these results, Berger and Mitchell (1976), on the basis of changes in phrenic nerve activity following carotid sinus nerve stimulation, have concluded that "carotid sinus nerve afferents may not directly excite inspiratory units of the dorsal respiratory nucleus." The net conclusion to be drawn from these studies is that carotid chemoreceptor afferents are undoubtedly distributed to medullary sites, possibly in close proximity to respiratory units (see Fig. 3).

G. Partitioning between Tidal Volume and Frequency of Ventilation

To this point, those processes within the respiratory control system which might be responsible for the definition of tidal volume and frequency of ventilation have been considered. What these considerations have not established is how ventilation is partitioned between tidal volume and frequency. To state this differently: Under normal conditions or in response to increased ventilatory drive, how does the respiratory controller define which portion of the total ventilatory output should be in terms of frequency and which in terms of tidal volume alterations? This question has concerned respiratory physiologists for a long period of time. Such factors as maintaining the work of the respiratory muscles at a minimum in overcoming both elastic and resistive elements have been invoked to explain how tidal volume and frequency are partitioned (see, e.g., Mead, 1960). In a series of studies, beginning in 1972, von Euler and his colleagues (Bradley *et al.*, 1974a,b, 1975; Clark and von Euler, 1972;

von Euler *et al.*, 1976; von Euler and Trippenbach, 1976) have maintained that the partitioning of tidal volume and frequency is an intrinsic function of the nervous system respiratory controller. They base this conclusion on the observation, in pentobarbital-anesthetized animals (Clark and von Euler, 1972), that there is a strict relationship between the tidal volume that an animal exhibits, both under normal conditions and in response to increased ventilatory drive, and the duration of the inspiratory phase of the respiratory cycle (T_I). In this system as described by Clark and von Euler (1972), inspiration is terminated at the point at which the lung volume reaches a threshold value; this threshold value decreases with time after the beginning of inspiration. It is thus evident that with inspiratory efforts beginning at the same point, larger tidal volumes will have a shorter duration than smaller tidal volumes. Another factor arising from this work of Clark and von Euler is that the duration of the inspiratory phase is directly related to the duration of the succeeding expiratory phase. Therefore, in this system, if the tidal volume as well as the durations of the inspiratory and expiratory phases are all set simultaneously, then, obviously, both the tidal volume and the frequency of ventilation will be simultaneously defined. This strict interdependence of V_T and T_I, noted above, has been found to be dependent upon intact vagal nerves, for, subsequent to bilateral vagotomy, alterations in tidal volume occur with little or no change in T_I (Clark and von Euler, 1972).

Assembling data from the work in their laboratory and that of other investigators, Bradley *et al.* (1975) have constructed a model for the definition of inspiratory cutoff and, by extension, for the simultaneous determination of V_T and f. In this model, inspiratory activity is generated at some undefined site within the brainstem controller. This inspiratory activity proceeds in two directions: (1) to the respiratory motoneurons of the spinal cord, and (2) to a pool where this activity is combined with activity from vagal afferent fibers. This summed activity then impinges upon a "switch neuronal pool." The absolute threshold of these switch neurons is defined by inputs from other structures, such as the pneumotaxic center and thermal sensors of the hypothalamus (both lowering threshold) and from chemoreceptor afferents (elevation of threshold). Thus, once the threshold level of these switch neurons is reached, off-switch will be activated and inspiratory activity terminated. Some components of this model have since been examined by von Euler and his colleagues (1976), again in pentobarbital-anesthetized cats. One striking result of these studies was the demonstration that apneusis may be replaced by a rhythmic respiratory pattern subsequent to less than a 2°C elevation of the body temperature of the experimental animal. As noted above, an elevation of body temperature would be predicted to lower the threshold of the switch neurons. Likewise, von Euler and Trippenbach (1976) found that the stimulus strength required to effect inspiratory off-switch by stimulation of the pneumotaxic center "was high early in inspiration and fell steeply with time." Other strengths of the Bradley *et al.* (1975) model and experimental evidence in support of their concepts are detailed in the recent review by Wyman (1977).

However, there are also some experimental observations which appear to directly conflict with the concepts of Bradley *et al.* and which, tend to cast some doubt upon their model system as one which can be generally applied to explain the partitioning between tidal volume and frequency of ventilation. These studies involve the examination of ventilatory activity in unanesthetized subjects or in animals at different levels of anesthesia. Thus, for example, in the 1972 paper of Clark and von Euler, which served as the basis for the later work noted above, it was reported that, in unanesthetized man, V_T varies inversely with T_I over only a small portion of the total tidal volume range. Likewise, in the same context, Cunningham and Gardner (1972) have reported that hypercapnia-induced changes in the respiratory frequency of unanesthetized man are accomplished primarily by a shortening of the expiratory duration (T_E); T_I remained constant in most of their subjects as V_T increased. Moreover, Gautier (1976) has recently shown that there is no seeming interdependence between V_T and T_I or T_I and T_E when unanesthetized cats are examined in response to hypercapnia. Gautier has further reported, however, that the "typical" inverse V_T–T_I and direct T_I–T_E interdependencies, as described by Clark and von Euler, were obtained if these same cats were anesthetized with pentobarbital. While the Bradley *et al.* (1975) model is indeed very attractive for explaining the partitioning of ventilation between its tidal volume and frequency components, additional experimentation is required involving examinations of unanesthetized subjects and subjects anesthetized with anesthetic agents other than the barbiturates, before the concepts of this model may be considered generally applicable.

IV. SUMMARY

As should be evident from the preceding discussion, considerable progress has been made toward an understanding of those neural processes controlling ventilation since Lumsden's classic work on the respiratory centers was published in 1923. It should be equally evident that considerable further experimentation is required not only to fill the gaps in existing knowledge, but to provide knowledge concerning those processes about which only scant firm information is presently available. Those processes responsible for the neurogenesis of the respiratory rhythm undoubtedly remain as the most significant unknown phenomenon. Thus, I would agree with Hugelin and Bertrand's (1973) conclusions as to the status of the understanding of the neural control of ventilation: "The specification and the function of structures generating the respiratory rhythm have long challenged the experimenter. As the result of research combining localized destructions with recordings of respiratory units, one now better knows the localization of these structures. In contrast, the mechanisms responsible for the periodic production of spike trains which cause the alternate contractions of inspiratory and expiratory muscles remains yet in the domain of hypotheses" (Author's translation from original French).

V. AFTERWORD: THE "PROBLEM OF ANESTHESIA"

A recurring theme throughout this chapter has been the "problem of anesthesia" in studies of ventilatory control. Although the meaning of the term "problem of anesthesia" is perhaps evident in the context of this chapter, I believe that a clear definition is imperative. The "problem of anesthesia" is that, in studies of ventilatory control, the investigator should consider and evaluate carefully the direct effect of the anesthetic agent per se upon the respiratory control system and the manner in which the use of this anesthetic or changes in the level thereof might have prejudiced the results. One method of circumventing this "problem of anesthesia," and one which the author prefers, is to utilize the decerebrate preparation. A second method of overcoming this problem would, of course, be the use of nonanesthetized and nondecerebrate animals. It is my strong opinion that this latter alternative should not be undertaken without firm consideration. Thus, it is absolutely required that in studies using unanesthetized animals, the discomfort to the experimental subject should be made as minimal as absolutely possible. One method which fulfills this requirement to the highest degree is the total body plethysmograph, originally designed by Drorbaugh and Fenn (1955) and refined by Bartlett and Tenney (1970). In the plethysmograph system, accurate determinations of ventilation can be performed in completely unrestrained and surgically intact animals. In other studies, potentially traumatic procedures can be performed under general anesthesia and the animals evaluated at later time periods under nontraumatic conditions in the unanesthetized state. My overall conclusion is, therefore, that evaluations performed with unanesthetized subjects should be undertaken only with great care on the part of the investigator. Not only is the former absolutely required by the *Guiding Principles in the Care and Use of Animals* which accompanies the publications of the Federation of American Societies for Experimental Biology, but investigators have a responsibility to observe both the spirit as well as the letter of these declarations.

ACKNOWLEDGMENTS

The author wishes to express his appreciation to Dr. Donald Bartlett, Jr. for his review of this manuscript and helpful suggestions in the preparation thereof.

These manuscripts of the author which are noted in the bibliography represent research activities which are supported by Grant 20574 and RCDA HL 00346 from the National Heart, Lung and Blood Institute, National Institutes of Health.

REFERENCES

Bartlett, D., Jr., and S. M. Tenney (1970). Control of breathing in experimental anemia. *Respir. Physiol.* **10**, 384–395.

Batsel, H. L. (1964). Localization of bulbar respiratory center by microelectrode sounding. *Exp. Neurol.* **9**, 410–426.

Batsel, H. L. (1965). Some functional properties of bulbar respiratory units. *Exp. Neurol.* **11**, 341–366.

Berger, A. J., and R. A. Mitchell (1976). Lateralized phrenic nerve responses to stimulating respiratory afferents in the cat. *Am. J. Physiol.* **230**, 1314–1320.

Bertrand, F., and A. Hugelin (1971). Respiratory synchronizing function of nucleus parabrachialis medialis: Pneumotaxic mechanisms. *J. Neurophysiol.* **34**, 189–207.

Bertrand, F., A. Hugelin, and J. F. Vibert (1973). Quantitative study of anatomical distribution of respiration related neurons in the pons. *Exp. Brain Res.* **16**, 383–399.

Bertrand, F., A. Hugelin, and J. F. Vibert (1974). A stereologic model of pneumotaxic oscillator based on spatial and temporal distributions of neuronal bursts. *J. Neurophysiol.* **37**, 91–107.

Bianchi, A. L. (1971). Localisation et étude des neurones respiratoires bulbaires. Mise en jeu antidromique par stimulation spinale ou vagale. *J. Physiol. (Paris)* **63**, 5–40.

Bianchi, A. L., and J. C. Barillot (1975). Activity of medullary respiratory neurones during reflexes from the lungs in cats. *Respir. Physiol.* **25**, 335–352.

Bjurstedt, A. G. H. (1946). Interaction of centrogenic and chemoreflex control of breathing during oxygen deficiency at rest. *Acta Physiol. Scand.* **12**, Suppl. 38, 1–88.

Bradley, G. W., C. von Euler, I. Marttila, and B. Roos (1974a). Transient and steady state effects of CO_2 on mechanisms determining rate and depth of breathing. *Acta Physiol. Scand.* **92**, 341–350.

Bradley, G. W., C. von Euler, I. Marttila, and B. Roos (1974b). Steady state effects of CO_2 and temperature on the relationship between lung volume and inspiratory duration (Hering–Breuer threshold curve). *Acta Physiol. Scand.* **92**, 351–363.

Bradley, G. W., C. von Euler, I. Marttila, and B. Roos (1975). A model of the central and reflex inhibition of inspiration in the cat. *Biol. Cybern.* **19**, 105–116.

Breckenridge, C. G., and H. E. Hoff (1950). Pontine and medullary regulation of respiration in the cat. *Am. J. Physiol.* **160**, 385–394.

Brodie, D. A. (1957). Doctoral dissertation, Department of Pharmacology, University of Utah, Salt Lake City.

Brodie, D. A., and H. L. Borison (1956). Analysis of central control of respiration by the use of cyanide. *J. Pharmacol. Exp. Ther.* **118**, 220–229.

Burns, B. D., and G. C. Salmoiraghi (1960). Repetitive firing of respiratory neurones during their burst activity. *J. Neurophysiol.* **23**, 27–46.

Clark, F. J., and C. von Euler (1972). On the regulation of depth and rate of breathing. *J. Physiol. (London)* **222**, 267–295.

Cohen, M. I. (1968). Discharge patterns of brain-stem respiratory neurons in relation to carbon dioxide tension. *J. Neurophysiol.* **31**, 142–165.

Cohen, M. I. (1969). Discharge patterns of brain-stem respiratory neurons during Hering–Breuer reflex evoked by lung inflation. *J. Neurophysiol.* **32**, 356–374.

Cohen, M. I. (1970). How respiratory rhythm originates: Evidence from discharge patterns of brainstem respiratory neurones. *In* "Breathing: Hering–Breuer Centenary Symposium" (R. Porter, ed.), pp. 125–150. Churchill, London.

Cohen, M. I. (1971). Switching of the respiratory phases and evoked phrenic responses produced by rostral pontine electrical stimulation. *J. Physiol. (London)* **217**, 133–158.

Cohen, M. I., and S. C. Wang (1959). Respiratory neuronal activity in pons of cat. *J. Neurophysiol.* **22**, 33–50.

Cohen, M. I., M. F. Piercey, P. M. Gootman, and P. Wolotsky (1974). Synaptic connections between medullary inspiratory neurons and phrenic motoneurons as revealed by cross-correlation. *Brain Res.* **81**, 319–324.

Cunningham, D. J. C., and W. N. Gardner (1972). The relation between tidal volume and inspiratory and expiratory times during steady-state CO_2 inhalation in man. *J. Physiol. (London)* **227**, 50P.

Davies, R. O., and M. W. Edwards, Jr. (1973). Distribution of carotid body chemoreceptor afferents in the medulla of the cat. *Brain Res.* **64**, 451–454.

Davies, R. O., and M. W. Edwards, Jr. (1975). Medullary relay neurons in the carotid body chemoreceptor pathway of cats. *Respir. Physiol.* **24**, 69–79.

Drorbaugh, J. E., and W. O. Fenn (1955). A barometric method for measuring ventilation in newborn infants. *Pediatrics* **16**, 81–87.

Duffin, J. (1971). The chemical regulation of ventilation. *Anaesthesia* **26**, 142–154.

Feldman, J. L., M. I. Cohen, and P. Wolotsky (1976). Powerful inhibition of pontine respiratory neurons by pulmonary afferent activity. *Brain Res.* **104**, 341–346.

Fitzgerald, R. S. (1973). Relationships between tidal volume and phrenic nerve activity during hypercapnia and hypoxia. *Acta Neurobiol. Exp.* **33**, 419–425.

Florez, J., and H. L. Borison (1967). Tidal volume in CO_2 regulation: Peripheral denervations and ablation of area postrema. *Am. J. Physiol.* **212**, 985–991.

Fukuda, Y., and Y. Honda (1976). pH sensitivity of cells located at the ventrolateral surface of the cat medulla oblongata *in vitro. Pfluegers Arch.* **364**, 243–247.

Gautier, H. (1975). Effects of hypoxia or hypercapnia on ventilatory pattern of chronic cats before and after vagotomy. *Bull. Physio-Pathol. Respir.* **11**, 89–90.

Gautier, H. (1976). Pattern of breathing during hypoxia or hypercapnia of the awake or anesthetized cat. *Respir. Physiol.* **27**, 193–206.

Gautier, H., and F. Bertrand (1975). Respiratory effects of pneumotaxic center lesions and subsequent vagotomy in chronic cats. *Respir. Physiol.* **23**, 71–85.

Haber, E., K. W. Kohn, S. H. Ngai, D. A. Holaday, and S. C. Wang (1957). Localization of spontaneous respiratory neuronal activities in the medulla oblongata of the cat: A new location of the expiratory center. *Am. J. Physiol.* **190**, 350–355.

Haldane, J. S., J. C. Meakins, and J. G. Priestley (1919). The respiratory response to anoxaemia. *J. Physiol. (London)* **52**, 420–432.

Hassen, A. H., W. M. St. John, and S. C. Wang (1976). Selective respiratory depressant action of morphine compared to meperidine in the cat. *Eur. J. Pharmacol.* **39**, 61–70.

Henderson, V. E., and T. A. Sweet (1929). On the respiratory centre. *Am. J. Physiol.* **91**, 94–102.

Hilaire, G., and R. Monteau (1975). Participation des différents types de neurones bulbaires a l'élaboration de l'activité respiratoire. *J. Physiol. (Paris)* **70**, 759–777.

Hilaire, G., and R. Monteau (1976). Connexions entre les neurones inspiratoires bulbaires et les motoneurones phréniques et intercostaux. *J. Physiol. (Paris)* **72**, 987–1000.

Hildebrandt, J. R. (1974). Intracellular activity of medullary respiratory neurons. *Exp. Neurol.* **45**, 298–313.

Hoff, H. E., and C. G. Breckenridge (1949). The medullary origin of respiratory periodicity in the dog. *Am. J. Physiol.* **158**, 157–172.

Hugelin, A., and F. Bertrand (1973). Le système pneumotaxique. *Arch. Ital. Biol.* **111**, 527–545.

Hukuhara, T. (1973). Neuronal organization of the central respiratory mechanisms in the brainstem of the cat. *Acta Neurobiol. Exp.* **33**, 219–244.

Hukuhara, T., S. Nakayama, S. Baba, and R. Odanaka (1951). On the localization of the respiratory center. *Jpn. J. Physiol.* **2**, 44–49.

Johnson, F. H., and G. V. Russell (1952). The locus coeruleus as a pneumotaxic center. *Anat. Rec.* **112**, 348.

Kahn, N., and S. C. Wang (1967). Electrophysiologic basis for pontine apneustic center and its role in integration of the Hering–Breuer reflex. *J. Neurophysiol.* **30**, 301–318.

Karczewski, W. A. (1973). Some effects of anesthetics on the functional organization of the bulbo-pontine respiratory complex. *Acta Neurobiol. Exp.* **9**, 731–738.

Lee, L.-Y., and H. T. Milhorn, Jr. (1975). Central ventilatory responses to O_2 and CO_2 at three levels of carotid chemoreceptor stimulation. *Respir. Physiol.* **25**, 319–333.

Lipscomb, W. T., and L. L. Boyarsky (1972). Neurophysiological investigations of medullary chemosensitive areas of respiration. *Respir. Physiol.* **16**, 362–376.

Lipski, J., R. M. McAllen, and A. Trzebski (1976). Carotid baroreceptor and chemoreceptor inputs onto single medullary neurones. *Brain Res.* **107**, 132–136.

Loeschcke, H. H. (1973). Respiratory chemosensitivity in the medulla oblongata. *Acta Neurobiol. Exp.* **33**, 97–112.

Loeschcke, H. H., R. A. Mitchell, B. Katsaros, J. F. Perkins, Jr., and A. Konig (1963). Interaction of intracranial chemosensitivity with peripheral afferents to the respiratory centers. *Ann. N.Y. Acad. Sci.* **109**, 651–660.

Lumsden, T. (1923). Observations on the respiratory centres in the cat. *J. Physiol. (London)* **57**, 153–160.

Marckwald, M. (1888). "The Movements of Respiration and their Innervation in the Rabbit" (transl. by T. A. Haig). Blackie and Son, London.

Mead, J. (1960). Control of respiratory frequency. *J. Appl. Physiol.* **15**, 325–336.

Merrill, E. G. (1974). Finding a respiratory function for the medullary respiratory neurons. *In* "Essays on the Nervous System" (G. Bellaris and E. Gary, eds.), pp. 451–486. Oxford Univ. Press (Clarendon), London and New York.

Mitchell, R. A., and A. J. Berger (1975). Neural regulation of respiration. *Am. Rev. Respir. Dis.* **111**, 206–224.

Mitchell, R. A., and D. A. Herbert (1974). The effect of carbon dioxide on the membrane potential of medullary respiratory neurons. *Brain Res.* **75**, 345–349.

Mitchell, R. A., H. H. Loeschcke, W. H. Massion, and J. W. Severinghaus (1963a). Respiratory responses mediated through superficial chemosensitive areas on the medulla. *J. Appl. Physiol.* **18**, 310–313.

Mitchell, R. A., H. H. Loeschcke, J. W. Severinghaus, B. W. Richardson, and W. H.

Massion (1963b). Regions of respiratory chemosensitivity on the surface of the medulla. *Ann. N.Y. Acad. Sci.* **109**, 661–681.

Nesland, R. S., F. Plum, J. R. Nelson, and H. D. Siedler (1966). The graded response to stimulation of medullary respiratory neurons. *Exp. Neurol.* **14**, 57–76.

Ngai, S. H. (1957). Pulmonary ventilation studies on pontile and medullary cats. Changes in O_2 consumption, in arterial blood pH, CO_2 tension and O_2 saturation and in response to CO_2 and cyanide. *Am. J. Physiol.* **190**, 356–360.

Ngai, S. H., and S. C. Wang (1957). Organization of central respiratory mechanisms in the brain stem of the cat: Localization by stimulation and destruction. *Am. J. Physiol.* **190**, 343–349.

Pappenheimer, J. R., V. Fencl, S. F. Heisey, and D. Held (1965). Role of cerebral fluids in control of respiration as studied in unanesthetized goats. *Am. J. Physiol.* **208**, 436–450.

Pitts, R. F. (1946). Organization of the respiratory center. *Physiol. Rev.* **26**, 609–630.

Pitts, R. F., H. W. Magoun, and S. W. Ranson (1939). The origin of respiratory rhythmicity. *Am. J. Physiol.* **127**, 654–670.

Pokorski, M. (1976). Neurophysiological studies on central chemosensor in medullary ventrolateral areas. *Am. J. Physiol.* **230**, 1288–1295.

Richter, D. W., F. Heyde, and M. Gabriel (1975). Intracellular recordings from different types of medullary respiratory neurons of the cat. *J. Neurophysiol.* **38**, 1162–1171.

Rosenstein, R., L. E. McCarthy, and H. L. Borison (1974). Influence of hypoxia on tidal volume response to CO_2 in decerebrate cats. *Respir. Physiol.* **20**, 239–250.

St. John, W. M. (1973a). Characterization of the tidal volume regulating function of the pneumotaxic center. *Respir. Physiol.* **18**, 64–79.

St. John, W. M. (1973b). Comparison of ketamine and pentobarbital depression of feline respiratory response to hypercapnia. *IRCS Libr. Compend.* **4**, 7–1–2.

St. John, W. M. (1975). Differing responses to hypercapnia and hypoxia following pneumotaxic center ablation. *Respir. Physiol.* **23**, 1–9.

St. John, W. M., and S. C. Wang (1976). Integration of chemoreceptor stimuli by caudal pontile and rostral medullary sites. *J. Appl. Physiol.* **41**, 612–622.

St. John, W. M., and S. C. Wang (1977a). Response of medullary respiratory neurons to hypercapnia and isocapnic hypoxia. *J. Appl. Physiol.* **43**, 812–822.

St. John, W. M. and S. C. Wang (1977b). Alteration from apneusis to more regular rhythmic respiration in decerebrate cats. *Respir. Physiol.* **31**, 91–106.

St. John, W. M., R. L. Glasser, and R. A. King (1971). Apneustic breathing after vagotomy in cats with chronic pneumotaxic center lesions. *Respir. Physiol.* **12**, 239–250.

St. John, W. M., R. L. Glasser, and R. A. King (1972). Rhythmic respiration in awake vagotomized cats with chronic pneumotaxic center lesions. *Respir. Physiol.* **15**, 233–244.

St. John, W. M., G. C. Bond, and J. N. Pasley (1975). Integration of chemoreceptor stimuli by rostral brainstem respiratory areas. *J. Appl. Physiol.* **39**, 209–214.

Salmoiraghi, G. C., and B. D. Burns (1960a). Localization and patterns of discharge of respiratory neurones in brain-stem of cat. *J. Neurophysiol.* **23**, 2–13.

Salmoiraghi, G. C., and B. D. Burns (1960b). Notes on mechanism of rhythmic respiration. *J. Neurophysiol.* **23**, 14–26.

Schlaefke, M. E. (1973). "Specific" and "non-specific" stimuli in the drive of respiration. *Acta Neurobiol. Exp.* **33**, 149–154.

Schlaefke, M. E., W. R. See, and H. H. Loeschcke (1970). Ventilatory response to alterations of H^+ ion concentration in small areas of the ventral medullary surface. *Respir. Physiol.* **10**, 198–212.

Schlaefke, M. E., H. Folgering, and A. Herker (1973). Separation of peripheral and central chemosensitive drives in anesthetized and unanesthetized cats. *Bull. Physio-Pathol. Respir.* **9**, 603–604.

Schlaefke, M. E., M. Polorski, W. E. See, R. K. Prill, and H. H. Loeschcke (1975). Chemosensitive neurons on the ventral medullary surface. *Bull. Physio-Pathol. Respir.* **11**, 277–284.

Severinghaus, J. W., and C. P. Larson (1965). Respiration in anesthesia. *Handb. Physiol. Sect. 3: Respir.* **2**, 1219–1264.

Sørensen, S. C. (1971). The chemical control of ventilation. *Acta Physiol. Scand., Suppl.* **361**, 1–72.

Tang, P. C. (1953). Localization of the pneumotaxic center in the cat. *Am. J. Physiol.* **172**, 645–652.

Tang, P. C. (1967). Brain stem control of respiratory depth and rate in the cat. *Respir. Physiol.* **3**, 349–366.

Tenney, S. M. and L. C. Ou (1977). Ventilatory response of decorticate and decerebrate cats to hypoxia and CO_2. *Respir. Physiol.* **29**, 81–92.

Vibert, J. F., F. Bertrand, M. Denavit-Saubié, and A. Hugelin (1976a). Discharge patterns of bulbo-pontine respiratory unit populations in cat. *Brain Res.* **114**, 211–225.

Vibert, J. F., F. Bertrand, M. Denavit-Saubié, and A. Hugelin (1976b). Three dimensional representation of bulbo-pontine respiratory networks architecture from unit density maps. *Brain Res.* **114**, 227–244.

von Baumgarten, R., and E. Kanzow (1958). The interaction of two types of inspiratory neurons in the region of the tractus solitarius of the cat. *Arch. Ital. Biol.* **96**, 361–373.

von Baumgarten, R., A. von Baumgarten, and K.-P. Schaefer (1957). Beitrag zur lokalisationsfrage bulboreticulärer respiratorischer neurone der katze. *Pfluegers Arch.* **264**, 217–227.

von Euler, C., and T. Trippenbach (1976). Excitability changes of the inspiratory off-switch mechanism tested by electrical stimulation in nucleus parabrachialis in the cat. *Acta Physiol. Scand.* **97**, 175–188.

von Euler, C., F. Herrero, and I. Wexler (1970). Control mechanisms determining rate and depth of respiratory movements. *Respir. Physiol.* **10**, 93–108.

von Euler, C., J. N. Hayward, I. Marttila, and R. J. Wyman (1973a). Respiratory neurones of the ventrolateral nucleus of the solitary tract of cat: Vagal input, spinal connections and morphological identification. *Brain Res.* **61**, 1–22.

von Euler, C., J. N. Hayward, I. Marttila, and R. J. Wyman (1973b). The spinal connections of the inspiratory neurones of the ventrolateral nucleus of the cat's tractus solitarius. *Brain Res.* **61**, 23–33.

von Euler, C., I. Marttila, J. E. Remmers, and T. Trippenbach (1976). Effects of lesions in the parabrachial nucleus on the mechanisms for central and reflex termination of inspiration in the cat. *Acta Physiol. Scand.* **96**, 324–337.

Wang, S. C., and L. F. Nims (1948). The effect of various anesthetics and decerebration on the CO_2 stimulating action on respiration in cats. *J. Pharmacol. Exp. Ther.* **92**, 187–195.

Wang, S. C., S. H. Ngai, and M. J. Frumin (1957). Organization of central respiratory mechanisms in the brain stem of the cat: Genesis of normal respiratory rhythmicity. *Am. J. Physiol.* **190**, 333–342.

Webber, C. L., Jr. (1974). Doctoral dissertation, Loyola University, Chicago, Illinois.

Webber, C. L., Jr., and C. N. Peiss (1972). Barbiturate-induced apneusis in the cat. *Physiologist* **15**, 299.

Widdicombe, J. G. (1964). Respiratory reflexes. *Handb. Physiol. Sect. 3: Respir.* **I**, 584–631.

Wyman, R. J. (1977). Neural generation of the breathing rhythm. *Annu. Rev. Physiol.* **39**, 417–448.

CHAPTER 2

Ventilatory Response to Muscular Exercise

SANFORD LEVINE

I. INTRODUCTION

The increase in ventilation which accompanies muscular exercise is influenced by the intensity, type, and phase of muscular activity as well as the environmental conditions under which exercise is performed.

a. Intensity of Exercise. The intensity of muscular exercise is usually quantitated by the aerobic metabolic rate, i.e., oxygen consumption ($\dot{V}_{O_2}$)

31

Regulation of Ventilation and Gas Exchange
Copyright © 1978 by Academic Press, Inc.
ISBN 0-12-204650-1

or carbon dioxide production ($\dot{V}_{CO_2}$). *Anaerobic threshold* (Wasserman *et al.*, 1973) is defined as the metabolic rate above which metabolic acidosis (*i.e.*, lactic acidosis) develops during exercise. *Moderate exercise* is the term used to designate exercise levels below the anaerobic threshold, whereas *severe exercise* (or heavy exercise) is the term used to designate exercise intensities above the anaerobic threshold. During moderate exercise, ventilation is linearly related to metabolic rate (Asmussen, 1965; Comroe, 1965; Dejours, 1964; Gray, 1950; Grodins, 1950; Kao, 1963), but a curvilinear relationship between ventilation and metabolic rate is observed in severe exercise (Asmussen, 1965; Comroe, 1965; Dejours, 1964; Grodins, 1950; Wasserman *et al.*, 1967; Wasserman and Whipp, 1975) (see Fig. 1).

b. Type of Exercise. *Dynamic exercise* (i.e., exercise characterized by limb movements) elicits predictable relationships between ventilation and oxygen consumption (Fig. 1), whereas *static exercise* (i.e., exercise characterized by an absence of limb movement) elicits variable relationships between ventilation and oxygen consumption. The literature indicates that at a given level of oxygen consumption, the increase in $\dot{V}_E$ elicited by static exercise may be greater than (Bedfort *et al.*, 1933; Myhre and Andersen, 1971; Wiley and Lind, 1971), less than (Dejours, 1964), or similar to (Asmussen, 1967) that elicited by dynamic exercise; the absence of a steady state (see Section I,c) in static exercise (Asmussen and Hansen, 1938; Bedfort *et al.*, 1933; Myhre and Andersen, 1971; Wiley and Lind, 1971) may account for these discrepant observations.

The muscles involved in carrying out a particular exercise protocol also influence the ventilatory response; e.g., at a given level of oxygen consumption, ventilation is higher in arm exercise than in leg exercise (As-

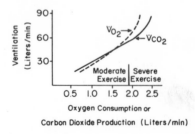

Figure 1. Steady-state relationships (in humans) between ventilation ($\dot{V}_E$) and metabolic rate during various intensities of dynamic muscular exercise. Over the range of moderate exercise, ventilation is linearly related to both oxygen consumption ($\dot{V}_{O_2}$) and carbon dioxide production ($\dot{V}_{CO_2}$), whereas curvilinear relationships are noted during severe exercise. The $\dot{V}_E$–$\dot{V}_{E_{O_2}}$ relationship becomes curvilinear at lower exercise intensities than the $\dot{V}_E$–$\dot{V}_{E_{O_2}}$ relationship. (Reprinted from Wasserman and Whipp, 1975; courtesy of the authors and the *American Review of Respiratory Disease.*)

mussen, 1965, 1967; Asmussen and Nielsen, 1946; Dejours, 1964). Additionally, Koyal and colleagues (1976) have demonstrated that at similar levels of oxygen consumption, bicycle exercise elicited greater increases in $\dot{V}_E$ than treadmill exercise.

c. **Phase of Muscular Exercise.**   An abrupt increase in ventilation usually occurs at the initiation of muscular exercise (Dejours, 1964, 1967; Harrison *et al.*, 1932; Krogh and Lindhard, 1913); however, ventilation continues to increase over the first several minutes of exercise (Davies *et al.*, 1965; Dejours, 1964, 1967; Matell, 1963). A steady state with respect to ventilation is usually attained after several minutes of dynamic exercise (Davies *et al.*, 1965; Dejours, 1964; Kao, 1963; Matell, 1963; Morgan *et al.*, 1955), whereas ventilation occasionally increases throughout the duration of static exercise (Asmussen and Hansen, 1938; Bedfort *et al.*, 1933; Myhre and Andersen, 1971; Wiley and Lind, 1971). Figure 2 depicts ventilation during various phases of dynamic muscular exercise.

d. **Environmental Conditions.**   Hypercapnic (Asmussen, 1965, 1967; Asmussen and Nielsen, 1957; Craig, 1955; Kao *et al.*, 1963, 1967; Luft *et al.*, 1974; Menn *et al.*, 1970; Rizzo *et al.*, 1976; Sinclair *et al.*, 1971) and

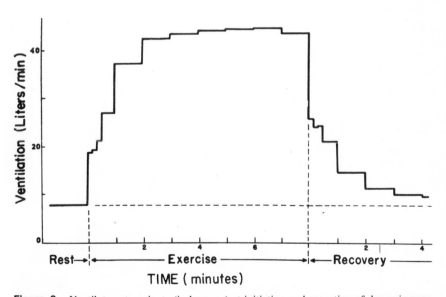

Figure 2.   Ventilatory transients (in humans) at initiation and cessation of dynamic exercise. Ventilation gradually increases during the first few minutes of exercise until a steady state is achieved. (Reprinted from Dejours, 1964; courtesy of the author and the American Physiological Society.)

hypoxic (Asmussen, 1965; 1967; Asmussen and Nielsen, 1957; Astrand, 1954; Bhattacharyya *et al.*, 1970; Cunningham *et al.*, 1968; Dejours, 1962, 1964; Dejours *et al.*, 1963; Kao *et al.*, 1967; Lahiri, 1976; Masson and Lahiri, 1974) environments augment the ventilatory response to muscular exercise (see Section III of this chapter). Ambient conditions characterized by increased heat and increased humidity (i.e., tropical environments) are also thought to augment the ventilatory response to muscular exercise (Dejours, 1964; Lahiri *et al.*, 1976), but the literature does not contain systematic data on this point (Dejours, 1964).

Because of space restraints, this chapter is limited to a consideration of ventilation (i.e., respiratory minute volume) during steady state dynamic exercise.

II. MODERATE EXERCISE

A. Overview of Ventilatory Control

Respiratory physiologists commonly utilize the following relationships between pulmonary ventilation and tissue metabolism to quantitatively assess the steady-state ventilatory response to muscular exercise: (a) the ventilatory equivalent for oxygen ($\dot{V}_{E_{O_2}}$)—the amount of ventilation per unit of oxygen consumption; (b) the ventilatory equivalent for carbon dioxide ($\dot{V}_{E_{CO_2}}$)—the amount of ventilation per unit of carbon dioxide production; and (c) arterial P_{CO_2}—the ratio between alveolar ventilation and CO_2 production.* During steady-state dynamic exercise in healthy man and animals, $\dot{V}_{E_{O_2}}$, $\dot{V}_{E_{CO_2}}$, and arterial P_{CO_2} are not significantly changed from the resting state (Comroe, 1965; Grodins, 1950; Kao *et al.*, 1967; Wasserman *et al.*, 1967; Wasserman and Whipp, 1975). In this chapter, the term *complete* (or *full*) ventilatory response to exercise indicates that $\dot{V}_{E_{O_2}}$ and $\dot{V}_{E_{CO_2}}$ are not decreased from resting measurements (i.e., control), and that arterial P_{CO_2} is not increased from control. The term *incomplete* (or *partial*) ventilatory response indicates that $\dot{V}_{E_{O_2}}$ and $\dot{V}_{E_{CO_2}}$ are decreased from control while arterial P_{CO_2} is increased from control.†

* Strictly speaking, assuming equality between arterial and alveolar P_{CO_2},

$$\text{Arterial } P_{CO_2} \text{ (in mm Hg)} = \frac{\dot{V}_{CO_2} \times 0.863}{\text{alveolar ventilation}}$$

where $\dot{V}_{CO_2}$ (CO_2 production) is stated in ml/min STPD and alveolar ventilation is stated in ml/min BTPS (Comroe *et al.*, 1962).

† This paragraph implies that three parameters are necessary to assess the completeness

The term *exercise stimulus* (Grodins, 1950; Kao, 1963) refers to the stimulus or combination of stimuli which act to elicit the hyperpnea of muscular exercise. Since the precise nature of the exercise stimulus is not known, its magnitude can only be assessed by the ventilatory response to exercise; i.e., a complete ventilatory response implies that a complete exercise stimulus is operative, whereas a partial ventilatory response suggests the presence of an incomplete exercise stimulus.‡ Since $\dot{V}_{E_{O_2}}$ and $\dot{V}_{E_{CO_2}}$ during steady-state exercise are unchanged from rest, Gray (1950), Grodins (1950), and others (Comroe, 1965; Kao, 1963; Wasserman *et al.*, 1967) have emphasized that during moderate exercise the exercise stimulus correlates with the increment in aerobic metabolic rate,** but this correlation does not imply a causal relationship.

B. Role of Peripheral Tissues in Initiating the Exercise Stimulus

In attempts to evaluate the role of the peripheral (i.e., extracranial) tissues in initiating the exercise stimulus, many investigators have devised techniques for inducing muscular exercise in man (Asmussen *et al.*, 1943; Krogh and Lindhard, 1917) and animals (Kao, 1963; Kao and Suckling, 1963; Levine and Huckabee, 1975) by direct electrical stimulation of limb muscles. Muscular exercise induced by these methods elicits complete increases in ventilation. Therefore, these observations suggest that the complete exercise stimulus can arise in working extremities. Since the efferent limb of the ventilatory response to exercise is presumed to originate in the respiratory center (Dejours, 1964; Kao, 1963), the exercise stimulus must be transmitted from working extremities to the respiratory center. Figure 3 indicates that both neural and humoral pathways exist for communication of this stimulus to the respiratory center.

---

of steady-state ventilatory adjustments to exercise (and other hypermetabolic states). However, many papers referred to in this review do not contain measurements of all three parameters (i.e., oxygen consumption, carbon dioxide production, arterial P_{CO_2}). In those instances in which limited data are contained in a communication, completeness of ventilatory response is still evaluated on the basis of available data.

‡ This analysis assumes (a) that both the respiratory controller and afferent pathways to the respiratory controller are functioning in a normal manner and (b) that ventilation adequately reflects the output of the respiratory controller. Abnormalities in the mechanical properties of the lungs, airways, or chest wall may invalidate the latter assumption (Cherniack, 1965; Eldridge and Davis, 1959; Lynne-Davies *et al.*, 1971; Milic-Emili and Tyler, 1963).

** Wasserman and colleagues (1967, 1973; Wasserman, 1976) have attempted to determine the measure of aerobic metabolic rate (i.e., $\dot{V}_{O_2}$ or $\dot{V}_{CO_2}$) with which ventilation is best correlated; their studies indicate that ventilation is best correlated with carbon dioxide production.

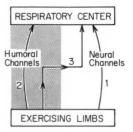

Figure 3. Two types of channels exist for communication of the peripheral exercise stimulus to the respiratory center: neural and vascular. The white area represents neural channels, while the shaded area represents humoral channels. Pathway 1 utilizes neural channels exclusively; pathway 2 utilizes vascular channels exclusively; and pathway 3 depicts a blood-borne change transduced by a receptor which communicates this information to the respiratory center via neural channels. In this review, pathway 1 is discussed in Section II,C, whereas pathways 2 and 3 are arbitrarily grouped under humoral pathway and discussed in Section II,D.

C. Role of Neural Pathways in Transmission of the Exercise Stimulus to the Respiratory Center

1. Overview

Literature on the role of neural pathways in transmission of the exercise stimulus focuses on the results of two types of experiments: regional perfusion experiments and analysis of ventilatory transients.

a. Regional Perfusion Experiments. To assess the role of neural pathways in transmission of the exercise stimulus to the respiratory center, Kao (1963; Kao *et al.*, 1963) attempted to abolish all humoral communication between exercising extremities and the respiratory center. Therefore, he completely perfused the lower body of an experimental dog (i.e., neural dog) with blood from a second dog (i.e., humoral dog); the neural dog's spinal cord remained intact and was intended to represent the sole communication between lower and upper body in the neural dog. Figure 4 presents a schematic diagram of the vascular connections between neural and humoral dogs. Kao noted that electrically induced exercise of the neural dog's hindlimbs consistently stimulated $\dot{V}_E$ in the neural dog; but, the increase in $\dot{V}_E$ per unit of lower-body oxygen consumption was less than that noted in intact animals. However, upper-body arterial P_{CO_2} decreased in these neural animals during hindlimb exercise, whereas muscular exercise in intact animals was accompanied by no change in arterial P_{CO_2}. Because arterial P_{CO_2} represents a tonic stimulus to $\dot{V}_E$, Kao (1963) calculated that the decreases in arterial P_{CO_2} observed in the neural

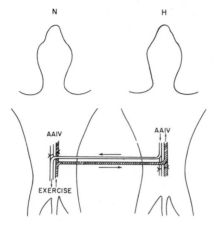

Figure 4. Lower body perfusion of Kao. The lower body of the neural dog (N) is completely perfused with blood from the humoral dog (H); this perfusion is accomplished by anastomosing the abdominal aorta and inferior vena cava of the two dogs at the fourth lumbar level. Therefore, the body of the humoral dog receives all venous blood from the exercising limbs of the neural dog. (Reprinted from Kao, 1963; courtesy of the author and Blackwell Scientific Publications Ltd.)

dog accounted for the difference in ventilatory responses between neural and intact animals. Accordingly, Kao concluded that a neural pathway can account for transmission of the *full* exercise stimulus to the respiratory center.

To confirm the role of intraspinal afferent pathways in transmission of the exercise stimulus, Kao (1963) completely transected the lumbar spinal cord of his neural dog at the third lumbar level; hindlimb muscular exercise no longer elicited increases in $\dot{V}_E$ in these spinal transected neural dogs. In subsequent experiments, Kao (1963) demonstrated that an intraspinal lesion localized to the lateral funiculus also completely eliminated the ventilatory response of his neural dog to hindlimb exercise. Accordingly, he concluded that the lateral columns of the spinal cord transmit the entire exercise stimulus (induced by hindlimb exercise) to the respiratory center.

In attempts to elucidate the peripheral neural pathway responsible for exercise hyperpnea, Kao (1963) and others (Bessou *et al.*, 1959; Koizumi *et al.*, 1961) have demonstrated that electrical stimulation of afferent fibers from muscle receptors elicits increases in ventilation; the magnitude of these increases is directly proportional to the strength of the stimulating current (Kao, 1963). While these observations demonstrate that muscle receptors can elicit increases in $\dot{V}_E$ via a neural pathway, they do not indicate that this pathway is operative during muscular exercise.

b. Analysis of Ventilatory Transients. Krogh and Lindhard (1913), Harrison and colleagues (1932), Dejours (1964), and others (Asmussen, 1965; Cunningham, 1967) have indicated that an abrupt increase in $\dot{V}_E$ occurs at the initiation of dynamic muscular exercise and that a similar abrupt decrease in $\dot{V}_E$ occurs at the cessation of dynamic muscular exercise (see Fig. 2). Because of the rapidity of these changes, these workers have concluded that a neural mechanism must account for them, and they have suggested that this neural mechanism plays an important role in transmission of the exercise stimulus to the respiratory center. Wasserman and colleagues (1974) have recently demonstrated that humoral pathways can also elicit rapid increases in $\dot{V}_E$; therefore, analysis of transients does not constitute a proper technique for distinguishing between neural and humoral mechanisms.

2. Receptors That Initiate Neural Transmission of the Exercise Stimulus

Receptors located in working extremities must initiate the peripheral exercise stimulus which is transmitted to the respiratory center via neural pathway(s). These receptors may be stimulated by mechanical, chemical, thermal, or metabolic changes associated with exercise.

a. Mechanoreceptors. Harrison and colleagues (1932) and others (Comroe and Schmidt, 1943; Dejours, 1964, 1967) have demonstrated that passive manipulation of the extremities of man and animals elicits increases in ventilation. These increases in $\dot{V}_E$ are not modified by occluding the circulation to the limbs (Comroe and Schmidt, 1943; Harrison et al., 1932), but spinal nerve section (Comroe and Schmidt, 1943) and spinal cord section (Comroe and Schmidt, 1943; Harrison et al., 1932) abolish them. Therefore, these observations demonstrate that limb receptors effect the hyperpnea of passive movement via a neural pathway. Dejours (1964, 1967) and others (Harrison et al., 1932) have hypothesized that this neural pathway may play an important role in exercise hyperpnea.

Comroe and Schmidt (1943) attempted to discern the relative roles of muscle and joint proprioceptors in the ventilatory response to passive movement. They noted that surgical division of the periarticular muscle did not eliminate increases in $\dot{V}_E$ elicited by passive limb movement, whereas local injection of anesthesia into the joint region did abolish these increases in $\dot{V}_E$. These observations led Comroe and Schmidt (1943) to conclude that articular receptors mediate the increase in $\dot{V}_E$ elicited by passive movement. However, Dejours (1967) believes that this conclusion may not be fully warranted since these authors did not eliminate the possibility that receptors outside of the joint region were exposed to the local anesthetic, nor did they preclude the possibility that the surgical division of the periarticular muscles exposed pain fibers to subsequent stimulation by movement.

In order to assess the influence of proprioceptor activity on the ventilatory response to exercise, Sipple and Gilbert (1966) measured ventilation during fast and slow bicycle pedaling; they noted that ventilation was uniquely related to oxygen consumption independent of pedaling speed. Therefore, Sipple and Gilbert (1966) concluded that the frequency of limb movement does not influence the ventilatory response to exercise. However, they correctly indicated that their data do not eliminate the possibility that the combination of frequency and force may constitute an important proprioceptive stimulus to $\dot{V}_E$ during exercise.

Some investigators (Bessou et al., 1959; Flandrois et al., 1967; Gautier et al., 1969; Leitner and Dejours, 1971) have systematically explored the possibility that muscle spindles are the receptors which provide the proprioceptive stimulus to ventilation. First, Bessou and colleagues (1959) and Koizumi and associates (1961) have demonstrated that electrical stimulation of afferent fibers originating in muscle spindles and in Golgi receptors elicits increases in ventilation. Second, Gautier and co-workers (1969) have demonstrated that succinylcholine, a chemical stimulus to muscle spindles (Granit et al., 1953), elicits increases in $\dot{V}_E$ via spinal afferent pathways. Third, Leitner and Dejours (1971) have demonstrated that vibration, a powerful stimulus to muscle spindles, elicits increases in $\dot{V}_E$ in cats. [However, Hodgson and Matthews (1968) and others (Kao, 1963) have failed to demonstrate that vibration stimulates $\dot{V}_E$ via muscle afferents. The possibility exists that differences in experimental protocol may account for these discrepant observations.] Fourth, Flandrois et al. (1967) have demonstrated that Ba 2288, a pharmacological depressant of muscle spindle activity (Bein and Fehr, 1962), diminishes the increase in $\dot{V}_E$ elicited by passive movement in the dog. In summary, these observations demonstrate that excitation of muscle spindles can stimulate ventilation, but the role of muscle spindles in eliciting the hyperpnea of muscular exercise still remains uncertain.

Kalia et al. (1972) have shown that stretching, pressing, or squeezing the gastronemius muscle of the dog elicits increases in $\dot{V}_E$. These workers have also demonstrated that these stimuli still elicit increases in $\dot{V}_E$ following blockade of Groups I, II, and III afferent nerve fibers [which are all medullated (Brinley, 1974)]. Because muscle spindles are innervated exclusively by Groups I and II fibers, these observations suggest that receptors other than muscle spindles mediate the increases in $\dot{V}_E$ elicited by stretching, pressing, or squeezing. Kalia and colleagues (1972) have hypothesized that the nonmedullated region of sensory nerve endings in muscle mediate these increases in V_E. The possibility exists that these sensory nerve endings in muscle may also play a role in eliciting the hyperpnea of muscular exercise.

b. Chemoreceptors.   During muscular exercise, decreases in P_{O_2}, increases in P_{CO_2}, and increases in $[H^+]$ are presumed to occur in working muscles (Kao, 1963). To assess the possibility that muscle chemoreceptors responsive to these changes stimulate $\dot{V}_E$, Comroe and Schmidt (1943) and Kao (1963) have perfused vascularly isolated limbs of animals with hypoxemic, hypercapnic, and acidemic blood; despite intactness of the nerve supply to these limbs, no increases in $\dot{V}_E$ were observed. These observations demonstrate that muscle chemoreceptors (if they do exist) do not stimulate $\dot{V}_E$ in response to usual chemical stimuli (i.e., P_{O_2}, P_{CO_2}, or $[H^+]$) and therefore, that muscle chemoreceptors for these substances do not play a role in eliciting the hyperpnea of muscular exercise. However, the possibility exists that muscle chemoreceptors for other substances may play a role in eliciting the hyperpnea of muscular exercise.

c. Thermoreceptors.   Moderate increases in muscle temperature (i.e., $1°-2°C$) occur in muscular exercise (Asmussen, 1965; Morgan et al., 1955). Morgan et al. (1955) have demonstrated that the increase in $\dot{V}_E$ noted during exercise (in the anesthetized dog) is linearly related to the temperature in exercising muscles. However, these same authors have demonstrated that similar increments in muscle temperature effected by microwave heating (in the absence of exercise) did not stimulate ventilation. These latter observations of Morgan et al. (1955) suggest that muscle thermoreceptors do not play a major role in eliciting the hyperpnea of muscular exercise.

d. Metabolic Receptors.   Increases in muscle metabolic rate occur in muscular exercise; therefore, in attempts to elucidate mechanisms underlying exercise hyperpnea, many investigators (Bailen and Horvath, 1959; Huch et al., 1969; Levine and Huckabee, 1975; Liang and Hood, 1973; Ramsay, 1955, 1959; Williams et al., 1958) have evaluated ventilatory responses to tissue hypermetabolism induced by 2,4-dinitrophenol (2,4-DNP)—an uncoupler of mitochondrial oxidative phosphorylation.* All workers have demonstrated that *full* increases in $\dot{V}_E$ accompany 2,4-DNP-induced tissue hypermetabolism. Since the increases in $\dot{V}_E$ which

---

* A description of mechanisms by which uncouplers of oxidative phosphorylation elicit increases in metabolic rate is contained in standard textbooks of biochemistry (Lehninger, 1970; McGilvery, 1970; White et al., 1973).

followed 2,4-DNP infusion occurred in the absence of movement, these observations raise the possibility that metabolic receptors account for the *complete* ventilatory response to moderate muscular exercise.

To assess the possibility that stimulation of ventilation and stimulation of oxygen consumption represented independent actions of 2,4-DNP, Levine (1977b) evaluated ventilatory and metabolic responses of the anesthetized dog to three different congeners of dinitrophenol. Figure 5 presents the structural formulas of these isomers, and Fig. 6 summarizes the steady-state increases in oxygen consumption and ventilation elicited by these drugs. Figure 6 indicates that three congeners of dinitrophenol exhibit similar structure–activity relationships with respect to both stimulation of ventilation and stimulation of oxygen consumption. These

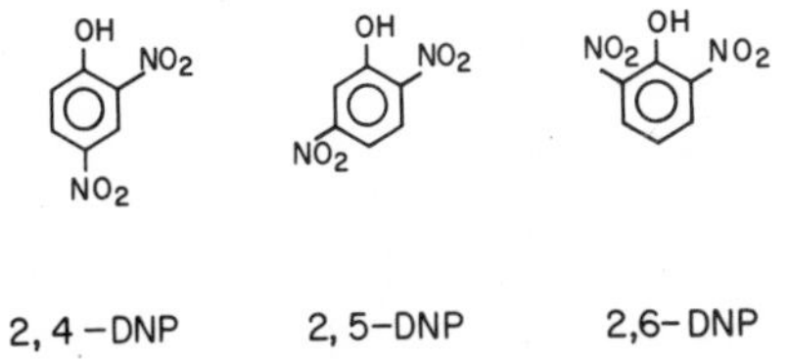

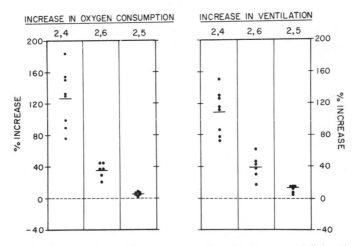

Figure 5. Isomers of dinitrophenol (DNP): 2,4-dinitrophenol (2,4-DNP); 2,5-dinitrophenol (2,5-DNP), and 2,6-dinitrophenol (2,6-DNP). (Reprinted from Levine, 1977b, through the courtesy of the *Journal of Applied Physiology*.)

Figure 6. Ventilatory and metabolic responses elicited by isomers of dinitrophenol. All isomers elicited significant increases in both ventilation and oxygen consumption. However, the isomers differed significantly with respect to both increases in ventilation and increases in oxygen consumption. (Reprinted from Levine, 1977b; courtesy of the *Journal of Applied Physiology*.)

observations are consistent with the hypothesis that stimulation of ventilation by dinitrophenols is related to tissue hypermetabolism.

In an attempt to obtain additional information on the relationship between stimulation of ventilation and stimulation of oxygen consumption by uncouplers of oxidative phosphorylation, Levine and Huckabee (1975) evaluated ventilatory responses of anesthetized dogs to tissue hypermetabolism induced by ethyl methylene blue (EMB)—another uncoupler of oxidative phosphorylation (see Fig. 7). They noted that full increases in $\dot{V}_E$ also accompanied tissue hypermetabolism induced by EMB. Since EMB differs from the dinitrophenols in chemical structure, these observations are consistent with the notion that stimulation of $\dot{V}_E$ by uncouplers is related to tissue hypermetabolism and not to the drugs per se.

In order to ascertain whether cephalic (i.e., carotid body and intracranial receptors) or extracephalic receptors mediate increases in ventilation elicited by uncouplers of oxidative phosphorylation (i.e., 2,4-DNP or EMB), Levine and Huckabee (1975) devised a perfusion technique for achieving complete vascular separation between cephalic and extracephalic regions in the dog (see Fig. 8). Utilizing this preparation, they demonstrated that these uncouplers (i.e., 2,4-DNP and EMB) elicit rather modest increases in ventilation (i.e., 21%) by excitation of cephalic receptors, whereas excitation of extracephalic receptors by these drugs elicits twofold increases in $\dot{V}_E$. In subsequent experiments, Levine and Huckabee (1975) demonstrated that these extracephalic receptors are poorly responsive to usual chemical stimuli in arterial blood (i.e., increments in P_{CO_2}, increments in $[H^+]$, or decrements in oxygen saturation).

To assess the possibility that these extracephalic receptors are located in the extremities, Liang and Hood (1976) perfused the isolated hindlimbs of experimental dogs with blood from support dogs. To ensure completeness of vascular separation between the isolated extremity and the remainder of the experimental animal, all articular, muscular, and cutaneous tissues joining the two regions were severed; the sciatic nerve remained intact and was intended to represent the sole communication between isolated hindlimb and the remainder of the experimental animal. These investigators demonstrated that selective administration of a large dose of 2,4-DNP (i.e., 6 mg/kg) to the isolated limb elicited nearly twofold

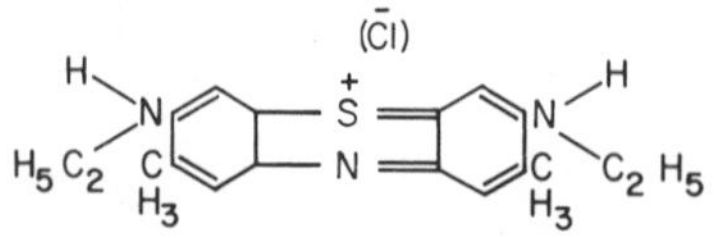

Figure 7.   Ethyl methylene blue (EMB). This uncoupler differs from the dinitrophenols in chemical structure.

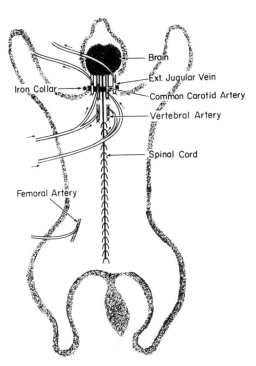

Figure 8. Diagram of a head-perfused animal. The head of the experimental dog was entirely perfused from a support dog with blood of unvarying gas composition via both carotid and both vertebral arteries. To ensure completeness of vascular separation between the body and the head of the experimental animal (i.e., head-perfused animal) all extraspinal nerves, muscles, and blood vessels in the neck were cut and tied, and an occlusive collar was placed around the bony spine. The cervical spinal cord remained intact and was intended to constitute the sole communication between the body and the head of the experimental dog. (Reprinted with modification from Levine and Huckabee, 1975; courtesy of the *Journal of Applied Physiology.*)

increases in ventilation; following section of the sciatic nerve, $\dot{V}_E$ of the experimental animal returned to control values. These observations of Liang and Hood [although differing from earlier reports (Bailen and Horvath, 1959)] demonstrate that limb receptors can initiate some portion of the increase in $\dot{V}_E$ elicited by 2,4-DNP. Accordingly, the possibility exists that these receptors may play an important role in eliciting the hyperpnea of muscular exercise. [The reader must realize that neither the experiments of Liang and Hood (1976) nor those of Levine and Huckabee (1975) preclude the possibility that 2,4-DNP per se or tissue metabolites released by 2,4-DNP also stimulate $\dot{V}_E$ by excitation of receptors in the central circulation.]

D. Role of Humoral Pathways in Transmission of the Exercise Stimulus to the Respiratory Center

1. Overview

At the present time, controversy regarding the role of humoral pathways in transmission of the exercise stimulus to the respiratory center focuses on the results of two types of experiments: spinal transection experiments and cross-circulation experiments. The spinal transection experiments support the notion that a humoral pathway exists for transmission of the exercise stimulus to the respiratory center, whereas the cross-circulation experiments have been interpreted as evidence against the existence of a humoral pathway for transmission of the exercise stimulus to the respiratory center. (In this chapter all pathways containing humoral components are termed *humoral* pathways, even though some of the pathways may contain neural elements, e.g., pathway 3 in Fig. 3.)

a. Spinal Transection Experiments.   In attempts to discern the existence of a humoral pathway for transmission of the exercise stimulus to the respiratory center, many investigators (Geppert and Zuntz, 1888; Grodins and Morgan, 1950; Kramer and Gauer, 1941; Lamb, 1968–1969; Levine 1976a, b) have studied the ventilatory response of lumbar spinal cord transected animals to hindlimb exercise. All workers have demonstrated that exercise of the denervated hindlimbs elicits increases in $\dot{V}_E$, and the data of Lamb (1968–1969) and others (Levine, 1976b) indicate that these increases in $\dot{V}_E$ occur in the absence of conventional chemical stimuli in arterial blood (i.e., increments in P_{CO_2}, increments in $[H^+]$, or decrements in oxygen saturation). Kramer and Gauer (1941) noted that muscular exercise in the lumbar spinal cord transected animal was accompanied by decreases in arterial blood pressure, and they suggested that these decreases in arterial blood pressure (by unloading of arterial baroreceptors) accounted for the lumbar spinal cord transected animal's ventilatory response to hindlimb exercise. However, the data of Lamb (1968–1969) demonstrate that the spinal transected animal can exhibit a *complete* ventilatory response to exercise of denervated extremities in the absence of significant decrements in mean arterial blood pressure. In summary, the spinal transected animal experiments demonstrate that a humoral pathway exists for transmission of the exercise stimulus to the respiratory center, but the precise nature of the humoral stimulus as well as the receptors in this pathway remain uncertain (see Sections II,D,2 and II,D,3 of this chapter).

b. Cross-Circulation Experiments. Kao (1963) utilized cross-circulation techniques to evaluate the role of humoral factors in the stimulation of $\dot{V}_E$ by muscular exercise. First, he demonstrated that perfusion of the head of a head-perfused animal (see Fig. 8) with arterial blood from an exercising support dog did not stimulate ventilation in the head-perfused animal. Kao concluded from these experiments that arterial blood of an exercising animal does not contain humoral agents which elicit increases in ventilation via excitation of intracranial receptors; however, this conclusion is not fully warranted, as it assumes that the cross-perfusion apparatus did not inactivate some labile humoral substance. Second, Kao noted that coincident with muscular exercise of the hindlimbs of the neural dog (see lower body perfusion, Fig. 4), increases in both ventilation and arterial P_{CO_2} were noted in the humoral dog; therefore, these experiments support the concept of a humoral exercise stimulus. However, since muscular exercise in the intact animal elicits increases in $\dot{V}_E$ in the absence of increases in arterial P_{CO_2}, Kao correctly concluded (in the opinion of this author) that these experiments demonstrating humoral transmission of an exercise stimulus were not relevant to exercise hyperpnea. Third, Kao noted that by experimentally excluding extrathoracic receptors in the humoral dog from contact with venous blood draining the neural dog's exercising extremities (see triad preparation, Fig. 9), he was able to eliminate the increase in ventilation in the humoral dog. These triad experiments of Kao suggest that exercise-released humoral agents in venous blood do not stimulate $\dot{V}_E$ by

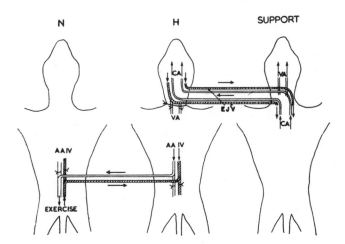

Figure 9. Triad preparation of Kao. The neural (N) and humoral (H) dogs are anastomosed in the same manner as the lower body perfusion (see legend to Fig. 4). However, in the triad preparation, the head of the humoral dog is completely perfused with blood from a third dog (support dog). Since the abdominal aorta (AA) and inferior vena cava (IV) of the humoral dog are ligated, only thoracic receptors in the humoral dog are exposed to venous blood draining from the exercising extremities of the neural dog. (Reprinted from Kao, 1963; courtesy of the author and Blackwell Scientific Publications Ltd.)

excitation of thoracic receptors. However, the possibility exists that the humoral dog of the triad preparation may not have been responsive to any ventilatory stimulus. Therefore, Kao's triad experiments may not have constituted an adequate evaluation of the roles of both exercise-released humoral agents and thoracic receptors in exercise hyperpnea. In summary (in the opinion of this author), Kao's cross-perfusion experiments regarding humoral transmission of the exercise stimulus do not permit one to draw definitive conclusions.

2. Nature of the Humoral Exercise Stimulus

Attempts to define the humoral exercise stimulus* have focused on the following parameters: chemical changes in arterial blood; chemical changes in mixed-venous blood; chemical changes in intracranial fluid compartments; pressure changes in the central circulation; temperature changes in arterial blood; and rate of carbon dioxide delivery to the lung.

a. Chemical Changes in Arterial Blood.   Arterial P_{O_2} during moderate exercise is usually unchanged from rest. However, some workers have noted that small increments in arterial P_{CO_2} and small increments in arterial [H+] occur during steady-state moderate exercise [see Dejours (1964) for review of these data]. Cunningham (1961, 1967) has calculated that these changes in arterial P_{CO_2} and arterial [H+] can account for an appreciable portion of the increase in $\dot{V}_E$ noted during moderate muscular exercise. However, most workers have failed to demonstrate that increments in mean arterial P_{CO_2} or increments in mean arterial [H+] accompany moderate muscular exercise in man (Comroe, 1965; Davies et al., 1965; Forster and Klausen, 1973; Wasserman, 1976; Wasserman and Whipp, 1975) or animals (Kao, 1956, 1963; Levine and Huckabee, 1975; Wagner et al., 1977). Accordingly, this author concludes that under special circumstances increments in arterial P_{CO_2} and increments in arterial [H+] may augment the ventilatory response to exercise (see Sections III,B and III,C of this chapter), but a *complete* ventilatory response to muscular exercise can occur independent of these changes.

b. Chemical Changes in Mixed-Venous Blood.   Increments in mixed-venous P_{CO_2} occur in muscular exercise, and Armstrong and colleagues (1961) and Riley et al. (1963) have noted that ventilation during exercise is linearly related to mixed-venous P_{CO_2}. Accordingly, these observations

---

* An adequate description of a humoral pathway must characterize both (a) the humoral stimulus and (b) the receptors which mediate increases in $\dot{V}_E$ elicited by this stimulus. In this review, Section II,D,2 describes humoral pathways in which the stimulus has been identified, whereas Section II,D,3 describes humoral mechanisms in which the stimulus has not been identified.

raised the possibility that increments in mixed-venous P_{CO_2} elicit the hyperpnea of muscular exercise by excitation of chemoreceptors in the right heart or pulmonary artery. However, Cropp and Comroe (1961) have demonstrated that increments in mixed-venous P_{CO_2} do not stimulate $\dot{V}_E$ by a mechanism independent of increments in arterial P_{CO_2} and, therefore, mixed-venous P_{CO_2} per se does not constitute the humoral exercise stimulus.

Decrements in mixed-venous P_{O_2} occur in muscular exercise, and the possibility exists that these decreases in P_{O_2} may stimulate $\dot{V}_E$ by excitation of chemoreceptors in the right heart or pulmonary artery. The data of Duke and associates (1963) suggest that chemoreceptors for oxygen do exist in the pulmonary artery of the cat; however, the experiments of Coleridge and colleagues (1967) are not consistent with this notion. Kollmeyer and Kleinman (1975) have demonstrated that decrements in mixed-venous P_{O_2} stimulate $\dot{V}_E$ in the newborn puppy, but they failed to detect a similar phenomenon in the adult dog. In summary, this author believes that the evidence suggesting a causal relationship between mixed-venous P_{O_2} and the humoral exercise stimulus is not definitive.

c. Chemical Changes in Intracranial Fluid Compartments.

Intracranial chemoreceptors responsive to [H^+] as well as other chemical substances can elicit increases in $\dot{V}_E$ (Leusen, 1965, 1972; Pappenheimer, 1967; Winterstein, 1961). Therefore, the possibility exists that these chemoreceptors may play a role in mediating the hyperpnea of muscular exercise. However, Leusen (1965) and Kao *et al.* (1965) have demonstrated that exercise hyperpnea is usually accompanied by no significant change in cerebrospinal fluid (CSF) [H^+]. Moreover, the observations of Kao *et al.* (1965) indicate that muscular exercise does not effect any change in sensitivity of the hypothetical CSF [H^+] receptors. Therefore, intracranial chemoreceptors which are responsive to CSF [H^+] do not appear to play a role in eliciting the increased ventilation of muscular exercise. However, the possibility exists that intracranial chemoreceptors which are responsive to chemical substances other than CSF [H^+] may play a role in eliciting the hyperpnea of muscular exercise.

d. Pressure Changes in the Central Circulation.

Increments in central venous pressure occur during exercise. Harrison and colleagues (1932) have reported that increments in central venous pressure (or increments in right heart intracardiac pressures) can elicit large increments in $\dot{V}_E$ by excitation of receptors innervated by the vagus nerve. Since Phillipson *et al.* (1970) and Lahiri and colleagues (1975) have demonstrated that the bilateral vagotomized animal still manifests a complete ventilatory response to muscular exercise, this mechanism of Harrison and colleagues does not play an obligatory role in eliciting the hyperpnea of muscular exercise.

Increases in pulmonary capillary pressure accompany muscular exercise (Ekelund and Holmgren, 1967), and these increases may effect increases in pulmonary interstitial volume (Paintal, 1970). Since Paintal and colleagues (1970, 1973) have demonstrated that increases in pulmonary interstitial volume stimulate ventilation by excitation of J receptors, some authors have hypothesized that these receptors may play an important role in eliciting exercise hyperpnea. However, J receptors stimulate $\dot{V}_E$ via vagal pathways; therefore, the studies of Phillipson *et al.* (1970) and of Lahiri and colleagues (1975) (see above) suggest that these vagally mediated receptors do not play a major role in effecting the hyperpnea of muscular exercise.

e. Temperature Changes in Arterial Blood. Small increments in the temperature of arterial blood (i.e., 1°–2°C) occur in moderate muscular exercise (Asmussen, 1965; Holmgren and McIlroy, 1964; Morgan *et al.*, 1955). These increments in blood temperature may stimulate $\dot{V}_E$ by the following mechanisms: (a) excitation of hypothalamic thermoregulatory neurons which in turn stimulate the medullary respiratory center (Bligh, 1966); (b) thermal-induced increases in the sensitivity of peripheral arterial chemoreceptors (Bernthal and Weeks, 1939); and (c) thermal-induced changes in the physicochemical properties of blood which effect increases in both arterial [H^+] and arterial P_{CO_2} (Holmgren and McIlroy, 1964). In summary, mechanisms exist whereby increments in blood temperature can stimulate $\dot{V}_E$, but the quantitative contribution of these mechanisms to exercise hyperpnea remains uncertain.

f. Rate of Carbon Dioxide Delivery to the Lung. Muscular exercise is accompanied by an increase in the rate of carbon dioxide delivery to the lung. Since no increase in mean arterial P_{CO_2} accompanies steady-state muscular exercise (Comroe, 1965; Forster and Klausen, 1973; Kao, 1956, 1963; Kao *et al.*, 1967; Wasserman *et al.*, 1967; Wasserman and Whipp, 1975), the increment in (alveolar) ventilation elicited by exercise must be precisely proportional to the increment in rate of carbon dioxide delivery to the lung. Therefore, some workers (Fordyce *et al.*, 1976; Lamb, 1966; Lewis, 1972; Mueller *et al.*, 1974; Wasserman *et al.*, 1974, 1975a; Yamamoto and Edwards, 1960) have investigated the hypothesis that increments in the rate of carbon dioxide delivery to the lung constitute the humoral exercise stimulus. Data which support and data which refute this hypothesis will now be presented.

(1) Evidence that rate of CO_2 delivery to the lung constitutes the humoral exercise stimulus. More than a decade ago, Yamamoto and Edwards (1960) interposed an extracorporeal gas exchanger into a surgically created arteriovenous fistula in rats in order to vary the rate of carbon dioxide delivered to the lungs. They noted that up to sixfold increases in carbon dioxide flow rate to the lung (i.e., six times metabolic CO_2 production) elicited proportional increases in ventilation in the absence of any increment in mean arterial P_{CO_2}. Wasserman and colleagues (1975a) have recently made similar observations in the dog. These observations of Yamamoto and Edwards (1960) and of Wasserman and colleagues (1975a) suggest that increments in rate of CO_2 delivery to the lung constitute the humoral exercise stimulus.

Because the flow rate of carbon dioxide to the lungs is determined by the product of cardiac output and mixed-venous CO_2 content, Wasserman and colleagues (1974) evaluated the ventilatory response to acute increments in cardiac output (effected by either isoproteronol infusion or cardiac pacing). They noted that increases in $\dot{V}_E$ consistently accompanied acute increases in cardiac output, and they also noted that these increases in $\dot{V}_E$ were accompanied by no change in end-tidal P_{CO_2}. Accordingly, these observations of Wasserman *et al.* (1974) are consistent with the notion that increments in rate of CO_2 delivery to the lung constitute the humoral exercise stimulus.

The experiments of Yamamoto and Edwards (1960) and of Wasserman and colleagues (1974, 1975a) did not localize the receptors which relate ventilation to rate of CO_2 delivery to the lung. Yamamoto and Edwards (1960) correctly indicated that a sensor responsive to the CO_2 tension of mixed-venous blood could correlate $\dot{V}_E$ to pulmonary CO_2 delivery only if an additional receptor transmitted information concerning cardiac output to the respiratory controller. However, CO_2 tension receptors located in pulmonary alveoli might possibly relate $\dot{V}_E$ to the rate of CO_2 delivery to the lung. Yamamoto and Edwards (1960) also raised the intriguing possibility that arterial chemoreceptors (location unspecified) might account for the hyperpnea elicited by venous CO_2 loading (i.e., increments in rate of CO_2 delivery to the lung). Based on mathematical considerations (Yamamoto, 1960; Yamamoto and Edwards, 1960), they suggested that venous CO_2 loading increases the oscillation of P_{CO_2} in arterial blood; they hypothesized that this increase in P_{CO_2} oscillation might stimulate arterial chemoreceptors even though mean arterial P_{CO_2} remained constant. The studies of Band *et al.* (1969a,b) support the notion that venous CO_2 loading increases the oscillation of P_{CO_2} in arterial blood, and the studies of Dutton and Permutt (1968) and Riley *et al.* (1963) suggest that P_{CO_2} oscillations may constitute a stimulus to $\dot{V}_E$ independent of mean arterial P_{CO_2}. The studies of Cunningham and associates (1973) demonstrate that ventilatory chemoreceptors are able to discriminate among small differences in time patterns of alveolar (and presumably arterial) P_{CO_2}.

(2) Evidence that rate of CO_2 delivery to the lung does not constitute the humoral exercise stimulus. The increase in $\dot{V}_E$ elicited by the breathing of high CO_2 gas mixtures (i.e., $> 1\%$) is invariably accompanied by increments in mean arterial P_{CO_2}. As stated above, the studies of Yamamoto and Edwards and of Wasserman and colleagues demonstrate that venous CO_2 loading elicits increases in $\dot{V}_E$ in the absence of increments in mean arterial P_{CO_2}. Therefore, their work implies that the route of CO_2 delivery to the lung (i.e., airway vs. venous blood) affects the ventilatory response. Lamb (1966) tested this hypothesis in cats by comparing the ventilatory response to airway and venous CO_2 loading. He noted that both methods of CO_2 administration elicited increments in $\dot{V}_E$ and increments in mean arterial P_{CO_2}; the relationship between $\dot{V}_E$ and mean arterial P_{CO_2} was similar in both types of experiments. The experiments of Lewis (1972) in monkeys also demonstrate that similar relationships between $\dot{V}_E$ and arterial P_{CO_2} follow airway and venous CO_2 loading. The experiments of Lamb (1966) and Lewis (1972) indicate that increments in mean arterial P_{CO_2} can completely account for increases in $\dot{V}_E$ elicited by venous CO_2 loading; these observations therefore suggest that increments in the rate of CO_2 delivery to the lung do not constitute the humoral exercise stimulus.

(3) Conclusions regarding the relationship between rate of CO_2 delivery to the lung and the humoral exercise stimulus. Conflicting data exist on ventilatory responses elicited by venous CO_2 loading. These discrepant observations on ventilatory responses to venous CO_2 loading may be accounted for by physiological differences in the animal preparations utilized in the different studies (i.e., differences in animal species, depths of anesthesia, and ventilatory responsiveness to increments in arterial P_{CO_2}). Technical differences between studies (e.g., position of catheter utilized for venous CO_2 loading) may also account for some portion of the discrepant results. Fordyce and colleagues (1976) have suggested that differences in the sequence of administration of experimental stimuli (i.e., venous or airway CO_2 loading) may fully explain the discrepant results. In summary, the precise relationship between the rate of CO_2 delivery to the lung and the humoral exercise stimulus remains uncertain. Further work is necessary to clarify this matter.

3. Receptors That Mediate Increases in $\dot{V}_E$ Elicited by the Humoral Exercise Stimulus

The receptors which mediate increases in $\dot{V}_E$ elicited by exercise-released humoral agents have not been definitively identified (see discussion of spinal transection experiments, Section II,D,1). Therefore, in order to clarify the role of peripheral arterial chemoreceptors in mediating these increases in $\dot{V}_E$, Levine (1976a) denervated the carotid and aortic chemoreceptors of animals who had previously undergone complete transection of the spinal cord at the second lumbar level (L-2). He noted that muscular exercise of the denervated hindlimbs in these chemodenervated spinal transected animals still elicited twofold increases in ventilation. Coincident with these increases in $\dot{V}_E$, arterial P_{CO_2} and arterial oxygen saturation were unchanged from control measurements, but small increments in arterial [H$^+$] (i.e., 5 nmole/liter) were noted. In subsequent experiments, Levine (1976a) demonstrated that comparable increments in arterial [H$^+$] effected by lactic acid infusion (under isocapnic conditions) could not account for the chemodenervated L-2 spinal transected animal's ventilatory response to exercise of denervated extremities. Therefore, these observations of Levine confirm previous work (Grodins and Morgan, 1950; Lamb, 1968–1969) that muscular exercise can stimulate $\dot{V}_E$ by a humoral mechanism other than usual chemical stimuli in arterial blood. Moreover, Levine's results indicate that receptors other than the carotid and aortic bodies can mediate the major portion of the increase in $\dot{V}_E$ elicited by exercise-released humoral agents.

To assess the possibility that extracranial receptors mediate increases in $\dot{V}_E$ elicited by exercise-released humoral agents, Levine (1976b) evaluated the ventilatory response of head-perfused L-2 spinal transected animals (i.e., preparation shown in Fig. 8 with spinal cord transected at the second lumbar level) to muscular exercise of the denervated hindlimbs. Coincident with hindlimb exercise (characterized by twofold increases in oxygen consumption), these head-perfused L-2 spinal transected animals exhibited twofold increases in ventilation. Accordingly, these preliminary observations suggest that extracranial (i.e., thoracic or upper abdominal) receptors can account for the major portion of the increase in $\dot{V}_E$ elicited by exercise-released humoral agents. These extracranial receptors may respond directly to exercise-released humoral agents* or they may respond to some cardiovascular change (e.g., pulmonary blood flow) effected by exercise-released humoral agents.

---

* The possibility exists that these receptors are stimulated by intrapulmonary CO_2 or [H$^+$] tensions or gradients (Bartoli et al., 1974; Filley, 1976; Whipp et al., 1975). However,

E.   Role of the Brain in Processing the Exercise Stimulus

1. Cerebral Mechanisms

Neurophysiological studies (see Plum, 1970, for review) have demonstrated that excitation of certain sites in the cerebral hemispheres elicits increases in ventilation, whereas excitation of other regions inhibits ventilation. The relevance of these observations to exercise hyperpnea remains uncertain, but it is known that cerebral mechanisms may augment or attenuate the ventilatory response to muscular exercise (e.g., exercise hyperventilation of neurocirculatory asthenia, exercise breath holding of trained sprint runners).

2. Brainstem Mechanisms

Some recent work by Eldridge (1973, 1976, 1977) suggests that intracranial amplification of the peripheral exercise stimulus may play a role in the ventilatory response to muscular exercise. Eldridge (1976) elicited "active" increases in ventilation in unanesthetized decerebrate cats by electrical stimulation of a carotid sinus nerve (CSN). During these increases in $\dot{V}_E$, he held arterial P_{CO_2} and arterial pH constant, and he noted that following cessation of CSN stimulation, increases in ventilation persisted for up to 30 seconds' duration. In an attempt to explain these observations, Eldridge (1973, 1976, 1977) hypothesized that increases in breathing induced by a variety of ventilatory stimuli (e.g., CSN stimulation, exercise) may elicit a facilitory feedback process in the brainstem, and he suggested that this "central reverberation" mechanism may contribute to both the increase in $\dot{V}_E$ which accompanies the ventilatory stimulus and the increase in $\dot{V}_E$ which persists after cessation of the ventilatory stimulus. Accordingly, Eldridge's hypothesis implies that intracranial amplification of a primary extracranial exercise stimulus may account for a portion of the increase in $\dot{V}_E$ noted during steady-state exercise (Eldridge, 1977).

The experiments of Asmussen and colleagues (Asmussen and Nielsen, 1964; Asmussen et al., 1965) on humans support the notion that central processing of a peripheral exercise stimulus may constitute an important determinant of the ventilatory response to muscular exercise. First, these workers (Asmussen and Nielsen, 1964) demonstrated that occlusion of the blood flow to exercising extremities augments the increase in $\dot{V}_E$ elicited by exercise. Second, they (Asmussen et al., 1965) demonstrated that small doses of curare also increased the ventilatory response to a standard exercise protocol. In an attempt to explain their data, Asmussen and

---

Levine's results are also consistent with the notion that these receptors are stimulated by substances other than carbon dioxide or hydrogen ion.

associates (Asmussen and Nielsen, 1964; Asmussen *et al.*, 1965) hypothesized that muscular exercise in both experimental conditions (i.e., during circulatory occlusion and after curare administration) involved the activation of an increased number of motor units, and they suggested that this increase in active motor units increased the transmission of afferent information from muscle spindles to the brainstem. They hypothesized that this increase in transmission of information to the brainstem caused an amplification of the peripheral exercise stimulus (Burns, 1963). While this hypothesis adequately explains the experimental results of Asmussen and colleagues (Asmussen and Nielsen, 1964; Asmussen *et al.*, 1965), their data do not preclude the possibility that their experimental conditions directly increased the extracranial component of the exercise stimulus.

III. INTERACTION OF MODERATE EXERCISE WITH OTHER VENTILATORY STIMULI

Numerous workers have extensively investigated the interaction between muscular exercise and the following ventilatory stimuli: oxygen, carbon dioxide, and metabolic acidosis.

A. Oxygen

Altitude (Asmussen *et al.*, 1965; Dejours, 1964; Dejours *et al.*, 1963; Lahiri, 1976; Pugh *et al.*, 1964) or the breathing of hypoxic gas mixtures (Asmussen, 1967; Asmussen and Nielsen, 1957; Bhattacharyya *et al.*, 1970; Cunningham *et al.*, 1968; Dejours, 1964; Kao *et al.*, 1967; Lahiri, 1976; Masson and Lahiri, 1974) augments the ventilatory response to muscular exercise. Figure 10 indicates that exercising man exhibits a linear relationship between ventilation ($\dot{V}_E$) and oxygen consumption ($\dot{V}_{O_2}$) at an arterial P_{O_2} of 100, whereas a curvilinear relationship exists at an arterial P_{O_2} of 45. Figure 10 shows that this curvilinearity is easily demonstrated under isocapnic conditions (triangles), but it can even be demonstrated at arterial CO_2 tensions below the normal resting level (open circles). In an attempt to elucidate the interaction between exercise and arterial hypoxemia, Cunningham *et al.* (1968) abruptly changed the inspired gas mixture of exercising human subjects from hypoxic gas mixtures to 100% oxygen; they noted that a decrease in ventilation occurred after a breath or two of 100% oxygen. Cunningham *et al.* (1968) concluded from this rapid decrease in $\dot{V}_E$ that a neural mechanism responsive to arterial oxygen tension (or to arterial oxygen saturation) accounts for the

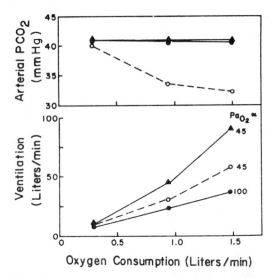

Figure 10.   Effect of arterial P_{O_2} on steady-state ventilation–oxygen consumption relationships (in humans) during muscular exercise. Closed circles, arterial P_{O_2} (Pa_{O_2}) of 100 mm Hg; open circles, Pa_{O_2} of 45 mm Hg without addition of CO_2 to inspired air; closed triangles, Pa_{O_2} of 45 mm Hg with addition of CO_2 to inspired air. (Reprinted with modification from Lahiri, 1976; courtesy of the author and Interprint Publications.)

multiplicative interaction between muscular exercise and arterial hypoxemia. Therefore, Davies and Lahiri (1973) explored the possibility that mean carotid chemoreceptor activity accounted for the excess ventilation of hypoxic exercise. These workers reported that muscular exercise failed to elicit increases in mean carotid chemoreceptor activity at all levels of arterial P_{O_2}. While these observations of Davies and Lahiri (1973) demonstrate that mean carotid chemoreceptor activity cannot account for the excess ventilation of hypoxic exercise, they do not eliminate the possibility that oscillations in carotid chemoreceptor activity account for this phenomenon (Lahiri, 1976). In summary, the precise mechanism underlying the interaction between arterial hypoxemia and muscular exercise has not been elucidated. Further work is necessary to resolve this important question.

B. Carbon Dioxide

Many investigators (Asmussen, 1965, 1967; Asmussen and Nielsen, 1957; Craig, 1955; Kao *et al.*, 1963, 1967; Luft *et al.*, 1974; Menn *et al.*, 1970; Rizzo *et al.*, 1976; Sinclair *et al.*, 1971) have demonstrated that a hypercapnic environment augments the ventilatory response to muscular exercise. Asmussen and Nielsen (1957; Asmussen, 1967), Kao (Kao *et al.*, 1963, 1967), and others have demonstrated that (low intensities of) arterial hypercapnia and moderate muscular exercise interact in an additive manner with respect to stimulation of ventilation (see Fig. 11).

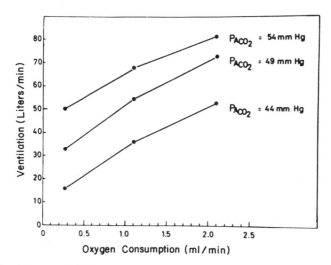

Figure 11. Effect of alveolar P_{CO_2} on steady-state ventilation–oxygen consumption relationships (in humans) during muscular exercise. Alveolar P_{O_2} was 100 mm Hg in all experiments. (Reprinted with modification from Asmussen, 1967; courtesy of the author and the American Heart Association.)

C. Metabolic Acidosis

Exercise-induced metabolic acidosis augments the ventilatory response to muscular exercise. In this chapter, this point is discussed in Section IV below. Additionally, the literature suggests that muscular exercise initiated during resting metabolic acidosis elicits an increased ventilatory response (Dennig *et al.*, 1930; Forster and Klausen, 1973; Refsum, 1961), but data regarding this point are sparse.

IV. SEVERE EXERCISE

A. Overview of Ventilatory Control

During steady-state severe exercise, the increase in ventilation is curvilinearly related to the increase in aerobic metabolic rate (see Fig. 1). Accordingly, both $\dot{V}_{E_{O_2}}$ and $\dot{V}_{E_{CO_2}}$ are increased from the resting state, while arterial P_{CO_2} is decreased from the resting state. *Excess ventilation* (Koyal *et al.*, 1976) is the term used to designate the amount by which ventilation exceeds that predicted by the aerobic metabolic rate (see Fig. 12). Since the combination of ventilatory stimuli operative during moder-

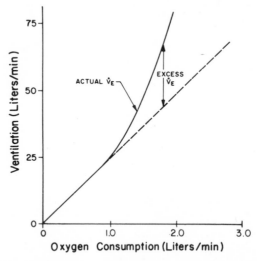

Figure 12. Definition of term *excess ventilation*. Solid line represents the relationship (in humans) between measured ventilation and oxygen consumption during various intensities of muscular exercise. Dashed line represents the relationship between ventilation and oxygen consumption at a ventilatory equivalent for oxygen ($\dot{V}_{E_{O_2}}$) which is constant and unchanged from rest. Excess ventilation is the difference between solid and dashed lines (i.e., vertical arrow). (Reprinted with modification from Koyal *et al.*, 1976; courtesy of the author and the *Journal of Applied Physiology*.)

ate exercise (i.e., the exercise stimulus) elicits increases in $\dot{V}_E$ which are proportional to the aerobic metabolic rate, additional stimuli have been invoked to explain the excess ventilation noted in severe exercise. (However, the possibility exists that ventilatory stimuli operative during moderate exercise may relate to the metabolic rate in a curvilinear manner, and therefore additional mechanisms need not be invoked to account for the excess ventilation of severe exercise.)

B.   Mechanisms Underlying the Excess Ventilation of Severe Exercise

The following mechanisms have been proposed to account for portions of the excess ventilation noted in severe exercise: metabolic acidosis (Comroe, 1965; Dejours, 1964; Grodins, 1950; Koyal *et al.*, 1976; Wasserman, 1976; Wasserman *et al.*, 1967, 1975b), increase in ventilatory responsiveness to oxygen (Asmussen, 1965; Asmussen and Nielsen, 1946, 1958; Bannister and Cunningham, 1954; Dejours, 1964; Hickam *et al.*, 1951), catecholamines (Dejours, 1964), increases in body temperature (Comroe, 1944; Wagner *et al.*, 1977), and unspecified humoral factors (Asmussen and Nielsen, 1950).

1. Metabolic Acidosis

Metabolic acidosis occurs in severe exercise, and increments in arterial lactate concentration largely account for its occurrence (Dejours, 1964; Grodins, 1950; Koyal *et al.*, 1976; Leusen, 1965; Wasserman *et al.*, 1967, 1975b; Wasserman and Whipp, 1975). In an attempt to elucidate the relationship between the excess ventilation of severe exercise and metabolic acidosis, Koyal and colleagues (1976) have noted that the excess ventilation of severe exercise is linearly related to the decrements in arterial bicarbonate concentration (see Fig. 13). This observation of Koyal *et al.* suggests that some aspect of metabolic acidosis may completely account for the excess ventilation of severe exercise.

In order to discern the role of the carotid bodies in mediating the excess ventilation of severe exercise, Wasserman and colleagues (1975b) have studied the ventilatory response of carotid body resected (CBR) human subjects to severe exercise. They noted that CBR subjects did not exhibit excess ventilation coincident with the metabolic acidosis of severe exercise. Therefore, these observations suggest that the carotid bodies play an important role in mediating the excess ventilation of severe exercise.

In order to gain further insight into the relationship between lactic acidosis and ventilation, Levine (1975) has studied the ventilatory response of anesthetized dogs to cyanide-induced lactic acidosis. He has

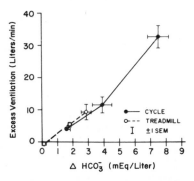

Figure 13. Relationship (in humans) between excess ventilation of severe exercise and decrease in arterial bicarbonate concentration (i.e., ΔHCO_3^-). The excess ventilation of severe exercise is linearly related to the decrease in arterial bicarbonate concentration. (Reprinted with modification from Koyal *et al.*, 1976; courtesy of the author and the *Journal of Applied Physiology*.)

demonstrated that cyanide-induced lactic acidosis stimulates $\dot{V}_E$ by excitation of extracranial receptors (other than the carotid and aortic bodies). The possibility exists that these extracranial receptors may play some role in eliciting the excess ventilation of severe exercise.

2. Increase in Ventilatory Responsiveness to Oxygen

Decrements in arterial P_{O_2} do not usually accompany most forms of severe exercise (Asmussen, 1965; Dejours, 1964; Holmgren and McIlroy, 1964; Wasserman et al., 1967; Wasserman and Whipp, 1975). Nonetheless, in order to evaluate the interaction between oxygen-induced ventilatory drive and intensity of exercise, many investigators (Asmussen, 1965; Asmussen and Nielsen, 1946, 1958; Bannister and Cunningham, 1954; Dejours, 1964; Hickam et al., 1951) have increased the oxygen concentration of the inspired gas mixture being breathed by human subjects during various intensities of exercise. These investigators have noted that decrements in $\dot{V}_E$ accompanied the breathing of high O_2 gas mixtures (Asmussen, 1965; Asmussen and Nielsen, 1946; Bannister and Cunningham, 1954; Dejours, 1964; Hickam et al., 1951); the magnitude of these hyperoxia-induced decrements in $\dot{V}_E$ varied directly with the aerobic metabolic rate (Asmussen, 1965; Asmussen and Nielsen, 1946, 1958; Dejours, 1964). These results indicate that an increased oxygen drive to $\dot{V}_E$ exists during severe exercise (i.e., high aerobic metabolic rates), and they suggest that this increased oxygen drive may account for a significant portion of the increase in $\dot{V}_E$ noted in severe exercise. The precise mechanism underlying this increased oxygen drive to $\dot{V}_E$ is not fully understood.

3. Catecholamines

The concentrations of epinephrine and norepinephrine in blood, as well as the excretion rate (and presumably the secretion rate) of these compounds, increase during heavy exercise (von Euler, 1974; Gray and Beetham, 1957; Holmgren, 1956). Because intravenous infusion of these catecholamines elicits increases in $\dot{V}_E$ in man (Barcroft et al., 1957; Heistad et al., 1972; Stone et al., 1973) and in animals (Joels and White, 1968; Young, 1957), the increase in blood concentration of these compounds may account for some portion of the excess ventilation noted in severe exercise. In attempts to elucidate the mechanism underlying stimulation of ventilation by catecholamines, some workers have demonstrated that injection of these compounds directly into the verebral arteries of man (Coles et al., 1956) or animals (Young, 1957) does not elicit immediate increases in ventilation. These observations suggest that catecholamines do not stimulate $\dot{V}_E$ by direct excitation of the respiratory center. Stimulation of $\dot{V}_E$ by these compounds (in the cat) is eliminated by denervation of the carotid and aortic chemoreceptors; therefore, Joels and White (1968) concluded that peripheral arterial chemoreceptors mediate the major portion of the increase in $\dot{V}_E$ elicited by catecholamines (i.e., epinephrine or norepinephrine). Heistad and colleagues (1972) have reported that a β-adrenergic mechanism (presumably located in the peripheral arterial chemoreceptors) mediates increases in $\dot{V}_E$ effected by norepinephrine, but the data of Stone and associates (1973) do not support this notion.

4. Increases in Body Temperature

Several investigators have noted that some species (e.g., dogs) manifest large increments (i.e., 2°–3°C) in rectal temperature during severe exercise (Wagner *et al.*, 1977; Young *et al.*, 1959). Because comparable changes in rectal temperature effected by external heating are associated with large increases in $\dot{V}_E$ (Bligh, 1966; Hales *et al.*, 1970), increments in body temperature may account for an appreciable portion of the excess ventilation noted during severe exercise in certain species. While the precise mechanism by which large increments in body temperature stimulate $\dot{V}_E$ remains uncertain, extracephalic as well as cephalic thermoreceptors appear to play an important role (Bligh, 1966; Hales *et al.*, 1970).

5. Unspecified Humoral Agents

Asmussen and Nielsen (1950) carried out endogenous infusion experiments in humans in an attempt to demonstrate that humoral agents released by severe exercise stimulate $\dot{V}_E$. These workers inflated thigh tourniquets at the cessation of severe exercise and thereby trapped "work blood" in the lower extremities. After ventilation had returned to control levels, they released the thigh tourniquets and noted large increases in $\dot{V}_E$. These increases in $\dot{V}_E$ were accompanied by increases in alveolar P_{CO_2} and by decreases in arterial blood pressure. In an attempt to discern the relationship between ventilation and these changes, they produced comparable increments in alveolar P_{CO_2} and comparable decrements in arterial blood pressure in the subjects at rest; the resultant increases in $\dot{V}_E$ were appreciably smaller than those noted following postexercise tourniquet release. While these observations of Asmussen and Nielsen (1950) demonstrate that humoral agents released by severe exercise can stimulate $\dot{V}_E$, they neither specify the nature of these humoral stimuli nor do they localize the receptors which mediate increases in $\dot{V}_E$ elicited by "severe exercise-released humoral agents."

V. SUMMARY AND CONCLUSIONS

A. Moderate Exercise

The relationships between ventilation and tissue metabolism during steady-state moderate exercise have been firmly established: $\dot{V}_{E_{O_2}}$, $\dot{V}_{E_{CO_2}}$, and arterial P_{CO_2} are unchanged from rest. Accordingly, a high degree of correlation exists between the sum of all ventilatory stimuli operative during moderate muscular exercise (i.e., the exercise stimulus) and the aerobic metabolic rate (i.e., $\dot{V}_{O_2}$, $\dot{V}_{CO_2}$).

The increased activity of the respiratory muscles during exercise is presumed to originate in the medullary respiratory center. Therefore, information concerning the exercise stimulus must be transmitted to the respiratory center.

Although supramedullary portions of the brain may in certain circumstances initiate or amplify the ventilatory response to muscular exercise, the complete steady-state stimulus to $\dot{V}_E$ can arise in exercising extremities.

Animal experiments have demonstrated that under specified experimental circumstances, either neural or humoral pathways can completely account for transmission of the full exercise stimulus to the respiratory center. However, in the intact organism, the precise manner in which neural and humoral pathways interact is not fully understood.

Receptors located in exercising extremities initiate a neural pathway; however, the precise nature of these receptors (i.e., mechanoreceptors or metaboreceptors) is not known. These unspecified receptors transmit information to the respiratory center via peripheral nerves and intraspinal afferent pathways.

The exercise-released humoral stimulus to $\dot{V}_E$ correlates with the rate of carbon dioxide delivery to the lung. However, the precise nature of this humoral stimulus is not known.

The receptors which mediate increases in $\dot{V}_E$ elicited by exercise-released humoral agents have not been definitively identified.

B. Severe Exercise

The following ventilation–metabolism relationships have been established for steady-state severe exercise: both $\dot{V}_{E_{O_2}}$ and $\dot{V}_{E_{CO_2}}$ are increased above the resting state, while arterial P_{CO_2} is decreased below resting levels.

Because of the fact that the combination of ventilatory stimuli operative during moderate exercise (i.e., the exercise stimulus) elicits increases in $\dot{V}_E$ which are proportional to the aerobic metabolic rate, additional mechanisms have been invoked to explain the excess ventilation noted in severe exercise.

Metabolic acidosis, catecholamines, and an increase in ventilatory responsiveness to oxygen contribute to the excess ventilation noted in severe exercise. Increases in body temperature and unspecified humoral factors may also contribute to the excess ventilation noted in severe exercise.

ACKNOWLEDGMENTS

The advice and help of Dr. Susan Levine is gratefully acknowledged. I am also indebted to my colleagues Drs. Richard Levinson and Michael Magno for a critical review of this manuscript. Ms. Geraldine Hill and Mrs. Bernice Richlin provided invaluable assistance in the preparation of this manuscript.

I thank Drs. Asmussen, Dejours, Kao, Koyal, Lahiri, and Wasserman for permission to reproduce illustrations from their publications. I am also indebted to the *American Review of Respiratory Disease, the Journal of Applied Physiology,* the American Physiologic Society, Blackwell Scientific Publications Ltd., and Interprint Publications for granting me permission to reproduce illustrations.

REFERENCES

Armstrong, B. W., H. H. Hurt, R. W. Blide, and J. M. Workman (1961). The humoral regulation of breathing. A concept based on the physicochemical composition of mixed venous and arterial blood is presented. *Science* **133**, 1897–1906.
Asmussen, E. (1965). Muscular exercise. *Hand. Physiol. Sect. 3 Respir.* **2**, 939–978.
Asmussen, E. (1967). Exercise and the regulation of ventilation. *Circ. Res.* **20**, Suppl., 1132–1145.
Asmussen, E., and O. Bøje (1945). Body temperature and capacity for work. *Acta Physiol. Scand.* **10**, 1–22.
Asmussen, E., and E. Hansen (1938). Ueber den einfluss statischer muskelarbeit auf atmung und kreislauf. *Skand. Arch. Physiol.* **78**, 283–303.
Asmussen, E., and M. Nielsen (1946). Studies on the regulation of respiration in heavy work. *Acta Physiol. Scand.* **12**, 171–188.
Asmussen, E., and M. Nielsen (1950). The effect of auto-transfusion of "work blood" on the pulmonary ventilation. *Acta Physiol. Scand.* **20**, 79–87.
Asmussen, E., and M. Nielsen (1957). Ventilatory response to CO_2 during work at normal and at low oxygen tensions. *Acta Physiol. Scand.* **39**, 27–35.
Asmussen, E., and M. Nielsen (1958). Pulmonary ventilation and effect of oxygen breathing in heavy exercise. *Acta Physiol. Scand.* **43**, 365–378.
Asmussen, E., and M. Nielsen (1964). Experiments on nervous factors controlling respiration and circulation during exercise employing blocking of the blood flow. *Acta Physiol. Scand.* **60**, 103–111.
Asmussen, E., M. Nielsen, and G. Weith-Pedersen (1943). Cortical or reflex control of respiration during muscular work? *Acta Physiol. Scand.* **6**, 168–175.
Asmussen, E., S. H. Johansen, M. Jørgensen, and M. Nielsen (1965). On the nervous factors controlling respiration and circulation during exercise. Experiments with curarization. *Acta Physiol. Scand.* **63**, 343–350.
Åstrand, P.-O. (1954). The respiratory activity in man exposed to prolonged hypoxia. *Acta Physiol. Scand.* **30**, 343–368.
Bailen, H. N., and S. M. Horvath (1959). Evaluation of neurogenic and metabolic influences from a perfused leg on respiration exchanges. *Am. J. Physiol.* **196**, 467–469.

Band, D. M., I. R. Cameron, and S. J. G. Semple (1969a). Oscillations in arterial pH with breathing in the cat. *J. Appl. Physiol.* **26**, 261–267.

Band, D. M., I. R. Cameron, and S. J. G. Semple (1969b). Effect of different methods of CO$_2$ administration on oscillations of arterial pH in the cat. *J. Appl. Physiol.* **26**, 268–273.

Bannister, R. G., and D. J. C. Cunningham (1954). The effects on the respiration and performance during exercise of adding oxygen to the inspired air. *J. Physiol. (London)* **125**, 118–137.

Barcroft, H., V. Basnayake, O. Celander, A. F. Cobbold, D. J. C. Cunningham, M. G. M. Jukes, and I. M. Young (1957). The effect of carbon dioxide on the respiratory response to noradrenaline in man. *J. Physiol. (London)* **137**, 365–373.

Bartoli, A., B. A. Cross, A. Guz, S. K. Jain, M. I. M. Noble, and D. W. Trenchard (1974). The effect of carbon dioxide in the airways and alveoli on ventilation; a vagal reflex studied in the dog. *J. Physiol. (London)* **240**, 91–109.

Bedfort, J., H. M. Vernon, and C. G. Warner (1933). The influence of static effort on the respiration and on the respiratory exchange. *J. Hyg.* **22**, 118–150.

Bein, H. J., and H. V. Fehr (1962). Depression of muscle spindle activity: New type of pharmacological action. *Br. J. Pharmacol. Chemother.* **19**, 375–384.

Bernthal, T., and W. F. Weeks (1939). Respiratory and vasomotor effects of variations in carotid body temperature: Study of the mechanisms of chemoreceptor stimulation. *Am. J. Physiol.* **127**, 94–105.

Bessou, P., P. Dejours, and Y. Laporte (1959). Effects ventilatoires réflexes de la stimulation de fibres afférentes de grand diametre d'origine musculaire, chez le chat. *C. R. Seances Soc. Biol. Ses Fil.* **153**, 477–481.

Bhattacharyya, N. K., D. J. C. Cunningham, R. C. Goode, M. G. Howson, and B. B. Lloyd (1970). Hypoxia, ventilation, P_{CO_2} and exercise. *Respir. Physiol.* **9**, 329–347.

Black, A. M. S., and R. W. Torrance (1971). Respiratory oscillations in chemoreceptor discharge in the control of breathing. *Respir. Physiol.* **13**, 221–237.

Bligh, J. (1966). The thermosensitivity of the hypothalamus and thermoregulation in mammals. *Biol. Rev. Cambridge Philos. Soc.* **41**, 317–367.

Bouverot, P. (1973). Vagal afferent fibres from the lung and regulation of breathing in awake dogs. *Respir. Physiol.* **17**, 325–335.

Brinley, F. J. (1974). Excitation and conduction in nerve fibers. *In* "Medical Physiology" (V. B. Mountcastle, ed.), I, pp. 34–76. Mosby, St. Louis, Missouri.

Burns, B. D. (1963). The central control of respiratory movements. *Br. Med. Bull.* **19**, 7–9.

Cherniack, R. M. (1965). Work of breathing and the ventilatory response to CO$_2$. *Handb. Physiol. Sect. 3: Respir.* **2**, 1469–1473.

Coleridge, H., J. C. G. Coleridge, and A. Howe (1967). A search for pulmonary arterial chemoreceptors in the cat, with a comparison of the blood supply of the aortic bodies in the new-born and adult animal. *J. Physiol. (London)* **191**, 353–374.

Coles, R. D., F. Duff, W. H. T. Shepherd, and R. F. Whelan (1956). The effect on respiration of infusions of adrenaline and noradrenaline into the carotid and vertebral arteries in man. *Br. J. Pharmacol. Chemother.* **11**, 346–350.

Comroe, J. H., Jr. (1944). The hyperpnea of muscular exercise. *Physiol. Rev.* **24**, 319–339.

Comroe, J. H., Jr. (1965). "Physiology of Respiration," p. 192. Yearbook Publ., Chicago, Illinois.

Comroe, J. H., Jr., and C. F. Schmidt (1943). Reflexes from the limbs as a factor in the hyperpnea of muscular exercise. *Am. J. Physiol.* **138**, 536–547.

Comroe, J. H., Jr., R. E. Forster, A. B. Dubois, W. A. Briscoe, and E. Carlsen (1962). "The Lung," 2nd ed., p. 342. Yearbook Publ., Chicago, Illinois.

Craig, F. N. (1955). Pulmonary ventilation during exercise and inhalation of carbon dioxide. *J. Appl. Physiol.* **7,** 467–471.

Cropp, G. J. A., and J. H. Comroe, Jr. (1961). Role of venous blood P_{CO_2} in respiratory control. *J. Appl. Physiol.* **16,** 1029–1033.

Cunningham, D. J. C. (1963). Some quantitative aspects of the regulation of human respiration in exercise. *Br. Med. Bull.* **19,** 25–30.

Cunningham, D. J. C. (1967). Regulation of breathing in exercise. *Circ. Res.* **20,** 1122–1131.

Cunningham, D. J. C., D. Spurr, and B. B. Lloyd (1968). Ventilatory drive in hypoxic exercise. *In* "Arterial Chemoreceptors" (R. W. Torrance, ed.), pp. 301–321. Blackwell, Oxford.

Cunningham, D. J. C., M. G. Howson, and S. B. Pearson (1973). The respiratory effects in man of altering the time profile of alveolar carbon dioxide and oxygen within each respiratory cycle. *J. Physiol. (London)* **234,** 1–28.

Davies, H., N. Gazetopoulos, and C. Oliver (1965). Ventilatory and metabolic response to graduated and prolonged exercise in normal subjects. *Clin. Sci.* **29,** 443–452.

Davies, R. O., and S. Lahiri (1973). Absence of carotid chemoreceptor response during hypoxic exercise in the cat. *Respir. Physiol.* **18,** 92–100.

Dejours, P. (1962). Chemoreflexes in breathing. *Physiol. Rev.* **42,** 335–358.

Dejours, P. (1964). Control of respiration in muscular exercise. *Handb. Physiol. Sect. 3: Respir.* **1,** 631–648.

Dejours, P. (1967). Neurogenic factors in the control of ventilation during exercise. *Circ. Res.* **20,** 1146–1153.

Dejours, P., R. H. Kellogg, and N. Pace (1963). Regulation of respiration and heart rate response in exercise during altitude acclimatization. *J. Appl. Physiol.* **18,** 10–18.

Denning, J., J. H. Talbott, H. T. Edwards, and D. B. Dill (1930). Effect of acidosis and alkalosis upon capacity for work. *J. Clin. Invest.* **9,** 601–613.

Duke, H. N., J. H. Green, P. F. Heffron, and V. W. J. Stubbens (1963). Pulmonary chemoreceptors. *Q. J. Exp. Physiol. Cogn. Med. Sci.* **48,** 164–175.

Dutton, R. E., and S. Permutt (1968). Ventilatory responses to transient changes in carbon dioxide. *In* "Arterial Chemoreceptors" (R. W. Torrance, ed.), pp. 373–384. Blackwell, Oxford.

Ekelund, L. G., and A. Holmgren (1967). Central hemodynamics during exercise. *Circ. Res.* **20,** 122–143.

Eldridge, F. L. (1973). Posthyperventilation breathing: Different effects of active and passive hyperventilation. *J. Appl. Physiol.* **34,** 422–430.

Eldridge, F. L. (1976). Central neural stimulation of respiration in unanesthetized decerebrate cats. *J. Appl. Physiol.* **40,** 23–28.

Eldridge, F. L. (1977). Neural drive mechanisms of central origin. *In* "Muscular Exercise and the Lung" (J. A. Dempsey and C. E. Reed, eds.), pp. 149–159. Univ. of Wisconsin Press, Madison.

Eldridge, F. L., and J. M. Davis (1959). Effect of mechanical factors on respiratory work and ventilatory responses to CO_2. *J. Appl. Physiol.* **14,** 721–726.

Filley, G. F. (1976). Blood gas disequilibria and exercise hyperpnea. *Trans. Am. Clinatol. (Clin.) Assoc.* **87,** 48–58.

Flandrois, R., J. R. Lacour, J. Islas-Maroquin, and J. Charlot (1967). Limbs mechanoreceptors inducing the reflex hyperpnea of exercise. *Respir. Physiol.* **2,** 335–343.

Fordyce, W. E., F. Gonzalez, and F. S. Grodins (1976). Ventilatory response to I. V. CO_2

loading in chloralose–urethane anesthetized dogs. *Fed. Proc., Fed. Am. Soc. Exp. Biol.* **35**, 718 (abstr.).

Forster, H. V., and K. Klausen (1973). The effect of chronic metabolic acidosis and alkalosis on ventilation during exercise and hypoxia. *Respir. Physiol.* **17**, 336–346.

Gautier, H., A. Lacaisse, and P. Dejours (1969). Ventilatory response to muscle spindle stimulation by succinylcholine in cats. *Respir. Physiol.* **7**, 383–388.

Geppert, J., and N. Zuntz (1888). Ueber die regulation der atmung. *Arch. Gesamte. Physiol. Menschen Tiere* **42**, 189–245.

Gonzalez, F., and W. E. Fordyce (1976). Evidence against a CO_2 mediated pulmonary chemoreflex in dogs. *Fed. Proc., Fed. Am. Soc. Exp. Biol.* **35**, 553 (abstr.).

Granit, R. (1955). "Receptors and Sensory Perception," pp. 237–276. Yale Univ. Press, New Haven, Connecticut.

Granit, R., S. Skoglund, and S. Thesleff (1953). Activation of muscle spindles by succinylcholine and decamethonium. The effects of curare. *Acta Physiol. Scand.* **28**, 134–151.

Gray, I., and W. P. Beetham (1957). Changes in plasma concentration of epinephrine and norepinephrine with muscular work. *Proc. Soc. Exp. Biol. Med.* **96**, 636–638.

Gray, J. S. (1950). "Pulmonary Ventilation and its Physiological Regulation," p. 82. Thomas, Springfield, Illinois.

Grodins, F. S. (1950). Analysis of factors concerned in regulation of breathing in exercise. *Physiol. Rev.* **30**, 220–239.

Grodins, F. S., and D. P. Morgan (1950). Regulation of breathing during electrically-induced muscular work in anesthetized dogs following transection of spinal cord. *Am. J. Physiol.* **162**, 64–73.

Hales, J. R. S., F. F. Kao, S. S. Mei, C. Wang, and M. Gretenstein (1970). Panting in heated cross-circulated dogs. *Am. J. Physiol.* **218**, 1389–1393.

Harrison, T. R., W. G. Harrison, J. A. Calhoun, and J. P. Marsh (1932). Congestive heart failure. XVII. The mechanism of dyspnea on exertion. *Arch. Intern. Med.* **50**, 690–720.

Heistad, D. D., R. C. Wheeler, A. L. Mark, P. G. Schmid, and F. M. Abboud (1972). Effects of adrenergic stimulation on ventilation in man. *J. Clin. Invest.* **51**, 1469–1475.

Heymans, C., J. Jacob, and G. Liljestrand (1947). Regulation of respiration during muscular work, as studied in the perfused isolated head. *Acta Physiol. Scand.* **14**, 86–101.

Hickam, J. B., W. W. Pryor, E. B. Page, and R. J. Atwell (1951). Respiratory regulation during exercise in unconditioned subjects. *J. Clin. Invest.* **30**, 503–516.

Hodgson, H. J. F., and P. B. C. Matthews (1968). The ineffectiveness of excitation of the primary endings of the muscle spindle by vibration as a respiratory stimulant in the decerebrate cat. *J. Physiol. (London)* **194**, 555–563.

Holmgren, A. (1956). Circulatory changes during muscular work in man with special reference to arterial and central venous pressures in the systemic circulation. *Scand. J. Clin. Lab. Invest.* **8**, Suppl. 24, 1–97.

Holmgren, A., and M. B. McIlroy (1964). Effect of temperature on arterial blood gas tensions and pH during exercise. *J. Appl. Physiol.* **19**, 243–245.

Huch, A., D. Kotter, R. Loerbroks, and J. Piiper (1969). O_2 transport in anesthetized dogs in hypoxia with O_2 uptake increased by 2:4-dinitrophenol. *Respir. Physiol.* **6**, 187–201.

Joels, N., and H. White (1968). The contribution of the arterial chemoreceptors to the stimulation of respiration by adrenaline and noradrenaline in the cat. *J. Physiol. (London)* **197**, 1–23.

Kalia, M., J. M. Senapati, B. Parida, and A. Panda (1972). Reflex increase in ventilation by muscle receptors with nonmedullated fibers (C Fibers). *J. Appl. Physiol.* **32**, 189–193.

Kao, F. F. (1956). Regulation of respiration during muscular activity. *Am. J. Physiol.* **185**, 145–151.

Kao, F. F. (1963). Experimental study of the pathways involved in exercise hyperpnoea employing cross-circulation techniques. *In* "Regulation of Human Respiration" (D. J. C. Cunningham and B. B. Lloyd, eds.), pp. 461–502. Blackwell, Oxford.

Kao, F. F., and E. E. Suckling (1963). A method for producing muscular exercise in anesthetized dogs and its validity. *J. Appl. Physiol.* **18**, 194–196.

Kao, F. F., C. C. Michel, S. S. Mei, and W. K. Li (1963). Somatic afferent influence on respiration. *Ann. N.Y. Acad. Sci.* **109**, 696–711.

Kao, F. F., C. W. Wang, S. S. Mei, and C. C. Michel (1965). Relationship of exercise hyperpnea to CSF pH. *In* "Cerebrospinal Fluid and the Regulation of Ventilation" (C. McC. Brooks, F. F. Kao, and B. B. Lloyd, eds.), pp. 269–275. Blackwell, Oxford.

Kao, F. F., S. Lahiri, C. Wang, and S. S. Mei (1967). Ventilation and cardiac output in exercise. Interaction of chemical and work stimuli. *Circ. Res.* **20**, 1179–1191.

Koizumi, K., J. Ushiyama, and C. McC. Brooks (1961). Muscle afferents and activity of respiratory neurons. *Am. J. Physiol.* **200**, 679–684.

Kollmeyer, K. R., and L. I. Kleinman (1975). A respiratory venous chemoreceptor in the young puppy. *J. Appl. Physiol.* **38**, 819–826.

Koyal, S. N., B. J. Whipp, D. Huntsman, G. Bray, and K. Wasserman (1976). Ventilatory responses to the metabolic acidosis of treadmill and cycle ergometry. *J. Appl. Physiol.* **40**, 864–867.

Kramer, K., and O. Gauer (1941). Uber die regelung der atmung bei muskelarbeit. *Pfluegers Arch. Gesamte Physiol. Menschen Tiere* **244**, 659–686.

Krogh, A., and J. Lindhard (1913). The regulation of respiration and circulation during the initial stages of muscular work. *J. Physiol. (London)* **47**, 112–136.

Krogh, A., and J. Lindhard (1917). A comparison between voluntarily and electrically induced muscular work in man. *J. Physiol. (London)* **51**, 182–201.

Lahiri, S. (1976). Control of ventilation during hypoxic exercise. *In* "Selected Topics in Environmental Biology" (B. Bhatia, G. S. Chhina, and B. Singh, eds.), pp. 243–246. Interprint, New Delhi.

Lahiri, S., S. S. Mei, and F. F. Kao (1975). Vagal modulation of respiratory control during exercise. *Respir. Physiol.* **23**, 133–146.

Lahiri, S., C. A. Weitz, J. S. Milledge, and M. C. Fishman (1976). Effects of hypoxia, heat, and humidity on physical performance. *J. Appl. Physiol.* **40**, 206–210.

Lamb, T. W. (1966). Ventilatory responses to intravenous and inspired carbon dioxide in anesthetized cats. *Respir. Physiol.* **2**, 99–104.

Lamb, T. W. (1968–1969). Ventilatory responses to hind limb exercise in anesthetized cats and dogs. *Respir. Physiol.* **6**, 88–104.

Lehninger, A. L. (1970). "Biochemistry," pp. 365–393. Worth, New York.

Leitner, L.-M. and P. Dejours (1971). Reflex increase in ventilation induced by vibrations applied to the triceps surae muscles in the cat. *Respir. Physiol.* **12**, 199–204.

Leusen, I. (1965). Aspects of the acid–base balance between blood and cerebrospinal fluid. *In* "Cerebrospinal Fluid and the Regulation of Ventilation" (C. McC. Brooks, F. F. Kao, and B. B. Lloyd, eds.), pp. 55–89. Blackwell, Oxford.

Leusen, I. (1972). Regulation of cerebrospinal fluid composition with reference to breathing. *Physiol. Rev.* **52**, 1–56.

Levine, S. (1975). Nonperipheral chemoreceptor stimulation of ventilation by cyanide. *J. Appl. Physiol.* **39**, 199–204.

Levine, S. (1976a). Ventilatory response to exercise of denervated extremities: Observations in peripheral chemodenervated dogs. *Physiologist* **19**, 268 (abstr.).

Levine, S. (1976b). Ventilatory response to muscular exercise: Role of humoral factors. *Am. Rev. Respir. Dis.* **113**, 218 (abstr.).

Levine, S. (1977a). Ventilatory response to drug-induced hypermetabolism: Possible relevance to exercise hyperpnea. *In* "Muscular Exercise and the Lung" (J. A. Dempsey and C. E. Reed, eds.), pp. 89–101. Univ. of Wisconsin Press, Madison.

Levine, S. (1977b). Role of tissue hypermetabolism in stimulation of ventilation by dinitrophenol. *J. Appl. Physiol.* **43**, 72–74.

Levine, S., and W. E. Huckabee (1975). Ventilatory response to drug-induced hypermetabolism. *J. Appl. Physiol.* **38**, 827–833.

Lewis, S. M. (1972). Awake baboon's ventilatory response to venous and inhaled CO_2 loading. *J. Appl. Physiol.* **39**, 417–422.

Liang, C.-S., and W. B. Hood, Jr. (1973). Comparison of cardiac output responses to 2,4-dinitrophenol-induced hypermetabolism and muscular work. *J. Clin. Invest.* **52**, 2283–2292.

Liang, C.-S., and W. B. Hood, Jr. (1976). Afferent neural pathway in the regulation of cardiopulmonary responses to tissue hypermetabolism. *Circ. Res.* **38**, 209–214.

Luft, V. C., S. Finkelstein, and J. C. Elliot (1974). Respiratory gas exchange, acid base balance, and electrolytes during and after maximal work breathing 15 mm Hg PI_{CO_2}. *In* "Carbon Dioxide and Metabolic Regulations" (G. Nahas and K. E. Schaefer, eds.), pp. 283–292. Springer-Verlag, Berlin and New York.

Lynne-Davies, P., J. Couture, L. D. Pengelly, and J. Milic-Emili (1971). Immediate ventilatory response to added inspiratory elastic loads in cats. *J. Appl. Physiol.* **30**, 512–516.

McGilvery, R. W. (1970). "Biochemistry," pp. 177–205. Saunders, Philadelphia, Pennsylvania.

Masson, R. G., and S. Lahiri (1974). Chemical control of ventilation during hypoxic exercise. *Respir. Physiol.* **22**, 241–262.

Matell, G. (1963). Time-courses of changes in ventilation and arterial gas tensions in man induced by moderate exercise. *Acta Physiol. Scand. Suppl.* **206**, 1–53.

Menn, S. J., R. D. Sinclair, and B. E. Welch (1970). Effect of inspired P_{CO_2} up to 30 mm Hg on response of normal man to exercise. *J. Appl. Physiol.* **28**, 663–671.

Milic-Emili, J., and J. M. Tyler (1963). Relation between work output of respiratory muscles and end-tidal CO_2 tension. *J. Appl. Physiol.* **18**, 497–504.

Morgan, D. P., F. Kao, T. P. K. Lim, and F. S. Grodins (1955). Temperature and respiratory responses in exercise. *Am. J. Physiol.* **183**, 454–458.

Mueller, J. V., S. M. Yamashiro, and F. S. Grodins (1974). Ventilatory response of anesthetized dogs to venous CO_2 loading at different RQ's and blood flows. *Fed. Proc., Fed. Am. Soc. Exp. Biol.* **33**, 438 (abstr.).

Myhre, K., and K. L. Andersen (1971). Respiratory responses to static muscular work. *Respir. Physiol.* **12**, 77–89.

Paintal, A. S. (1970). The mechanism of excitation of type J receptors and the J reflex. *In* "Breathing: Hering–Breuer Centenary Symposium" (R. Porter, ed.), pp. 59–76. Churchill, London.

Paintal, A. S. (1973). Vagal sensory receptors and their reflex effects. *Physiol. Rev.* **53**, 159–227.

Pappenheimer, J. R. (1967). The ionic composition of cerebral extracellular fluid and its relation to control of breathing. *Harvey Lect.* **61**, 71–94.

Phillipson, E. A., R. F. Hickey, C. R. Bainton, and J. A. Nadel (1970). Effect of vagal blockade on regulation of breathing in conscious dogs. *J. Appl. Physiol.* **29**, 475–479.

Plum, F. (1970). Neurological integration of behavioral and metabolic control of breathing. *In* "Breathing: Hering–Breuer Centenary Symposium" (R. Porter, ed.), pp. 159–174. Churchill, London.

Pugh, L. G.C.E., M. B. Gill, S. Lahiri, J. S. Milledge, M. P. Ward, and J. B. West (1964). Muscular exercise at great altitudes. *J. Appl. Physiol.* **19,** 431–440.

Ramsay, A. G. (1955). Muscle metabolism and the regulation of breathing. *J. Physiol. (London)* **127,** 30P (abstr.).

Ramsay, A. G. (1959). Effects of metabolism and anesthesia on pulmonary ventilation. *J. Appl. Physiol.* **14,** 102–104.

Refsum, H. E. (1961). Respiratory response to acute exercise in induced metabolic acidosis. *Acta Physiol. Scand.* **52,** 32–35.

Riley, R. L., R. E. Dutton, Jr., F. J. D. Fuleihan, S. Nath, H. H. Hurt, Jr., C. Yoshimoto, J. H. Sipple, S. Permutt, and B. Bromberger-Barnea (1963). Regulation of respiration and blood gases. *Ann N.Y. Acad. Sci.* **109,** 829–851.

Rizzo, A., M. Gimemez, P. Horsky, and C. Savnier (1976). Metabolism during exercise in young men breathing 4% CO_2. *Bull. Eur. Physiopathol. Respir.* **12,** 209–219.

Sinclair, R. D., J. M. Clark, and B. E. Welch (1971). Comparison of physiological responses of normal man to exercise in air and in acute and chronic hypercapnia. *In* "Underwater Physiology" (C. J. Lambertsen, ed.), pp. 409–417. Academic Press, New York.

Sipple, J. H., and R. Gilbert (1966). Influence of proprioceptor activity in the ventilatory response to exercise. *J. Appl. Physiol.* **21,** 143–146.

Stone, D. J., H. Keltz, T. K. Sarkar, and J. Singzon (1973). Ventilatory response to alpha-adrenergic stimulation and inhibition. *J. Appl. Physiol.* **34,** 619–623.

von Euler, U. S. (1974). Sympatho-adrenal activity in physical exercise. *Med. Sci. Sports* **6,** 166–173.

Wagner, J. A., S. M. Horvath, and T. E. Dahms (1977). Cardiovascular, respiratory, and metabolic adjustments to exercise in dogs. *J. Appl. Physiol.* **42,** 403–407.

Wasserman, K. (1976). Testing regulation of ventilation with exercise. *Chest* **70,** Suppl. 1, 173–178.

Wasserman, K., and B. J. Whipp (1975). Exercise physiology in health and disease. *Am. Rev. Respir. Dis.* **112,** 219–249.

Wasserman, K., A. L. Van Kessel, and G. G. Burton (1967). Interaction of physiological mechanisms during exercise. *J. Appl. Physiol.* **22,** 71–85.

Wasserman, K., B. J. Whipp, S. N. Koyal, and W. L. Beaver (1973). Anaerobic threshold and respiratory gas exchange during exercise. *J. Appl. Physiol.* **35,** 236–243.

Wasserman, K., B. J. Whipp, and J. Castagna (1974). Cardiodynamic hyperpnea: Hyperpnea secondary to cardiac output increase. *J. Appl. Physiol.* **36,** 457–464.

Wasserman, K., B. J. Whipp, R. Casaburi, D. J. Huntsman, J. Castagna, and R. Lugliani (1975a). Regulation of arterial P_{CO_2} during intravenous CO_2 loading. *J. Appl. Physiol.* **38,** 651–656.

Wasserman, K., B. J. Whipp, S. N. Koyal, and M. G. Cleary (1975b). Effect of carotid body resection on ventilatory and acid–base control during exercise. *J. Appl. Physiol.* **39,** 354–358.

Whipp, B. J., and K. Wasserman (1970). Effect of body temperature on the ventilatory response to exercise. *Respir. Physiol.* **8,** 354–360.

Whipp, B. J., D. J. Huntsman, and K. Wasserman (1975). Evidence for a CO_2-mediated pulmonary chemoreflex in dog. *Physiologist* **18,** 447 (abstr.).

White, A., P. Handler, and E. L. Smith (1973). "Principles of Biochemistry," pp. 360–370. McGraw-Hill, New York.

Wiley, R. L., and A. R. Lind (1971). Respiratory responses to sustained static muscular contractions in humans. *Clin. Sci.* **40,** 221–234.

Williams, T. F., R. W. Winters, J. R. Clapp, W. Hollander, Jr., and L. G. Welt (1958). Effects of 2,4-dinitrophenol on respiration in the dog. *Am. J. Physiol.* **193,** 181–188.

Winterstein, H. (1961). The actions of substances introduced into the cerebrospinal fluid and the problem of intracranial chemoreceptors. *Pharmacol. Rev.* **13,** 71–107.

Yamamoto, W. S. (1960). Mathematical analysis of the time course of alveolar CO_2. *J. Appl. Physiol.* **15,** 215–219.

Yamamoto, W. S., and M. W. Edwards, Jr. (1960). Homeostasis of carbon dioxide during intravenous infusion of carbon dioxide. *J. Appl. Physiol.* **15,** 807–818.

Young, D. R., R. Mosher, P. Erve, and H. Spector (1959). Energy metabolism and gas exchange during treadmill running in dogs. *J. Appl. Physiol.* **14,** 834–838.

Young, I. M. (1957). Some observations on the mechanism of adrenaline hyperpnoea. *J. Physiol. (London)* **137,** 374–395.

CHAPTER 3

Ammonia and the
Regulation of Ventilation

ROBERT E. DUTTON
ROBERT A. BERKMAN

I. INTRODUCTION

Although increasing attention is being paid to the high incidence of elevated ammonia levels in patients with chronic obstructive pulmonary

Regulation of Ventilation and Gas Exchange
Copyright © 1978 by Academic Press, Inc.
All rights of reproduction in any form reserved.
ISBN 0-12-204650-1

disease (COPD), little is known about the influence of ammonia on the course of the disease. This chapter explores the possible role of ammonia in the ventilatory depression observed in these patients. An emphasis is placed on the neural toxicity of ammonia, since similar neurological manifestations occur in hepatic failure and pulmonary insufficiency associated with ventilatory failure (Austen *et al.*, 1957). The level of consciousness in patients with either condition may diminish, and they may manifest a full spectrum of mental changes ranging from restlessness to unresponsive coma (Comroe *et al.*, 1950; Sherlock, 1960). Ammonia has been implicated as the compound responsible for initiating these syndromes.

Evidence that ammonia causes metabolic changes in glycolysis, Krebs cycle intermediate compounds, the $NADH-NAD^+$ system, and organic amine metabolism is presented in this chapter. All these changes may influence the respiratory control system if ammonia depresses neural function either by depleting these substances or by leading to an overproduction of depressant agents, or both.

A. Control of Ventilation in Hepatic Failure

Despite the frequent occurrence of a high resting ventilation, patients with liver failure have a reduced sensitivity to inspired carbon dioxide (Robin *et al.*, 1957). This depressed ventilatory response to inhaled carbon dioxide occurs even though its administration reverses the respiratory alkalosis of these patients (Posner and Plum, 1960). With the administration of 5% CO_2, the severity of the patients' neurological signs and symptoms becomes worse, with increased confusion, disorientation, dysarthria, and tremulousness. Hence, there is no improvement in their clinical state, and they develop higher arterial carbon dioxide tensions and lower arterial pH values than patients used as control subjects.

Recently, Stanley *et al.* (1975) determined the ventilatory response to carbon dioxide inhalation and measured the acid–base status of the cerebrospinal fluid in 12 patients with liver failure. They also induced liver failure in animals by daily injections of carbon tetrachloride. They found that liver failure in both man and animals is accompanied by respiratory alkalosis, manifested by an elevated cerebrospinal fluid pH and decreased P_{CO_2}. Nevertheless, the ventilatory response to carbon dioxide is reduced in both man and animals.

B. Control of Ventilation in Chronic Obstructive Pulmonary Disease

In comparison with control subjects, the ventilatory response to carbon dioxide inhalation of patients with advanced COPD is depressed. Resting hypoventilation may become severe, resulti.ig in arterial CO_2 tensions greater than 80 mm Hg (Ayres *et al.*, 1965; Williams and Zohman, 1959).

Several mechanisms which could account for a decreased CO_2 sensitivity in these patients have been suggested by Cherniack (1965): (a) an increased buffering capacity of the blood may occur secondary to renal bicarbonate retention as a result of the hypercapnia; (b) the chemoreceptor response to hypoxia may be active, but is reduced when alveolar oxygen tension rises during a CO_2 test; (c) altered respiratory mechanics may result in an increased work of breathing; (d) the narcotic properties of CO_2 may reduce ventilation; or (e) there may be adaptation to an elevated carbon dioxide tension.

A reduced sensitivity to carbon dioxide was suggested by Scott (1920) to be due to an elevated buffering capacity of the blood. Tenney (1954) supported this view, and Schaefer (1958) showed that chronic exposure of normal subjects to elevated environmental carbon dioxide is accompanied by an increase in buffering capacity of the blood. However, an increased buffering capacity achieved by oral administration of bicarbonate in normal man has been reported to elevate only the threshold to carbon dioxide stimulation without altering the slope of the response (Katsaros *et al.*, 1960). Therefore, bicarbonate retention may not be the sole reason that prolonged exposure to hypercapnia results in a depressed CO_2 response.

If a patient with COPD has hypoxemia, a hypoxic drive to ventilation exists which may be removed by the increase in alveolar P_{O_2} that occurs during carbon dioxide inhalation (Cherniack, 1965) and thereby leads to an apparent decrease in the sensitivity to carbon dioxide. This phenomenon of depression of ventilation by diminution of the hypoxic drive is common in patients with COPD (Davies and MacKinnon, 1949; Lopez-Majano and Dutton, 1973). However, despite the importance of the hypoxic drive in these patients, their ventilatory response to hypoxia still appears to be blunted (Flenley and Millar, 1967; Jones, 1966).

More recently, Cherniack and Chodirker (1972) demonstrated that, under circumstances where the hypoxic drive is suddenly removed but airway resistance maintained at an increased level, normal subjects will breathe less and tolerate hypercapnia in preference to increasing their work of breathing. Cherniack *et al.* (1956) and Brodovsky *et al.* (1960) have shown in patients with COPD that ventilation is depressed and, as a result of a mechanical limitation of the respiratory system, does not accurately reflect the neural output from the respiratory center.

Decreasing the hypoxic drive to ventilation by administration of oxygen to certain emphysematous patients results in immediate hypoventilation, rises in arterial carbon dioxide tension to narcotic levels, uncompensated decreases in arterial pH, worsening of the neurological symptoms, and eventually coma (Alexander *et al.*, 1955; Comroe *et al.*, 1950; Winslow and Grant, 1967). However, factors other than acidosis are involved in the ventilatory depression, since restoration of pH to normal by administration of trishydroxymethylaminomethane (THAM) leads to further hypoventilation (Massaro et al., 1962). This observation also implies that a residual hydrogen ion drive to respiration exists in CO_2 narcosis. Although there is no consistent relationship between the onset of neurological symptoms and arterial blood gas tensions in emphysematous patients (Gellhorn, 1953; Comroe et al., 1950), the critical level of arterial P_{CO_2} required to initiate mental aberration ($Pa_{CO_2} > 56$ mm Hg) and respiratory depression ($Pa_{CO_2} > 72$ mm Hg) is higher in normals than in patients with COPD; in the clinical studies of Comroe et al. (1950), no patient became somnolent unless the resting arterial oxygen saturation was initially below 90% and the resting Pa_{CO_2} above 50 mm Hg, and oxygen administration completely alleviated the hypoxemia.

It is evident from this discussion that the cause of the reduced ventilatory response to both hypoxia and hypercapnia observed in COPD patients as well as the mechanism by which ventilation is depressed in CO_2 narcosis have not been elucidated.

C. Ammonia and Its Metabolites in Chronic Obstructive Pulmonary Disease

The presence of asterixis in a patient with COPD prompted Austen et al. (1957) to measure the patient's venous ammonia level, which was elevated. The authors suggested that elevation of ammonia was responsible for the patient's neurological symptoms. However, the patient had cor pulmonale with right heart failure, and elevations of blood ammonia levels have been previously reported in congestive heart failure (Bessman and Evans, 1955). Therefore, to establish whether or not an elevation of ammonia occurs in COPD in the absence of cardiac failure, Dutton et al. (1959) measured venous ammonia levels in 34 patients with emphysema, but without either congestive heart failure or liver disease. The venous blood ammonia levels in these patients were significantly higher than in control subjects. These results led Renzetti et al. (1961) to test the effect of an induced elevation of ammonia on ventilation in 11 patients. Elevations of arterial ammonia concentrations to 20 times the control values resulted in metabolic stimulation and a ventilatory depression; i.e., arterial P_{CO_2} increased in conjunction with an increase in CO_2 production. In addition, in two patients tested, the ventilatory response to 5% CO_2 was decreased.

When ammonia is elevated, there is an increased output of glutamine by the brain (Clark and Eiseman, 1958). An increase in cerebrospinal fluid glutamine was found in every patient with chronic hypercapnia studied by Jaiken and Agrest (1969), although such a uniform elevation was not confirmed by Valero *et al.* (1971). Approximately half of the hypercapnic patients of Valero *et al.* (1971) had elevated glutamine levels. These patients were all drowsy, whereas those with no elevation of glutamine were alert. All of the drowsy patients also had hepatomegaly secondary to right heart failure, suggesting that the blood ammonia of these patients was elevated. In a subsequent report, Valero *et al.* (1974) confirmed their initial impression that hepatic congestion raised the blood ammonia level in COPD. Indeed, the blood and cerebrospinal fluid ammonia levels were extremely high in these patients, and were of the same magnitude as the non-COPD patients with hepatic encephalopathy included in the same study.

II. METABOLIC EFFECTS OF AMMONIA

Nonionized ammonia is more than 1200 times more soluble than CO_2 in water and is 14 times more soluble than CO_2 in lipids (Lawrence *et al.*, 1946). Diffusion of ammonia across the cell wall of the erythrocyte proceeds to equilibrium in 0.1 second (Klocke *et al.*, 1972). Despite the high diffusivity of ammonia, it does not freely diffuse across the blood–brain barrier. If free diffusion of the nonionized NH_3 molecule prevailed, the ammonia concentration should redistribute itself according to the pH gradient–drug distribution hypothesis (Rall *et al.*, 1959; Milne *et al.*, 1958), and be higher in the cerebrospinal fluid than in blood. Yet, ammonia is relatively excluded from the cerebrospinal fluid. Recent explanations for this phenomenon have invoked the charged membrane hypothesis (Wien effect) (Davies and Gurtner, 1973; Davies *et al.*, 1973; Dutton *et al.*, 1974). Nevertheless, when the concentration of hydrogen ions is altered in patients with high ammonia levels, the ammonia concentration redistributes itself between cerebrospinal fluid and blood in the direction (although not to the extent) predicted by the pH gradient–drug distribution hypothesis (Warren *et al.*, 1960; Moore *et al.*, 1963; Warren and Nathan, 1958; Stabenau *et al.*, 1959; Bromberg *et al.*, 1960). In general, cerebrospinal fluid concentrations of ammonia rise with increases in arterial blood ammonia. The following sections present the current status of our knowledge of the toxic effects of high ammonia levels on glycolysis, Krebs cycle intermediate compounds, the $NADH–NAD^+$ system, and organic amine metabolism. Results of ammonia infusion in dogs, and of similar metabolic changes in the cerebrospinal fluid of patients studied by the authors, are also presented.

A.   **Effect of Ammonia on Glucose and Pyruvate Metabolism**

Ammonia in toxic concentration initially stimulates glycolysis, resulting in decreases of brain glycogen and glucose (Muntz and Hurwitz, 1951a,b). This leads to increased concentrations of pyruvate and lactate. Clark and Eiseman (1958) found an increase in pyruvate concentration of the brain to 2.7 times control in dogs during infusion of sufficient 1% ammonia to produce coma. McKhann and Tower (1961) confirmed that there is an increase in pyruvate when cat brain slices are incubated with an elevated ammonia concentration. In their experiments, the decrease in pyruvate utilization by the ammonia-treated cortex paralleled the decrease in oxygen consumption. However, oxygen consumption was restored by the addition of succinate to the medium, and this led the authors to infer that ammonia primarily interferes with the oxidative decarboxylation of pyruvate and α-ketoglutarate. Katunuma et al. (1966) also observed an inhibition of oxidation of pyruvate in liver homogenates incubated with ammonia, but they did not ascribe a primary role to a block at this level because the oxidation of succinate was also interfered with.

Accompanying the rise in pyruvate, there is an even greater proportional rise in lactate (Schenker et al., 1967; Hindfelt and Siesjö, 1970). Hence, there is a rise in the lactate/pyruvate ratio.

B.   **Effect of Ammonia on the Conversion of Citrate to α-Ketoglutarate in the Krebs Cycle**

The citrate concentration in dog brain during ammonia infusion appears to be maintained despite ample evidence for an interference with brain energy metabolism (Prior et al., 1971). During the experiments, electroencephalograms showed large spikes in association with muscle twitching and dyskinetic movements of the experimental animal. Respiration became depressed. Similarly, Katunuma et al. (1966) observed elevated levels of citrate in liver homogenates incubated with ammonia. They also found elevated levels of isocitrate and depletion of α-ketoglutarate and suggested that oxidation of isocitrate to α-ketoglutarate is the reaction most affected by elevated ammonia levels. The enzyme located at this site in the Krebs cycle is isocitrate dehydrogenase, the normal activity of which requires normal levels of pyrimidine nucleotides. Prior et al. (1971) point out that citrate itself can inhibit phosphorylation of fructose 6-phosphate by feedback inhibition of phosphofructokinase. After an initial stimulation of the glycolytic pathways, this should result in decreased glucose utilization. Furthermore, there is evidence that isocitrate dehydrogenase catalyzes the rate-limiting reaction of the Krebs cycle (Plaut and Aogaichi, 1968; Chen and Plaut, 1963; Plaut, 1970; Lehninger, 1970; Coleman, 1975).

An increase in the ratio of citrate to α-ketoglutarate was noted by Folbergrová et al. (1972) in rats exposed to carbon dioxide without ammonia infusion, although the absolute citrate concentrations fell as inspired CO_2 was raised to the 40% level. They concluded that the enzyme isocitrate dehydrogenase was in some way inhibited by elevated carbon dioxide tensions. As will be seen below, this may have occurred as a result of an induced elevation of ammonia during the hypercapnia.

C.   Effect of Ammonia on α-Ketoglutarate and Organic Amines

In 1955, Bessman and Bessman postulated that ammonia taken up in brain tissue reacts with α-ketoglutarate to form glutamine according to the following reactions.

$$\alpha\text{-Ketoglutarate} + NH_3 + NADH + H^+ \xrightleftharpoons[\text{glutamic dehydrogenase}]{\text{HOH}} \text{glutamate} + NAD^+$$

and

$$\text{Glutamate} + NH_3 + ATP \xrightleftharpoons[\text{glutaminase}]{\text{glutamine synthetase}} \text{glutamine} + ADP$$

Subsequently, elevation of brain tissue and cerebrospinal fluid glutamine has been amply documented (Clark and Eiseman, 1958; Du Ruisseau et al., 1957; Peters and Tower, 1959; Tews et al., 1963). It was further postulated that depletion of α-ketoglutarate would reduce brain energy stores, since α-ketoglutarate is an essential component of the Krebs cycle and the reaction itself consumes ATP (Woodman and McIlwain, 1961).

Once formed, the increased levels of glutamine can be degraded via two pathways. Both of these pathways require reversion to glutamate. The first and major pathway normally used is transamination back to α-ketoglutarate (Lowry et al., 1956). However, in the presence of increased levels of ammonia, the kinetics of this reaction are inhibited. The second pathway is conversion of glutamate to succinate through the γ-aminobutyric acid shunt. The importance of this pathway in respiratory control is emphasized by the observation that γ-aminobutyric acid iontophoretically applied to both inspiratory and expiratory medullary respiratory neurons causes a decrease in firing rate or complete abolition of firing, dependent upon the dosage used. The response to application of glutamate was a marked stimulation of these cells (Toleikis *et al.*, 1976). Although Tews *et al.* (1963) failed to find an elevation of γ-aminobutyric acid during 45 minutes of ammonium chloride infusion in dogs, Weyne *et al.* (1976) did find elevated levels in rats chronically exposed to high levels of environmental CO_2.

The competitive inhibition of glutamine synthetase with methionine sulfoximine greatly reduced the formation of glutamine (Warren and Schenker, 1964). It was demonstrated that pretreatment rats given an intravenous LD_{50} dosage of ammonium chloride and methionine sulfoximine resulted in complete protection of the treated animals. The brain tissue failed to consume ammonia, and brain ammonia concentration doubled. The improved survival may have been due to a reduction in the drain of α-ketoglutarate or adenosine triphosphate (ATP) from the brain.

D.   Effect of Ammonia on Nucleic Acids of the Brain

Elevated blood levels of ammonia can produce substantial lowering of high-energy intermediate compounds in the brain (McKhann and Tower, 1961). These authors felt that the observed depletion of ATP stores in cat brain slices exposed to ammonia was secondary to a diminution in activity of the Krebs cycle, because of a depletion of available 4-carbon dicarboxylic acids and an increased use of ATP for glutamine formation. Worcel and Erecinska (1962) confirmed these observations and noted an inhibition of oxygen uptake to 50% of its maximum with ammonia concentration of only 20 nM/liter. However, Schenker *et al.* (1967) observed that during induction of coma by ammonia infusion in rats, adenosine triphosphate and phosphocreatine fell only at the base of the brain, and Hindfelt and Siesjö (1970) found no change at all in ATP concentration in rats after 15 minutes of ammonia infusion. On the other hand, the latter authors did find a decrease in phosphocreatine content in hepatectomized rats and an increase in cytoplasmic $NADH/NAD^+$ following both hepatectomy and ammonia infusion, which led them to propose that there is an interference with the electron transport system of the respiratory chain.

E.   Changes in Intermediate Metabolism in Dogs during
Ammonia Infusion

The present authors obtained cerebrospinal fluid (CSF) samples in order to measure brain tissue metabolites in 10 dogs before and after one hour of administration of a buffered ammonium chloride solution (Berkman *et al.*, 1976a). The infusion led to a fourfold elevation of arterial

ammonia that approximated levels found in hepatic failure and in some
patients with COPD (Valero *et al.*, 1974). The CSF ammonia and
glutamine concentrations rose (Fig. 1), as did pyruvate, lactate, and the
lactate/pyruvate ratio (Fig. 2). An elevation of CSF citrate concentration
occurred in the presence of a decrease in α-ketoglutarate (Fig. 3), implying the existence of a block in Krebs cycle energy metabolism located
between these two compounds. The location of the inhibitory effect of
ammonia is probably at the level of isocitrate dehydrogenase.

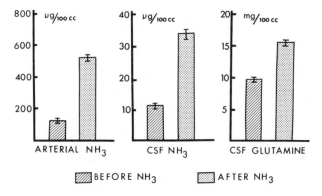

Figure 1. Alterations of arterial ammonia concentration, CSF ammonia concentration,
and CSF glutamine concentration induced by intravenous buffered ammonia administration
in ten dogs. The vertical bars indicate one standard error about the mean.

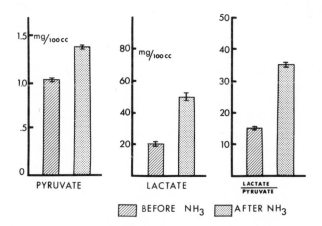

Figure 2. Alterations of CSF pyruvate and CSF lactate concentrations, and lactate/
pyruvate ratio induced by intravenous administration of buffered ammonia in ten dogs. The
vertical bars indicate one standard error about the mean.

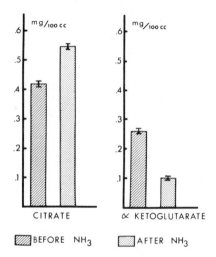

Figure 3. Alterations in CSF citrate and α-ketoglutarate concentrations induced by intra-venous buffered ammonia administration in ten dogs. The vertical bars indicate one standard error about the mean.

F. Changes in Intermediate Metabolism in Animals with Hypoxia, Hypercapnia, and Elevated Ammonia Levels

Several animal studies have been performed that pertain to the question of whether hypoxia and hypercapnia can cause elevations in ammonia in aminals with normal liver function. Flores et al. (1962) rendered anesthetized rats hypoxic and hypercapnic by placing them in a sealed beaker. A significant drop of liver ATP, from 1.02 to 0.07 μg/gm tissue, was found. Although ammonia and blood gases were not measured, the depletion of ATP was more marked the longer the rats were asphyxiated. Rats, inspiring 4–8% CO_2, have both significant elevations of their brain ammonia concentrations and reductions in the amount of ATP proportional to the degree of hypercapnia (Agrest et al., 1965).

An increase in inspired CO_2 to 10% in dogs result in significant increases of brain ammonia and glutamine and decreases in glutamate (Kazemi et al., 1973, 1976). Weyne et al. (1973) have also documented that there is an elevation of glutamine and a fall in glutamate in rat brain during hypercapnia (inspired 13% CO_2) and during hypoxia (inspired 10% O_2) as well. They extended their hypercapnic studies to three weeks and found that these changes persisted (Weyne et al., 1976). In addition, they observed a significant increase in ammonia and γ-aminobutyric acid and proposed that the excitatory neurotransmitter, glutamate, is removed from synaptic clefts at a time when the inhibitory neurotransmitter, γ-aminobutyric acid, is increasing. It is interesting to note here that two hypoxic ($Pa_{O_2} < 60$ mm Hg)–hypercapnic ($Pa_{CO_2} > 60$ mm Hg) patients with COPD exhibited elevated γ-aminobutyric acid levels (twice normal) at the time they were studied by the present authors (R. A. Berkman and R. Dutton, unpublished observations). The depressant effect of γ-aminobutyric acid on respiration observed by Toleikis et al. (1976) may have contributed to the hypoventilation of these patients.

G.   Cerebrospinal Fluid Intermediate Metabolites in Patients

Measurements of CSF ammonia, glutamine, lactate, pyruvate, α-ketoglutarate, citrate, and γ-aminobutyric acid were made by Berkman and Dutton (1976) in 47 patients. Twenty-eight patients were undergoing spinal anesthesia for elective surgery, and 19 patients had COPD. A positive correlation was found between the degree of hypoxia of arterial blood and both ammonia ($r = 0.68, P < 0.05$) and glutamine ($r = 0.60, P < 0.05$) in the CSF. A slightly lower correlation was observed between the level of hypercapnia and both ammonia ($r = 0.61, P < 0.05$) and glutamine ($r = 0.56, P < 0.05$) in the CSF.

The elective surgery patients, none of whom had CO_2 retention, were divided into two groups according to whether or not their arterial P_{O_2} exceeded 80 mm Hg. Krebs cycle intermediate compounds were measured in the CSF of these patients and in two patients with COPD (Table I). The CSF concentrations of citrate, α-ketoglutarate, lactate, pyruvate,

Table I. Cerebrospinal Fluid Concentrations (mg%) of Krebs Cycle Intermediate Compounds and Glycolytic Metabolites

	PATIENT DESCRIPTION		
	ELECTIVE SURGERY		COPD
	Normal blood gases	$P_{O_2} < 80$ mm Hg P_{CO_2} normal	$P_{O_2} < 80$ mm Hg $P_{CO_2} > 65$ mm Hg
Citrate	0.033	0.035	0.056
SE	±0.001	±0.008	
α-Ketoglutarate	0.029	0.032	0.013
SE	±0.001	±0.003	
Lactate	17.4	22.0	37.2
SE	±0.6	±1.6	
Pyruvate	1.422	1.791	0.548
SE	±0.360	±0.077	
Lactate/pyruvate ratio	12.5	12.2	67.8
SE	±0.7	±0.6	

and the lactate/pyruvate ratio were all changed in the direction that would be predicted for ammonia intoxication.

III. SOURCE OF AMMONIA

The organs in the body that influence ammonia levels are the gastrointestinal tract, liver, kidney, and, to a smaller extent, the brain. The lungs have been shown to exhale small amounts of ammonia (Jacquez *et al.*, 1959; Robin *et al.*, 1959). Glutamine has been proposed as a source of ammonia in the brain (Kazemi *et al.*, 1973; Kazemi, 1976) and in the kidney (Pitts, 1964). However, it now appears that glutamine is not an important source of ammonia in the brain during hypercapnia (Kazemi *et al.*, 1976), and in respiratory acidosis the kidney would be expected to excrete, not retain, ammonia (Pitts, 1964).

The gastrointestinal tract has long been known to be the source of ammonia that may precipitate hepatic encephalopathy in patients with liver disease (Philips *et al.*, 1952; White *et al.*, 1955). The ammonia produced from ingested nitrogenous products is absorbed into the portal circulation and detoxified in the liver by formation of urea. Patients with liver disease are postulated to have intrahepatic shunting of portal venous blood into the hepatic vein, for an elevation of hepatic vein ammonia occurs at a time when the maximum rate that the liver can form urea has not been exceeded (White *et al.*, 1955).

The present authors designed experiments to test the hypothesis that the gastrointestinal tract was the site of origin of the elevated ammonia concentration observed during hypercapnia and hypoxia (Berkman *et al.*, 1975; Berkman and Dutton, 1975). The effect of hypercapnia and hypoxia on liver blood flow (Dutton *et al.*, 1976) and on splanchnic and hepatic gas exchange (Meyer *et al.*, 1977) were also examined.

Inhalation of 6% CO_2 in the dog resulted in a 20% increase in hepatic blood flow, all the result of an increase in portal vein flow (Dutton *et al.*, 1975). This increase in blood flow was paralleled by an increase in the amount of ammonia presented to the liver secondary to an increased uptake from the gastrointestinal tract (Berkman *et al.*, 1975), and portal venous ammonia concentration remained stable despite the increased flow to the gastrointestinal tract. Thus, hypercapnia somehow increases the transport of ammonia from the lumen of the gastrointestinal tract into the blood.

In the presence of the elevated ammonia load during hypercapnia, liver uptake of ammonia rose, but not enough to match the increased ammonia inflow (Fig. 4). The reason for the inability of the liver to metabolize the increased load of ammonia is unknown. A possible explanation is that

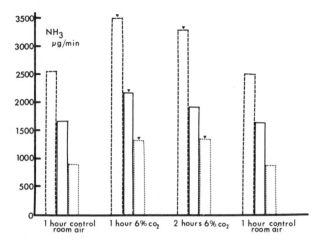

Figure 4. Changes in liver uptake of ammonia and transport of ammonia to and from the liver during room air control, at 1 and 2 hours of hypercapnia, and during return to room air control (1 hour). The bar on the left-hand side with a dashed line represents the total inflow of ammonia to the liver. The bar in the center with a solid outline is the liver uptake of ammonia. The bar on the right-hand side with a dotted line is the heptic vein contribution of ammonia to the systemic circuit. The solid triangles indicate a statistically significant difference ($P < 0.05$) from the first room air control by paired t test.

there was an increased shunting of blood in the liver with an increased portal vein pressure (tenHove and Leevy, 1973).

Inhalation of a hypoxic mixture sufficient to lower arterial P_{O_2} to 42 mm Hg led to a decreased uptake of ammonia from the gastrointestinal tract (Berkman and Dutton, 1975). There was a reduction of 6 mm Hg in mean P_{CO_2} of the arterial blood, and a decrease in hepatic blood flow. Nevertheless, the hepatic uptake of ammonia fell even more than the diminution in the amount of ammonia being presented to it via the portal vein (Fig. 5), resulting in increased hepatic vein ammonia.

The superimposition of hypercapnia on hypoxia resulted in an increase in portal vein blood flow to levels comparable to those of hypercapnia alone (Berkman and Dutton, 1975). The ammonia load to the liver from the gastrointestinal tract again increased above control levels, and liver uptake again rose. As before, this was inadequate to maintain normal hepatic vein ammonia levels (Fig. 5). The elevation of arterial ammonia in this situation was higher than that observed in either hypercapnia or hypoxia alone.

It is concluded from these experiments that the source of the elevated ammonia in hypoxia and hypercapnia is the gastrointestinal tract, and that this ammonia reaches the brain by transport in the systemic circulation and diffusion across the blood–brain barrier.

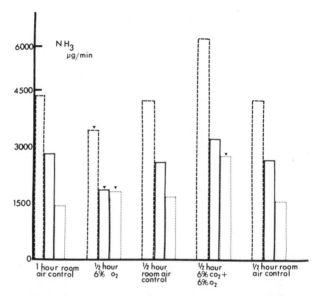

Figure 5. Changes in liver uptake of ammonia and transport of ammonia to and from the liver during room air control, at 30 minutes of hypoxia, at 30 minutes of combined hypoxia–hypercapnia, and at the end of two room air control periods ($\frac{1}{2}$ hours). The bar on the left-hand side with a dashed line is total inflow of ammonia into the liver. The center bar with a solid outline is liver ammonia uptake. The bar on the right-hand side with a dotted outline is hepatic vein ammonia contribution to the systemic circulation. The solid triangles above the bars indicate a significant difference ($P < 0.05$) from the test measurement made during the immediately preceding room air control period by paired t test.

IV. EFFECT OF AMMONIA ON CONTROL OF VENTILATION IN THE DOG

As in humans with hepatic encephalopathy, ammonia infusion in animals with intact respiratory control system most frequently causes an increase in resting ventilation and a drop in arterial P_{CO_2} (Roberts *et al.*, 1956; Hindfelt and Siesjö, 1970; Wichser and Kazemi 1974). Berkman *et al.* (1976a,b) undertook an alternative approach by testing the effect of infusion of a buffered ammonia solution on the ventilatory response to graded levels of hypercapnia and hypoxia in the anesthetized dog (sodium pentobarbital, 25 mg/kg i.v.).

Because the anesthetic level can alter the ventilatory response to hypoxia and hypercapnia, the sodium pentobarbital was given in a single dose in order to ensure that any decrease in the ventilatory response following the ammonia infusion could not be attributed to an anesthetic depression of the respiratory control system. Animals that required supplemental anesthesia upon approaching stage II anesthesia were not included in the results.

A. Ventilatory Response to Hypercapnia during Ammonia Infusion

The CO_2 responses to three levels of carbon dioxide (4, 6, and 10% CO_2 in air) obtained in 16 dogs before and 30 minutes after ammonia infusion were studied. In these animals, resting control hyperventilation was not observed despite an increase in arterial ammonia four times control value. There were also no statistically significant differences in the ventilatory response between the control and ammonia infusion state when 4% CO_2 was inhaled. However, during inhalation of 6% and 10% CO_2, there was a significant depression of the CO_2 response during ammonia infusion (Fig. 6). Thirty minutes following completion of the CO_2 response curve, but while the ammonia infusion was continued, arterial [HCO_3^-] had decreased by 4.9 mEq/liter, whereas no change had occurred in CSF [HCO_3^-], pH, or P_{CO_2}.

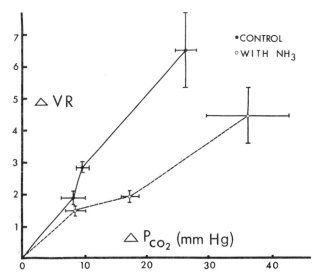

Figure 6. Changes in ventilation ratio vs. changes in arterial P_{CO_2} (ΔP_{CO_2}) during CO_2 breathing in 16 dogs before and after intravenous administration of a buffered ammonia solution. The solid line connects mean values obtained before ammonia infusion, whereas the dashed line connects mean values obtained during ammonia infusion. The vertical and horizontal bars indicate one standard error about the mean.

B. Ventilatory Response to Hypoxia during Ammonia Infusion

The ventilatory response to two levels of hypoxia (6.0 and 12.5% in N_2) was tested in eight additional dogs during successive five minute test periods before and 30 minutes after starting a continuous infusion of buffered ammonia solution. A significant decrease in the ventilatory response to both levels was observed in these animals during the ammonia infusion period (Fig. 7).

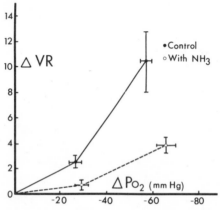

Figure 7. Changes in ventilation (ΔVR) vs. changes in arterial P_{O_2} (ΔP_{O_2}) during inhalation of 12.5% O_2 and 6% O_2 in ten dogs before and after intravenous administration of a buffered ammonia solution. The solid line connects mean values obtained before ammonia infusion, whereas the dashed line connects mean values obtained during ammonia infusion. The vertical and horizontal bars indicate one standard error about the mean. Control Pa_{O_2} was 87.9 ± 1.4 mm Hg before ammonia administration and 86.7 ± 4.6 mm Hg after ammonia administration.

C. Ventilatory Response to Carbon Dioxide during Ammonia Infusion in Sinoaortic Chemodenervated Animals

A third group of eight dogs had sinoaortic chemodenervation performed at least one week before CO_2 response curves were obtained. Elevation of the arterial ammonia concentration by a buffered ammonia infusion resulted in depression of the room air control ventilation in these animals. When tested with the same inspired hypercapnic mixtures that were used in the first group of dogs, their mean ventilatory response was even more depressed by the ammonia infusion (Fig. 8).

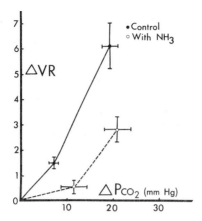

Figure 8.   Changes in ventilation ratio vs. changes in arterial P_{CO_2} effected by CO_2 breathing in sinoaortic chemodenervated dogs before and after intravenous administration of a buffered ammonia solution. The solid line connects mean values obtained before ammonia infusion, and the dashed line connects mean values obtained during ammonia infusion. The vertical and horizontal bars indicate one standard error about the mean.

Thus, in the absence of peripheral chemoreceptors, ammonia still depresses the ventilatory drive to hypercapnia. Although pointing to a central depression of ventilation that may be originating either in the central chemoreceptors or in the neurons of the respiratory center itself, these results do not entirely exclude the possibility that a peripheral chemoreceptor depression exists in the intact animal during ammonia infusion. Von Euler *et al.* (1939) and Eldridge (1972) have both observed a decrease or cessation of activity in the carotid sinus nerve following injection of ammonia into the blood supply of the carotid body.

V. SUMMARY

In this chapter, the current status of our knowledge about the metabolism of ammonia and the influence of these metabolites on the respiratory control system has been explored. Although there are many conflicting results, the likely sites of inhibition of Krebs cycle energy production by ammonia appear to be the entrance of pyruvate into the cycle by inhibition of phosphofructokinase, the conversion of isocitrate to α-ketoglutarate by inhibition of isocitrate dehydrogenase, and the depletion of α-ketoglutarate from the cycle by its conversion to glutamine (Fig. 9). Another possibility is that elevated levels of γ-aminobutyric acid in con-

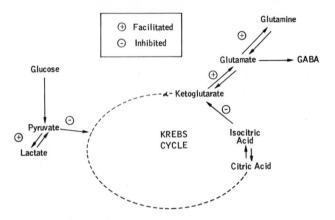

Figure 9. Diagram of the sites in the Krebs cycle that are influenced by an elevated ammonia concentration. A plus sign indicates facilitation; a minus sign indicates inhibition. The entrance of pyruvate into the cycle and the conversion of citric acid into α-ketoglutarate appear to be inhibited. The conversion of α-ketoglutarate and glutamate into glutamine appears to be facilitated. As a result of inhibition of Krebs cycle energy metabolism, the conversion of pyruvate to lactate is also facilitated.

junction with a depletion of glutamate may depress respiratory neural activity. All of these may contribute to the mental changes and decreased sensitivity to carbon dioxide observed in patients with chronic obstructive pulmonary disease.

As in hepatic failure, the source of an elevated ammonia during hypoxia and hypercapnia appears to be nitrogenous products in the gastrointestinal tract. In hypercapnia, the ammonia load to the liver appears to exceed the capacity for urea formation; in hypoxia, liver uptake of ammonia is depressed to the point that it cannot remove a reduced ammonia load from the gastrointestinal tract. Hypercapnia and hypoxia may act synergistically in elevating arterial ammonia.

Within a very short time after starting an ammonia infusion, the ventilatory responses to both hypoxia and hypercapnia are depressed. This depression appears to be accentuated in sinoaortic chemodenervated animals, suggesting that the respiratory depression induced by ammonia elevation is at least in part medullary in origin.

ACKNOWLEDGMENT

This research was supported by Grant HLB12564 of the U.S. Public Health Service.

REFERENCES

Agrest, A., C. de Bercovich, and S. Navon (1965). Ammonia and adenosinetriphosphate in the central nervous system of rats with dyspnoea and chronic hypercapnia. *Clin. Sci.* **28**, 401–405.

Alexander, J. K., J. R. West, J. A. Wood, and D. W. Richards (1955). Analysis of the respiratory response to carbon dioxide inhalation in varying clinical states of hypercapnia, anoxia, and acid–base derangement. *J. Clin. Invest.* **34**, 511–532.

Austen, F. K., M. W. Carmichael, and R. D. Adams (1957). Neurologic manifestations of chronic pulmonary insufficiency. *N. Engl. J. Med.* **257**, 579–590.

Ayres, S. M., S. Giannelli, Jr., A. Criscitiello, R. G. Armstrong, and M. E. Buehler (1965). Causes of arterial hypoxemia in patients with chronic obstructive pulmonary disease. *Am. J. Med.* **39**, 422–428.

Berkman, R. A., and R. E. Dutton (1975). Studies of factors resulting in ammonia elevation in hypoxia and superimposed hypercapnia. *Physiologist* **18**, 140.

Berkman, R. A., and R. E. Dutton (1976). Organic amines and oxidative metabolism of the brain as reflected in the cerebrospinal fluid of patients with chronic obstructive pulmonary disease and hypoxia. *Proc. East. Sect., Am. Thorac. Soc.* **3**, 8.

Berkman, R. A., M. D. Levtzky, and R. E. Dutton (1975). Portal blood flow and peripheral arterial NH_3 concentration during systemic hypercapnea. *Fed. Proc., Fed. Am. Soc. Exp. Biol.* **34**, 430.

Berkman, R. A., K. T. Meyer, A. G. Rosenberg, and R. E. Dutton (1976a). Depression of respiration and elevation of citric acid cycle components during ammonia infusion. *Fed. Proc., Fed. Am. Soc. Exp. Biol.* **35**, 718.

Berkman, R. A., A. G. Rosenberg, P. J. Feustel, and R. E. Dutton (1976b). Central depression of respiration by ammonia. *Physiologist* **19**, 126.

Bessman, A. M., and J. M. Evans (1955). The blood ammonia in congestive heart failure. *Am. Heart J.* **50**, 715–719.

Bessman, S. P., and A. M. Bessman (1955). The cerebral and peripheral uptake of ammonia in liver disease with an hypothesis for the mechanism of hepatic coma. *J. Clin. Invest.* **34**, 622–628.

Brodovsky, D., J. A. MacDonell, and R. M. Cherniack (1960). The respiratory response to carbon dioxide in health and in emphysema. *J. Clin. Invest.* **39**, 724–729.

Bromberg, P. A., E. D. Robin, and C. E. Forkner, Jr. (1960). The existence of ammonia in blood *in vivo* with observations on the significance of the NH_4^+–NH_3 system. *J. Clin. Invest.* **39**, 332–341.

Cavanagh, J. B., and M. H. Kyu (1971a). Type II alzheimer change experimentally produced in astrocytes in the rat. *Neurol. Sci.* **12**, 63–75.

Cavanagh, J. B., and M. H. Kyu (1971b). On the mechanism of Type I alzheimer abnormality in the nuclei of astrocytes: An essay in quantitative histology. *Neurol. Sci.* **12**, 241–261.

Chen, R. F., and G. W. E. Plaut (1963). Activation and inhibition of DPN-linked isocitrate dehydrogenase of heart by certain nucleotides. *Biochemistry* **2**, 1023–1032.

Cherniack, R. M. (1965). Work of breathing and the ventilatory response to CO_2. *Handb. Physiol. Sect. 3: Respir.* **2**, 1469–1473.

Cherniack, R. M., and W. B. Chodirker (1972). Hypercapnia with relief of hypoxia in normal individuals with increased work of breathing. *J. Appl. Physiol.* **33**, 189–192.

Clark, G. M., and B. Eiseman (1958). Studies in ammonia metabolism. Biochemical changes in brain tissue of dogs during ammonia-induced coma. *N. Engl. J. Med.* **259**, 178–180.

Coleman, R. (1975). Mechanisms for the oxidative decarboxylation of isocitrate: Implications for control. Adv. Enzyme Regul. **13**, 413–433.

Comroe, J. H., E. R. Bahnson, and E. O. Coates, Jr. (1950). Mental changes occurring in chronically anoxemic patients during oxygen therapy. J. Am. Med. Assoc. **143**, 1044–1048.

Davies, C. E., and J. Mackinnon (1949). Neurological effects of oxygen in chronic cor pulmonale. Lancet **2**, 883–885.

Davies, D. G., and G. H. Gurtner (1973). CSF acid–base balance and the Wien effect. J. Appl. Physiol. **34**, 249–254.

Davies, D. G., R. S. Fitzgerald, and G. H. Gurtner (1973). Acid–base relationships between CSF and blood during acute metabolic acidosis. J. Appl. Physiol. **34**, 243–248.

Du Ruisseau, J. P., J. P. Greenstein, M. Winitz, and S. M. Birnbaum (1957). Studies on the metabolism of amino acids and related compounds. VI. Free amino acid levels in the tissues of rats protected against ammonia toxicity. Arch. Biochem. Biophys. **68**, 161–171.

Dutton, R., M. Levitzky, and R. Berkman (1976). Carbon dioxide and liver blood flow. Bull. Eur. Physiopathol. Respir. **12**, 265–272.

Dutton, R. E., T. M. Harris, and D. G. Davies (1974). Distribution of ammonia between blood and cerebrospinal fluid in pulmonary emphysema. J. Appl. Physiol. **36**, 668–673.

Dutton, R., Jr., W. Nicholas, C. J. Fisher, and A. D. Renzetti, Jr. (1959). Blood ammonia in chronic pulmonary emphysea. N. Engl. J. Med. **261**, 1369–1373.

Eldridge, F. L. (1972). The importance of timing on the respiratory effects of intermittent carotid body chemoreceptor stimulation. J. Physiol. (London) **222**, 319–333.

Flenley, D. C., and J. S. Millar (1967). Ventilatory response to oxygen and carbon dioxide in chronic respiratory failure. Clin. Sci. **33**, 319–334.

Flores, G., A. Rosado, J. Torres, and G. Sobéron (1962). Liver enzyme activities in ammonia fixation by the rat. Am. J. Physiol. **203**, 43–48.

Folbergrová, J., V. MacMillan, and B. K. Siesjö (1972). The effect of hypercapnic acidosis upon some glycolytic and Krebs cycle-associated intermediates in the rat brain. J. Neurochem. **19**, 2507–2517.

Gellhorn, E. (1953). "Physiological Foundations of Neurology and Psychiatry," pp. 450–563. Univ. of Minnesota Press, Minneapolis.

Gibson, G. E., A. Zimber, L. Krook, and W. J. Visek (1971). Nucleic acids and brain and intestinal lesions in ammonia intoxicated mice. Fed. Proc., Fed. Am. Soc. Exp. Biol. **30**, 578.

Gibson, G. E., A. Zimber, L. Krook, E. Richardson, and W. Visek (1974). Brain histology and behavior of mice injected with urease. J. Neuropathol. Exp. Toxicol. **32**, 201–211.

Hindfelt, B., and B. K. Siesjö (1970). The effect of ammonia on the energy metabolism of the rat brain. Life Sci. **9**, 1021–1028.

Jacquez, J. A., J. W. Poppell, and R. Jeltsch (1959). Partial pressure of ammonia in alveolar air. Science **129**, 269–271.

Jaikin, A., and A. Agrest (1969). Cerebrospinal fluid glutamine concentration in patients with chronic hypercapnia. Clin. Sci. **36**, 11–14.

Jones, N. L. (1966). Pulmonary gas exchange during exercise in patients with chronic airway obstruction. Clin. Sci. **31**, 39–50.

Katsaros, B., H. H. Loeschcke, D. Lerche, H. Schönthal, and N. Hahn (1960). Wirkung der bicarbonat-alkalose auf die lungenbelüftung beim menschen bestimmung der teilwirkungen von pH und CO_2-druck auf die ventilation und vergleich mit den ergebnissen bei acidose. Pfluegers Arch. Gesamte Physiol. Menschen Tiere **271**, 732–747.

Katunuma, N., M. Okada, and Y. Nishii (1966). Regulation of the urea cycle and TCA cycle by ammonia. *Adv. Enzyme Regul.* **4**, 317–320.

Kazemi, H. (1976). Discussion. *Bull. Eur. Physiopathol. Respir.* **12**, 310–315.

Kazemi, H., N. S. Shore, V. E. Shih, and D. C. Shannon (1973). Brain organic buffers in respiratory acidosis and alkalosis. *J. Appl. Physiol.* **34**, 478–482.

Kazemi, H., J. Weyne, F. Van Leuven, and I. Leusen (1976). The CSF HCO_3^- increase in hypercapnia. Relationship to HCO_3^-, glutamate, glutamine and NH_3 in brain. *Respir. Physiol.* **28**, 387–401.

Klocke. R. A., K. K. Andersson, H. H. Rotman, and R. E. Forster (1972). Permeability of human erythrocytes to ammonia and weak acids. *Am. J. Physiol.* **222**, 1004–1013.

Lawrence, J. H., W. F. Loomis, C. A. Tobin, and F. H. Turpin (1946). Preliminary observations on the narcotic effect of xenon with a review of values for solubilities of gases in water and oils. *J. Physiol. (London)* **105**, 197–204.

Lehninger, A. (1970). "Biochemistry: The Molecular Basis of Cell Structure and Function," p. 348. New York: Worth Publ.

Lopez-Majano, V., and R. E. Dutton (1973). Regulation of respiration during oxygen breathing in chronic obstructive lung disease. *Am. Rev. Respir. Dis.* **108**, 232–240.

Lowry, O. H., N. R. Roberts, and C. Lewis (1956). The quantitative histochemistry of the retina. *J. Biol. Chem.* **220**, 879–892.

McKhann, G. M., and D. B. Tower (1961). Ammonia toxicity and cerebral oxidative metabolism. *Am. J. Physiol.* **200**, 420–424.

Massaro, D. J., S. Katz, and P. C. Luchsinger (1962). The use of a carbon dioxide buffer (trishydroxymethylaminomethane) in the treatment of respiratory acidosis. *Am. Rev. Respir. Dis.* **86**, 353–359.

Meyer, K. T., R. A. Berkman, and R. E. Dutton (1977). Gas exchange in the liver and intestines during hypoxia. *Bull. Eur. Physiopathol. Respir.* **13**, 541–550.

Miline, M. O., B. H. Scribner, and M. A. Crawford (1958). Non-ionic diffusion and the excretion of weak acids and bases. *Am. J. Med.* **24**, 709–729.

Moore, E. W., G. W. Strohmeyer, and T. C. Chalmers (1963). Distribution of ammonia across the blood–cerebrospinal fluid barrier in patients with hepatic failure. *Am. J. Med.* **35**, 350–362.

Muntz, J. A., and J. Hurwitz (1951a). Effect of potassium and ammonium ions upon glycolysis catalyzed by an extract of rat brain. *Arch. Biochem. Biophys.* **32**, 124–136.

Muntz, J. A., and J. Hurwitz (1951b). The effect of ammonium ions upon isolated reactions of the glycolytic scheme. *Arch. Biochem. Biophys.* **32**, 137–149.

Peters, E. L., and D. B. Tower (1959). Glutamic acid and glutamine metabolism in cerebral cortex after seizures induced by methionine sulphoximine. *J. Neurochem.* **5**, 80–90.

Philips, G. B., R. Schwartz, G. J. Gabuzda, Jr., and C. S. Davidson (1952). The syndrome of impending hepatic coma in patients with cirrhosis of the liver given certain nitrogenous substances. *N. Engl. J. Med.* **247**, 239–246.

Pitts, R. F. (1964). Renal production and excretion of ammonia. *Am. J. Med.* **36**, 720–724.

Plaut, G. W. E. (1970). DPN-linked isocitrate dehydrogenase of animal tissues. *Curr. Top. Cell. Reg.* **2**, 1–18.

Plaut, G. W. E., and T. Aogaichi (1968). Purification and properties of diphosphopyridine nucleotide-linked isocitrate dehydrogenase of mammalian liver. *J. Biol. Chem.* **243**, 5572–5583.

Posner, J. B., and F. Plum (1960). The toxic effects of carbon dioxide and acetazolamide in hepatic encephalopathy. *J. Clin. Invest.* **39**, 1246–1258.

Prior, R. L., A. J. Clifford, G. E. Gibson, and W. J. Visek (1971). Effects of insulin on glucose metabolism in hyperammonemic rats. *Am. J. Physiol.* **221**, 432–436.

Rall, D. P., J. R. Stabenau, and C. G. Zubrod (1959). Distribution of drugs between blood and cerebrospinal fluid: General methodology and effect of pH gradients. *J. Pharmacol. Exp. Ther.* **125**, 185–193.

Renzetti, A. D., Jr., B. A. Harris, and J. F. Bowen (1961). Influence of ammonia on respiration. *J. Appl. Physiol.* **16**, 703–708.

Roberts, K. E., F. G. Thompson, III, J. W. Poppell, and P. Vanamee (1956). Respiratory alkalosis accompanying ammonium toxicity. *J. Appl. Physiol.* **9**, 367–370.

Robin, E. D., R. D. Whaley, C. H. Crump, and D. M. Travis (1957). The nature of the respiratory acidosis of sleep and of the respiratory alkalosis of hepatic coma. *J. Clin. Invest.* **36**, 924.

Schaefer, K. E. (1958). Respiratory pattern and respiratory response to CO_2. *J. Appl. Physiol.* **3**, 1–14.

Schenker, S., D. W. McCandless, E. Brophy, and M. S. Lewis (1967). Studies on the intracerebral toxicity of ammonia. *J. Clin. Invest.* **46**, 838–848.

Scott, R. W. (1920). Observations on the pathologic physiology of chronic pulmonary emphysema. *Arch Intern. Med.* **26**, 544–560.

Sherlock, S. (1960). Hepatic coma. *Annu. Rev. Med.* **11**, 47–55.

Stabenau, J. R., D. S. Warren, and D. P. Rall (1959). The role of pH gradient in the distribution of ammonia between blood and cerebrospinal fluid, brain and muscle. *J. Clin. Invest.* **38**, 373–383.

Stanley, N. N., B. G. Salisbury, L. D. McHenry, Jr., and N. S. Cherniack (1975). Effect of liver failure on the response of ventilation and cerebral circulation to carbon dioxide in man and in the goat. *Clin. Sci. Mol. Med.* **49**, 157–169.

tenHove, W., and C. M. Leevy (1973). Hepatic circulation and portal hypertension. *Postgrad. Med.* **19**, 135–142.

Tenney, S. M. (1954). Ventilatory response to carbon dioxide in pulmonary emphysema. *J. Appl. Physiol.* **6**, 477–484.

Tews, J. K., S. H. Carter, P. D. Roa, and W. E. Stone (1963). Free amino acids and related compounds in dog brain: Post-mortem and anoxic changes, effects of ammonium chloride infusion and levels during seizures induced by picrotoxin and by pentylenetetrazol. *J. Neurochem.* **10**, 641–653.

Toleikis, J. R., L. D. L. Wang, and L. L. Boyarsky (1976). Effect of amino acids on the activity of medullary respiratory neurons. *Fed. Proc., Fed. Am. Soc. Exp. Biol.* **35**, 719.

Valero, A., G. Alroy, and A. Stein (1971). Cerebrospinal fluid glutamine, blood–CSF acid–base balance and their relation to neurologic symptoms in chronic hypercapnia. *Respiration* **28**, 137–147.

Valero, A., G. Alroy, B. Eisenkraft, and J. Itskovitch (1974). Ammonia metabolism in chronic obstructive pulmonary disease with special reference to congestive right ventricular failure. *Thorax* **29**, 703–709.

von Euler, U. S., G. Liljestrand, and Y. Zotterman (1939). Excitation mechanism of chemoreceptors of the carotid body. *Skand. Arch. Physiol.* **83**, 132–152.

Warren, K. S., and D. G. Nathan (1958). The passage of ammonia across the blood–brain barrier and its relation to blood pH. *J. Clin. Invest.* **37**, 1724–1728.

Warren, K. S., and S. Schenker (1964). Effect of an inhibitor of glutamine synthesis (methionine sulfoximine) on ammonia toxicity and metabolism *J. Lab. Clin. Invest.* **64**, 442–449.

Warren, K. S., F. L. Iber, W. Dölle, and S. Sherlock (1960). Effect of alterations in blood pH on distribution of ammonia from blood to cerebrospinal fluid in patients in hepatic coma. *J. Lab. Clin. Med.* **56**, 687–694.

Weyne, J., F. Van Leuven, and I. Leusen (1973). Glutamate and glutamine in the brain:

Influence of acute P_{CO_2} changes in normal rats and in rats under sustained hypercapnia or hypocapnia. *Life Sci.* **12,** 211–221.

Weyne, J., F. Van Leuven, and I. Leusen (1976). Brain organic acids during hypercapnia. *Bull. Eur. Physiopathol. Respir.* **12,** 285–291.

White, L. P., E. A. Phear, W. H. J. Summerskill, and S. Sherlock (1955). Ammonium tolerance in liver disease: Observations based on catheterization of the hepatic veins. *J. Clin. Invest.* **34,** 158–168.

Wichser, J., and H. Kazemi (1974). Ammonia and ventilation: Site and mechanism of action. *Respir. Physiol.* **20,** 393–406.

Williams, M., and L. Zohman (1959). Cardiopulmonary function in chronic obstructive pulmonary emphysema. *Am. Rev. Respir. Dis.* **80,** 689–695.

Winslow, A. H., and J. L. Grant (1967). Oxygen induced hypoventilation. *Am. Rev. Respir. Dis.* **95,** 225–232.

Woodman, R. J., and H. McIlwain (1961). Glutamic acid, other amino acids and related compounds as substrates for cerebral tissues: Their effects on tissue phosphates. *Biochem. J.* **81,** 83–93.

Worcel, A., and M. Erecinska (1962). Mechanism of inhibitory action of ammonia on the respiration of rat liver mitochondria. *Biochim. Biophys. Acta* **65,** 27–33.

CHAPTER 4

Respiratory Control
in Air-Breathing Ectotherms

DONALD C. JACKSON

I. INTRODUCTION

Because of the crucial importance of oxygen supply and acid–base balance, the control of gas exchange is an important physiological function in all higher animals. Among the vertebrates, the study of the topic has been largely confined to mammals because of the interest in human physiology. Yet despite this attention, large fundamental gaps still exist in our understanding of the mammalian control system.

Control in nonmammalian vertebrates is, of course, even less well understood, because of lack of both interest and adequate support. Much comparative research is still in the descriptive phase, as the comprehensive background data required for the analysis of mechanism are not yet

Regulation of Ventilation and Gas Exchange
Copyright © 1978 by Academic Press, Inc.
All rights of reproduction in any form reserved.
ISBN 0-12-204650-1

available. A major complicating factor in this area is the enormous diversity of animals, which precludes ready generalizations from the study of isolated species. Even limiting ourselves to air-breathing vertebrates, we must deal with animals ranging from those adapted to a strictly aquatic existence to arid-adapted desert species. Included among the adaptations to environments linking these extremes are striking adaptations of respiratory gas exchange and, presumably, of its control. As an example, consider the salamander, *Siren lacertina,* a large aquatic species native to the southern United States. This animal exchanges gas through three distinct surfaces: its skin, its gills, and its lungs (Guimond and Hutchison, 1973a). At 15°C, this animal loses at least 18% of its CO_2 through each of these three surfaces. How is the respiratory control system of such an animal organized in which the possibility exists for distinct physiological control of three separate exchangers?

Clearly, the comparative study of respiratory control is a complex topic which is still in its infancy. In this chapter I will summarize our present knowledge in this area with selected examples from the literature and also suggest some of the directions in which research in this field is heading. Hopefully, this endeavor will stimulate some students of mammalian respiratory control to appreciate the challenging problems in this area and possibly to seek insights into their particular problems among the "lower" vertebrates. I have chosen to omit the fishes and to confine my discussion to air-breathing vertebrates, with emphasis on the ectotherms. There is a recent comprehensive review of respiratory control in fish (Shelton, 1970), for those interested in this topic.

II. RESPIRATORY ADAPTATIONS OF VERTEBRATES

Before the specifics of comparative respiratory control are discussed, some of the particular adaptations of vertebrates which involve, or may involve, specializations of their respiratory control mechanisms will be considered. This discussion will raise questions rather than answer them, since most of the work in these areas has involved descriptions of the phenomena and little or nothing is known regarding the basic adaptations of the control systems.

A. Adaptations to Aquatic Life

Many air-breathing vertebrates spend much or all of their time in water, and many of their normal pursuits are conducted under the surface while breath-holding. Under normal circumstances, the animal surfaces periodically and engages in an episode of breathing before returning once again to its underwater endeavors. The particular pattern employed is variable and depends on the species and on its activity level. For example, among the turtles, the freshwater species characteristically exhibit rather long apneic periods, often lasting an hour or more, interrupted by a rapid series of breaths (Belkin, 1964; Lenfant et al., 1970; McCutcheon, 1943). This pattern persists even when the turtle is out of water. Sea turtles, on the other hand, such as the green turtle, *Chelonia mydas,* take single breaths at fairly regular intervals in the manner of marine mammals (Prange and Jackson, 1976). Episodic breathing is also typical of various amphibians and air-breathing fish.

How does respiratory control operate in an episodic breather? We may assume that the regulated variables of the system, P_{O_2}, P_{CO_2}, and pH, oscillate in relation to the breathing episodes, and that the initiation of breathing at the end of an apneic phase is due to these variables, in some unknown combination, causing a threshold stimulus. This pattern was observed experimentally by Lenfant et al. (1970) on the South American freshwater turtle, *Chelys fimbriata.* Blood gases and pH were measured at frequent intervals during a succession of breathing episodes, and these variables were found to oscillate predictably (Fig. 1). Breathing appeared to commence in each of the episodes depicted at about the same elevated P_{CO_2} and at the same lowered P_{O_2} and pH. This sluggish animal could remain apneic for 30 minutes, with a fall of Pa_{O_2} to only 50 torr. In my observations of the freshwater turtle, *Pseudemys scripta,* an increase in metabolic activity both shortened the apneic interval and increased the number and depth of the breaths within each breathing episode. It is tempting to speculate that the episode is the fundamental output unit of the respiratory center in these animals rather than the individual breath within the episode. This pattern of breathing presents a challenge to the investigator attempting to quantify a response to a respiratory stimulus, for the notion of respiratory frequency is difficult to apply unambiguously.

The normal respiratory control of the aquatic vertebrates may have a prepotent voluntary input which can suspend breathing and permit the regulated system to deviate far from its normal state. The most familiar example of this voluntary override is apneic diving, which is common to aquatic members of all vertebrate classes. Among the reptiles, the turtles are particularly noted for their ability to tolerate long periods of apnea (Belkin, 1963); forced experimental diving has demonstrated that these animals can survive dives which last long after internal O_2 stores have been exhausted (Belkin, 1962; Jackson, 1968; Robin et al., 1964) and which produce profound respiratory and metabolic acidosis (Berkson,

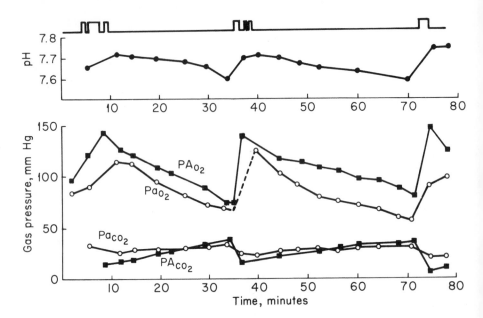

Figure 1.   Arterial and alveolar gas tensions and blood pH values sampled in association with three consecutive breathing episodes in the South American freshwater turtle, *Chelys fimbriata*. (From Lenfant *et al.*, 1970.)

1966; Jackson and Silverblatt, 1974). Fewer data are available on long-term voluntary diving, but Moberly (1968b) recorded dives lasting more than four hours in frightened green iguanas (*I. iguana*) with resulting anoxia and acidosis. In our laboratory, we have observed turtles undergoing marked respiratory stimulation (CO_2 breathing or cerebral ventricular perfusion) cease breathing entirely for 30 minutes when disturbed. Apparently, potent suprathreshold chemical stimuli to breathe can be tolerated by a stressed animal when survival is favored by not breathing.

Another feature of many aquatic vertebrates, already alluded to in Section I above, is the presence of bi- or trimodal gas exchange. Both branchial and aerial exchange are employed in many species of amphibians and fish and in these same groups, and in many aquatic reptiles, significant cutaneous exchange occurs as well. Furthermore, pulmonary ventilation is totally absent and all exchange is cutaneous and buccopharyngeal in the small lungless salamanders, the plethodonts (Whitford and Hutchison, 1965). Because effective respiratory control requires a coupling between the load on the system and the output of the exchanger, the organization of the control system promises to be rather complex in an animal with multiple exchange outputs. As suggested earlier, the trimodal breather, *Siren lacertina,* may respond to an elevated metabolic rate by increasing the rate of gas exchange through its lungs, gills, or skin.

We have recently obtained evidence, however, from studies of the bullfrog, *Rana catesbeiana,* that the cutaneous gas exchange mode in this species may be principally a passive, poorly controlled process. Three separate pieces of evidence favor this evaluation. First, the cutaneous CO_2 loss at constant temperature in normally respiring bullfrogs is nearly constant despite wide variation of total CO_2 loss rates in the individual frogs (Fig. 2). Thus, at low levels of activity, the loss through the skin is a much larger fraction of the total loss than at high levels of activity. The control of CO_2 loss is accomplished via the pulmonary exchange which accounts for more than 90% of an incremental increase in CO_2 loss at 10°, 20°, or 30°C (Jackson and Mackenzie, 1977). Second, in an apneic, normoxic bullfrog, cutaneous loss following submergence rises to equal the preapneic total loss (lung plus skin), but the arterial P_{CO_2} also rises proportionately (Gottleib and Jackson, 1976). This indicates that skin CO_2 loss is a passive function which is principally dependent on the P_{CO_2} difference across the skin, and that no active physiological control is involved. Third, there was no evidence for an adaptive increase in skin CO_2 loss when bullfrogs breathed CO_2-enriched air, although when the converse experiment was performed and CO_2 was administered across the skin, pulmonary ventilation increased markedly and kept Pa_{CO_2} within narrow limits (D. C. Jackson, B. A. Braun and J. Chertoff, unpublished observations). A final line of evidence pointing to the passive nature of cutaneous gas exchange concerns the frog's response to temperature, but this will be considered later.

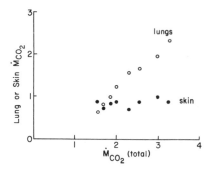

Figure 2. CO_2 loss from the lung and skin of the bullfrog, *Rana catesbeiana,* as a function of the total CO_2 loss. Eight separate experiments at 20°C are shown. (After Jackson and Mackenzie, 1977).

However, these observations on the bullfrog leave important questions unanswered. What is the effect of an increase or decrease in skin blood flow on cutaneous gas exchange? Unless the exchange is not perfusion limited, the increase in cardiac output presumably associated with increased metabolic rate and body temperature should increase skin blood flow and enhance skin gas exchange. Present data provide little evidence for a significant influence of skin flow under the circumstances tested. In a recent analysis of skin gas exchange in the lungless salamander *Desmognathus fuscus,* Piiper *et al.* (1975) calculated, on the basis of experimental inert gas kinetics, that O_2 and CO_2 exchange across the skin of this species is primarily diffusion, and not perfusion, limited. A second question concerns those amphibians which rely predominantly or exclusively on the skin for gas exchange. Do they not have active control over their respiratory exchange? If not, their internal gas tension should drift with changes in their metabolic rate. The small lungless plethodonts are the logical, but technically difficult, candidates for the study of this question. The large salamander, *Cryptobranchus alleganiensis,* the hellbender, has been shown by Guimond and Hutchison (1973b) to be an almost exclusive skin breather and may be more easily studied.

The more complex control problem may involve those animals which employ both gills and an aerial gas exchanger for their respiration. Studies of partitioning of gas exchange between these two modes have been carried out on gilled amphibians (Guimond and Hutchison, 1972, 1973a), but studies related to control of this dual process have been largely confined to the air-breathing fishes (see Johansen, 1970, for a detailed review). Here again, diversity is an overriding factor, since the air-breathing mode has emerged in many different lines, utilizing a variety of surfaces for exchange, including the swim bladder, the gastrointestinal (GI) tract, the oral cavity, and the lungs (Steen, 1971). The lungfish are of particular interest, as they represent an extant form probably similar to the transitional animals which linked the sarcopterygian fishes with the terrestrial tetrapods. The control of breathing in these species is relevant to the evolution of respiratory control in the terrestrial vertebrates but is not necessarily the same as the control in air-breathing fishes among the teleosts.

B. Altered Ambient Gas Composition

As air breathers, confined for the most part near sea level, we humans are accustomed to a very uniform environment with respect to gas concentration and partial pressures. The same is true for most air-breathing vertebrates, but certain circumstances or habitats do involve significant departures of P_{O_2} and P_{CO_2} from their usual ambient levels. Some of these will be noted and discussed in the context of respiratory control and homeostasis.

1. Water

Gas concentrations and pressures are inherently more variable in water than in air as a result of diffusion and mixing problems as well as local gas production and depletion (Krogh, 1941). Oxygen pressure may fall to low levels because of oxidation of organic matter by microorganisms or it may rise well above ambient air P_{O_2} in regions of intense photosynthetic activity. The P_{CO_2} will commonly change in the opposite direction, so that an aquatic animal may be subject to a combined stress of hypoxia and hypercarbia if it depends on the water for gas exchange. Some aquatic animals, such as the marine mammals and the large aquatic reptiles, are probably largely independent of aquatic gas tension variations for their own respiratory needs, because they rely chiefly on the air above the surface which has a stable composition. Other air-breathing vertebrates, however, including aquatic amphibians, reptiles, and air-breathing fish, exchange most of their respiratory gas through the skin; these animals are affected by changes in the gas composition of the water. The responses elicited by altered aquatic gas tensions may have profound evolutionary significance, for it is considered probable that air breathing was initiated in the Devonian period by fishes exposed to hypoxic conditions in search of a more reliable source of O_2. Studies of contemporary air-breathing fish have revealed adaptive responses to deoxygenated water (Johansen, 1970). For example, the Australian lungfish *Neoceratodus*, which relies chiefly on its gills for gas exchange, increases branchial pumping with only a slight rise in lung ventilation (Johansen et al., 1967). The bowfin, *Amia calva*, which uses its swim bladder as a gas exchanger, first increases gill ventilation when exposed to hypoxic water but eventually reduces gill ventilation in favor of an increase in air breathing (Johansen et al., 1970). The African lungfish, *Protopterus*, an obligate air breather, showed little response to hypoxic water because its gills are degenerate and of little importance.

Although attention is usually focused on O_2 availability, the accumulation of CO_2 in the water may also pose serious problems for bimodal breathers. In animals which exchange gas with both water and air, CO_2 loss to the water exceeds O_2 uptake from the water because of the more rapid diffusion of CO_2 in aqueous solution. What then is the consequence for an air-breathing fish or amphibian exposed to an aquatic environment which has both low P_{O_2} and high P_{CO_2}? It is likely that a greater reliance on air breathing can relieve the hypoxic stress; but because of the ease of

CO_2 penetration through the skin, a severe respiratory acidosis may ensue. An excellent animal for the study of the problem is again the large salamander, *Siren lacertina,* which inhabits ponds in the southern United States. According to Ultsch (1976), these animals, which weigh up to 700 gm and can survive indefinitely in air-equilibrated water at 25°C without access to air, are found in water hyacinth-covered ponds in which aquatic P_{CO_2} levels sometimes reach 40 torr. Although the blood status of *S. lacertina* has not yet been measured under these conditions, it is likely that high P_{CO_2} levels are readily tolerated, as individuals survived several days of experimental submergence in water having a P_{CO_2} of 200 torr or higher (Ultsch, 1976).

2. Air

The P_{O_2} of air may fall below normal either at altitude or in local microenvironments in which O_2 usage exceeds replacement from the surroundings. The P_{CO_2} may likewise rise in the latter situation. Altitude exposure probably does not impose a severe hypoxic stress on resident ectotherms because of their modest O_2 requirements and generally high tolerance to low O_2. The stresses of low temperature, desiccation, and inadequate food would probably restrict the ectotherm to altitudes below those where P_{O_2} would be a limitation (Hock, 1964). Birds, however, are of enormous interest in this regard, since they not only are found at high altitudes but even engage in demanding, flapping flight (Tucker, 1968). Evidence is accumulating which suggests that the bird's adaptation resides in its unusual lung design (Bretz and Schmidt-Nielsen, 1971). A cross-current flow occurs between gas and blood which permits a high extraction of inspired O_2 without compromising arterial P_{O_2} (Colacino *et al.*, 1977; Scheid and Piiper, 1972).

Altered gas composition may be encountered locally at lower altitudes in such artificial environments as submarines or poorly ventilated lecture halls or, perhaps more naturally, in animal burrows or nests (Hayward, 1966; Kay, 1977). Once again, however, this problem is more severe for endothermic species which utilize O_2 and produce CO_2 at a higher rate. Under similar conditions of ventilation and body size, the depletion of oxygen and the retention of CO_2 will be much more severe for an endotherm than an ectotherm because of differences in metabolic rate.

C.   Adaptations to Variable Body Temperature

The chief characteristic distinguishing ectothermic animals from endotherms is the absence of effective physiological or autonomic temperature-control mechanism in the former group. This is not to say that some ectotherms do not maintain a constant body temperature; indeed, certain aquatic species, such as those inhabiting the thermally stable Antarctic waters, experience much smaller deviations in body temperature than do typical endotherms. Our interest here, however, is with those ectotherms whose environment is not so uniform and which therefore must cope with significant daily and/or seasonal changes in body temperature. Some of these animals continue normal activity over a temperature range of 25°C or more, although many limit the extent of these excursions by behavioral thermoregulatory responses (Brattstrom, 1970; Templeton, 1970).

Because all the physical parameters concerned with gas exchange and gas transport are temperature dependent, and the metabolic processes concerned with the utilization of O_2 and the production of CO_2 are also temperature dependent, significant alterations in respiratory physiology may be expected when comparing animals at different temperatures. This is in fact the case, and experiments in recent years have not only succeeded in describing some of the adaptations involved but have challenged a basic assumption of mammalian respiratory physiology: namely, that $[H^+]$ and P_{CO_2} are the fundamental regulated variables of the control system. This topic will be discussed in detail later in this chapter.

III. BASES OF RESPIRATORY CONTROL

The existence of respiratory control in an animal is inferred from several standard experimental observations. First, the supposed regulated variables of the system (blood P_{CO_2}, pH, and/or P_{O_2}) are stable over time; second, the ventilation or gas exchange of the animal is matched in some consistent way to the metabolic rate of the animal; and third, the animal responds, in an appropriate way, to experimental disturbances in the regulated variables. On all counts, various ectothermic vertebrates have been shown to possess effective respiratory control systems.

A. Stability of Regulated Variables

To illustrate the stability of a prime regulated variable, arterial P_{CO_2}, a selection of recent data on a variety of species is presented in Table I. In the experimental collection of such data, certain precautions are essential if consistent results are to be obtained. The failure to observe these precautions in earlier studies delayed the appreciation of the accuracy of ectothermic control. First, samples must be taken from quiescent animals after adequate recovery from handling and catheterization stress. This is

Table I   Arterial P_{CO_2} Values of Selected Ectotherms[a]

Species	Temperature (°C)	Pa_{CO_2} (torr)	Reference
American alligator (*A. mississippiensis*)	25	17.9 ± 0.6 (13)	Davies and Kopetzky, 1976
Monitor lizard (*Varanus exanthematicus*)	25	17.1 ± 0.8 (9)	Wood *et al.*, 1977
Red-eared turtle (*Pseudemys scripta*)	20	22.7 ± 0.8 (13)	Jackson *et al.*, 1974
Snapping turtle (*Chelydra serpentina*)	20	25.2 ± 0.4 (13)	Howell *et al.*, 1970
Marine toad (*Bufo marinus*)	20	10.4 ± 0.2 (6)	Howell *et al.*, 1970
Bullfrog (*Rana catesbeiana*)	20	12.7 ± 1.0 (16)	Howell *et al.*, 1970

[a] Values are mean ± SEM, with number of observations in parentheses.

especially crucial in water-breathing species with their low, volatile P_{CO_2} and pH values (Rahn and Baumgardner, 1972), but it is also important for reptiles, which support vigorous bouts of struggling by anaerobic metabolism with consequent metabolic acidosis (Bennett, 1972; Gatten, 1974). The source of blood is also of importance, although in many studies it has been more convenient and feasible to obtain blood of questionable origin by heart puncture rather than to obtain true arterial blood. A final precaution that is of utmost importance concerns the animal's body temperature, since the regulated variables, P_{CO_2} and pH, are strongly temperature dependent (Howell *et al.*, 1970). In the studies cited in Table I, all animals in each group were kept at the indicated temperature for a day or more prior to sampling.

B.   Matching between Ventilation and Metabolic Rate

The constancy of arterial P_{CO_2} values in a population of animals or in the same animal at different times strongly indicates that a constant relationship exists between the gas-exchange mechanism (i.e., ventilation) and the metabolic rate. There are a few data of this kind available on ectotherms (Jackson, 1971; Wood *et al.*, 1977), and measurements from my laboratory on the turtle, *Pseudemys scripta,* are shown in Fig. 3. These are steady-state measurements, and each point represents the mean value for at least one hour in a single animal at 20°C. The variations in metabolic rate were spontaneous, and I consider these to be different levels of

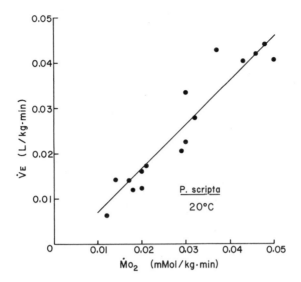

Figure 3. Paired values of ventilation and oxygen consumption of the turtle, *Pseudemys scripta*, at 20°C. Each point is a single steady-state value. (After Jackson, 1971.)

"resting," although not basal, metabolism. There may be no clear distinction, however, between these different levels of "resting" metabolism which cover a three- to fivefold range and frank physical exercise.

There has been considerable interest in recent years in the physiological correlates of exercise or induced activity in ectotherms. One result of these studies has been to reveal the heavy dependence of many animals on anaerobic metabolism during intense activity (Bennett, 1972; Gatten, 1974; Moberly, 1968a). Lower levels of activity, however, may be supported by the limited aerobic capacities of these animals (Moberly, 1968b). Certain reptiles, however, notably the varanid lizards and the marine turtles, are noted for their ability to sustain prolonged periods of activity supported largely by aerobic metabolism (Bennett, 1972; Prange, 1976). Recently, pulmonary ventilation has been measured in species of both groups, the lizard, *Varanus gouldii* (Bennett, 1973a) and the green turtle, *Chelonia mydas* (Prange and Jackson, 1976). Maximal activity was induced in the former by electrical stimulation, while the latter exercised spontaneously by being released and allowed to move about on land. Both species wore masks, and ventilation and gas exchange were measured simultaneously. In each case, ventilation increased generally in proportion to metabolic rate, although in *C. mydas* there was some evidence for hyperventilation as a result of mild metabolic (lactic) acidosis. An interesting difference between the two responses was that the increased ventilation in *V. gouldii* was almost entirely due to increased tidal volume, while in *C. mydas* the increase was due to a higher respiratory frequency. These studies certainly establish that a ventilatory response to activity occurs in reptiles; still, further studies in which ventilation and blood gas and acid–base variables are monitored during graded, "normal" exercise are needed.

C. ∼ Respiratory Chemoreceptors: Responses to Altered Inspired Gas

Considerable interest in respiratory control physiology centers on the respiratory receptors, or chemoreceptors, in terms of their location, their adequate stimuli, their central connections and effects, and their basic cellular characteristics. In the comparative field, this is an area which is just beginning to be explored. The existence of chemoreceptor structures in submammalian vertebrates has long been inferred from the respiratory responses of many species to alterations in inspired gas composition. Recently, local chemical stimulation and neurophysiological investigation have been carried out in several laboratories on both peripheral and central chemoreceptors.

1. *CO$_2$ Responses and Receptors*

There have been a considerable number of studies in which air-breathing ectotherms have been subjected to alterations in inspired gas composition. Unfortunately, the results of many of these studies are difficult to interpret or to reconcile with related studies because of the differences in experimental design and in the species studied. For example, let us consider selected studies of the ventilatory response to elevated inspired CO$_2$ in reptiles. The following responses have been elicited and reported: In the lizards, *Lacerta viridis* and *L. sicula,* Nielsen (1961) reported a slight increase in $\dot{V}_E$ with up to 3% CO$_2$ in the inspired gas and an inhibitory effect at higher CO$_2$ concentrations. The response consisted of an increase in tidal volume and a decrease in respiratory frequency; at the higher concentrations of CO$_2$, the frequency inhibition became dominant and accounted for the net decrease in $\dot{V}_E$. Similar responses have been reported to occur in the lizard, *Crotaphytus collaris,* by Templeton and Dawson (1963), and earlier in *Lacerta* by Boelaert (1941). In contrast, the green sea turtle, *Chelonia mydas,* responded markedly and in graded fashion to inspired CO$_2$ concentrations up to 7.5% primarily with an increase in frequency and with a small increase in tidal volume occurring at the highest concentration (Jackson and Prange, 1977). The freshwater turtle, *Pseudemys scripta,* on the other hand, increased ventilation progressively up to 6% CO_2 (the highest gas tested) by approximately equivalent increases in both frequency and depth (Jackson *et al.*, 1974). A similar response pattern has recently been observed in the American alligator, *A. mississippiensis*, by Davies and Kopetzky (1976), as illustrated in Fig. 4. To further confound this picture, there have been studies on some of the same species which produced quite different results. For

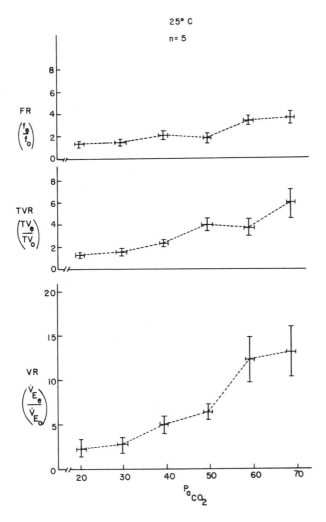

Figure 4. Ventilatory response to CO_2 in the alligator, *A. mississippiensis*, at 25°C. Frequency, tidal volume, and ventilation values are presented as ratios of the measured value to the value of the same animal breathing air. (After Davies and Kopetzky, 1976.)

example, Millen *et al.* (1964) reported that *P. scripta* responded only slightly to inhalation of 6% CO_2, a result which is difficult to reconcile with this author's repeated observation of a large, consistent respiratory response to this gas.

The explanation of these disparate results (although not the intraspecific disparities) should be found when the chemoreceptor structures of these animals have been described. A recent study on central chemoreceptors in the turtle, *Pseudemys scripta,* has made a promising start (Hitzig, 1977). Hitzig succeeded in stereotaxically implanting chronic needle catheters into the lateral and fourth ventricles of turtles and subsequently perfusing artificial cerebrospinal fluid (CSF) solutions through the ventricles while measuring ventilation. The physiological measurements were made on unanesthetized animals following recovery from the operation. The results were clear and dramatic. The turtles responded to decreases in the strong ion difference (i.e., $[HCO_3^-]$) of the perfusing fluid with a marked increase in ventilation. The normal $[HCO_3^-]$ of the turtle's CSF averaged 32 mEq/liter, and perfusion with a fluid having a concentration reduced to only 30 mEq/liter induced a fourfold increase in ventilation. Perfusion with normal concentrations had little or no effect. These results represent the first direct experimental proof for the existence of central chemoreceptors in a lower vertebrate. Their location and functional characteristics, at least as thus far defined, appear to be similar to the mammalian central chemoreceptors. It is remarkable that these receptors are so sensitive to small changes in the acid–base properties of the ventricular fluid, even when compared to mammalian receptors studied under similar experimental circumstances (Pappenheimer *et al.,* 1965). The sensitivity of the turtle, however, is consistent with responsiveness of this animal to inspired CO_2, as noted previously (Jackson *et al.,* 1974).

Although Hitzig studied only the central chemoreceptor response directly, he performed a series of experiments which produced results suggesting the existence of at least two distinct receptor systems within the turtle. The results of the experiment are summarized in Fig. 5. After a control measurement of frequency and tidal volume, the ventricles were perfused with artificial CSF with low $[HCO_3^-]$ (30 mEq/liter compared to the normal 32 mEq/liter). Ventilation increased primarily because of an elevation in frequency of breathing. While the perfusion was continued, the inspired gas was switched from air to 4.5% CO_2. This further stimulated ventilation, but the major contributing factor was an increase in tidal volume. Next, the $[HCO_3^-]$ of the perfusion fluid was increased to a supranormal 43 mEq/liter. This depressed ventilation back toward the control value by a sharp reduction in frequency, although tidal volume

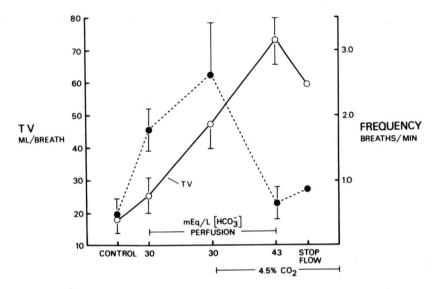

Figure 5. Tidal volume and respiratory frequency of turtles, *Pseudemys scripta*, during ventricular perfusion and CO_2 breathing. See text for details. (From Hitzig, 1977.)

was elevated still further. The interpretation of these data is as follows. There are at least two chemoreceptor populations: one in the brain, sensitive to changes in the CSF composition, which principally affects the frequency of breathing; and a second, peripheral to the brain (or at least to the direct influence of CSF), sensitive to arterial P_{CO_2} which principally affects the depth of breathing. It is possible that the lizards studied by Nielsen (1961) and by Templeton and Dawson (1963) lacked the first, or central receptor. Their peak response to CO_2 resembles that observed in the turtle during CO_2 breathing (peripheral stimulation) and high $[HCO_3^-]$ ventricular perfusion (central inhibition). Verification of this hypothesis will require assessment of central chemosensitivity in a lizard exhibiting this type of CO_2 response. The inhibition at high CO_2 levels exhibited by the lizards may have been due to receptors sensitive to CO_2 which depress ventilation by slowing the frequency. Both Nielsen (1961) and Templeton and Dawson (1963) postulated that, because of the rapid rate-inhibitory on-response and rapid rate-stimulatory off-response, these inhibitory receptors were not responding to changes in the blood.

Another possible group of respiratory chemoreceptors thought to be involved in the response to CO_2 is also found within the lung. These so-called *intrapulmonary* CO_2 receptors have been studied most extensively in birds, where they have been shown to be highly specific to CO_2

but unresponsive to stretch, changes in P_{O_2}, or to acetylcholine administration (Fedde and Peterson, 1970). Besides responding to the composition of gas flowing in the lung, these receptors are also responsive to the P_{CO_2} of the pulmonary artery blood (Banzett and Burger, 1977). The signal from these receptors actually inhibits respiratory activity, but since the activity of the receptors is raised by a decrease in P_{CO_2}, their effect is to stimulate breathing when P_{CO_2} is elevated. There is recent evidence that receptors possessing similar properties are present in the lungs of the lizard, *Tupinambis nigropunctatus* (Gatz et al., 1975), and the turtle, *Chrysemys picta* (Milsom and Jones, 1975). The receptors of the lizard have been subjected to a thorough investigation involving electrophysiological recording of single vagal afferents, and these studies confirm the functional similarity between the pulmonary receptors of the lizard and bird (Fedde *et al.*, 1977; Scheid *et al.*, 1977). These receptors in the lizard appear to be located on the surface of the saclike lung rather than in conducting airways (Scheid *et al.*, 1977).

In a recent study of the respiratory response to CO_2 in the green turtle, *Chelonia mydas* (Jackson and Prange, 1977), circumstantial evidence was obtained for the existence of airway receptors sensitive to CO_2 which stimulated ventilation. We found that three of five turtles tested, when switched from air to CO_2 mixture, gave an immediate and maximal ventilatory response following the first breath of CO_2 and immediately returned to control ventilation when air breathing was resumed (Fig. 6). Our interpretation that this indicates the presence of an airway receptor rather than a lung receptor is based on two factors: first, the rapidity of the

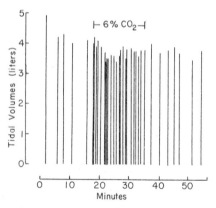

Figure 6. Respiratory response of a sea turtle, *Chelonia mydas*, to a period of CO_2 breathing. Each vertical line represents a single breath. Note rapid onset and cessation of the response. (After Jackson and Prange, 1977.)

response, which would have been delayed if the receptor were in the lung due to the dilution effect of the residual gas; and second, the fact that the respiratory cycle of the turtle terminates following inspiration, thus subjecting the airways to the pure inspired gas during the respiratory pause following the first breath of the gas. No electrophysiological investigation of this system has been attempted.

These studies suggest the existence of as many as five distinct respiratory chemoreceptors sensitive to CO_2 in reptiles (Table II). To date, only the intrapulmonary receptor of the lizard, *Tupinambus*, and the central chemoreceptor of the turtle, *Pseudemys*, can be considered to be experimentally verified. This potential array of receptor types and the numerous possible combinations that could be present in the various species provide a basis to account for the different response patterns and point the way toward a rational experimental strategy for explaining these differences.

2. Response to Lowered O_2

Hypoxia induced by breathing inspired gas deficient in O_2 has been consistently reported to cause increased ventilation in air-breathing vertebrates. It appears probable that this response can be attributed to receptor structures located near the carotid artery or aortic arch as in mammals. The evidence is stronger, however, for amphibians such as the frog, *Rana esculenta* (Smyth, 1939), and for birds such as the duck (Jones and Purves, 1970; Bouverot and Leitner, 1972) than for reptiles, where the only study of receptor mechanisms appears to be a preliminary investigation of the turtle, *Pseudemys scripta* (Frankel *et al.*, 1969). It is possible

Table II. Proposed respiratory CO_2 receptors in reptiles

Species	Location	Effect of CO_2	Reference
Turtles			
Pseudemys scripta	Brain	Frequency stimulation	Hitzig, 1977
Pseudemys scripta	Arterial (?)	Tidal volume stimulation	Hitzig, 1977
Lizards			
Crotaphytus collaris and *Lacerta*	Lungs or airways	Frequency inhibition	Templeton and Dawson, 1963; Nielsen, 1961
Tupinambus nigropunctatus	Lung surface	Ventilatory stimulation	Gatz *et al.*, 1975; Scheid *et al.*, 1977
Sea turtle			
Chelonia mydas	Airways (?)	Frequency stimulation	Jackson and Prange, 1977

that reptiles lack a distinct structure similar to the carotid and aortic bodies of mammals and that the distribution of receptor cells is more diffuse (Adams, 1958). Many reptiles possess O_2-sensitive receptors of some sort because, as shall be described, they are quite responsive to lowered ambient O_2.

Although there is considerable variability in the magnitude and in the threshold of the response to lowered O_2 among the various vertebrates, air breathers in general respond only slightly except to rather substantial decreases in inspired P_{O_2}. Dejours (1975) has suggested an evolutionary basis for understanding this relative insensitivity to hypoxia. He points out that fish, living as they do in a severely O_2-deficient environment (compared to air), are quite sensitive to changes in ambient O_2; gill ventilation usually increases when O_2 is lowered and decreases under hyperoxic conditions. The air-breathing descendants of fish (ourselves included) still possess the same basic respiratory control system as fish, but our normal respiratory environment, and our ventilatory activity within that environment are analogous to fish in hyperoxic water (Fig. 7). According to Dejours, our standard of reference for air breathers should

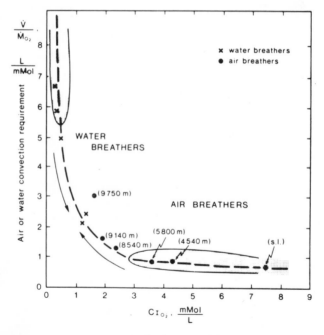

Figure 7. Air convection requirement ($\dot{V}_E/\dot{M}_{O_2}$) of water and air breathers as a function of the O_2 concentration of the ambient media. (From Dejours, 1975.)

be those living in an hypoxic environment, such as at high altitude, because under such conditions, chemoreceptor activity, and thus ventilation, vary directly with ambient P_{O_2}. This view gives preeminence to O_2 as the respiratory variable and leads to the conclusion that after all these years, we and our fellow air-breathing vertebrates are still only "fish out of water." The fact remains, however, that the hyperoxia of fish has become the normoxia of air breathers. Accurate control of ventilation exists in spite of the insensitivity to small increases or decreases in ambient P_{O_2}. Acid–base regulation appears to have supplanted O_2 supply as the principal routine controlling factor in the respiration of most air-breathing vertebrates. Low ambient O_2 is a potent stimulus to a variety of adaptive responses in mammals, however, such as lung development (Burri and Weibel, 1971), erythropoiesis (Hurtado, 1964), and tissue capillary density (Ou and Tenney, 1970). Chronic exposure to high CO_2 induces no such adaptive responses.

Progressive reductions in ambient O_2 eventually lead to a depression of metabolic rate. The P_{O_2} at which this occurs has been termed the *critical* P_{O_2} and represents the minimal $P_{I_{O_2}}$ at which the normal resting metabolic rate can be sustained (Prosser, 1973). There are quite large differences in critical P_{O_2} among air-breathing ectotherms. For example, Belkin (1965) found that the musk turtle, *Sternothaerus minor,* could maintain a resting metabolic rate down to an inspired P_{O_2} of 8 torr, while the snake, *Farancia abacura,* could only accomplish this down to $P_{I_{O_2}}$ of 40 torr. Bennett and Dawson (1976) state that the critical P_{O_2} of lizards, snakes, and crocodilians is generally much higher (ca. 70 torr) than in turtles (8–15 torr). The experimentally determined critical P_{O_2} depends on a number of factors, such as metabolic rate and body temperature. Thus, a metabolic rate above resting could elevate the measured critical P_{O_2} and obscure valid comparison between species.

What accounts for these differences in critical P_{O_2}? The limiting P_{O_2} at the mitochondrial level is quite low, probably 5 torr or less (Chance, 1957), and is probably not subject to much adaptive variation. The difference probably resides in the responses of the O_2 transport systems, the respiratory system, and the cardiovascular system to hypoxia. Boyer (1966) found that the snapping turtle, *Chelydra serpentina,* displayed a vigorous respiratory response to hypoxia and was much more resistant to hypoxia than were the desert iguana, *Dipsosaurus dorsalis,* the bullsnake, *Pituophis melanoleucus,* and the alligator, *A. mississippiensis,* none of which exhibited much respiratory response. Similarly, Nielsen (1962) observed little respiratory stimulation by 5% O_2 in the lizards *Lacerta viridis* and *Tarentola mauretanica,* and reported that these lizards grew limp breathing this gas at 30°C. The freshwater turtle, *Pseudemys scripta,* which was studied breathing low O_2 mixtures at various temperatures (Jackson, 1973), suffered metabolic depression and incapacitation only at the highest temperature and lowest inspired O_2 (30°C and 3% O_2). From these studies, therefore, it would appear that the magnitude of the ventilatory response to low O_2 correlates with the ability of various reptiles to tolerate low O_2 and may be a major factor determining the critical P_{O_2}. The turtles have a large ventilatory response to hypoxic gas mixtures and are noted for their low critical P_{O_2} values.

The turtles, as mentioned earlier, also possess the greatest capacity among the reptiles for tolerating and surviving prolonged anoxic diving. This seemingly paradoxical combination of hypoxic sensitivity and hypoxic tolerance may be due to this animal's adaptation to prolonged apneic diving. During diving, the turtle can maintain normal metabolic rate down to low internal P_{O_2} values before experiencing metabolic depression. Following the exhaustion of internal O_2 stores, the turtle can continue to survive solely on anaerobic metabolism (Jackson, 1968). Following the dive, when the turtle emerges into air, its sensitive chemoreceptor system promotes pronounced hyperventilation (Fig. 8), which rapidly restores normal blood gas and acid–base status (Jackson and Silverblatt, 1974). During the dive, the intense stimulation to breathe must somehow be suppressed to prevent the turtle from reaching the point which we term the *breaking point* in human breath-holding.

Body temperature is also an important factor influencing the ventilatory response to low O_2 in ectotherms. I measured ventilation and gas exchange in the turtle, *Pseudemys scripta*, at 10°, 20°, and 30°C (Jackson, 1973). The response was clearly temperature dependent. At 10°C, there

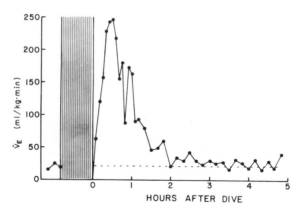

Figure 8. Ventilation of a turtle, *Pseudemys scripta,* before and after a 4-hour dive (stippled region) at 24°C. (From Jackson and Silverblatt, 1974.)

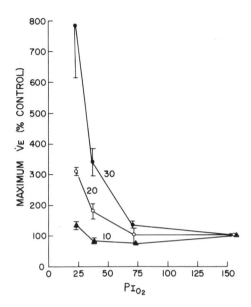

Figure 9. Maximal ventilatory response (shown as percent of the air-breathing control value) to various low O_2 breathing mixtures in the turtle, *Pseudemys scripta,* at 10°, 20°, and 30°C. (From Jackson, 1973.)

was little response even when 3% O_2 ($P_{I_{O_2}}$ = 23 torr) was breathed, whereas at 30°C, there was slight response to 10% O_2 and pronounced response to 5% O_2 ($P_{I_{O_2}}$ = 38 torr), as shown in Fig. 9. A major factor contributing to this temperature difference is the normal relationship that exists between ventilation and O_2 consumption at different temperatures in this animal and in many other air-breathing ectotherms. As this temperature–ventilation relationship will be discussed next, I will delay interpretation of the low O_2 response.

IV. TEMPERATURE AND RESPIRATORY CONTROL

A. Temperature and pH

The unique aspect of respiratory control in ectotherms is due to their variable body temperature and to the effect that temperature has upon the pH of the body fluids. It is now well documented that, within the normal temperature span of most ectothermic species—including both air breathers and water breathers—the pH of the body fluids decreases systematically with body temperature by about 0.016 units/°C. Because the prime regulated variable is temperature dependent, the physiological systems which act as acid–base controlling mechanisms are also of necessity temperature dependent. In this discussion, I will summarize current work on the pH–temperature relationship and then examine the consequences this relationship has for respiratory control of air-breathing ectotherms. An important symposium on this general topic, including contributions on intracellular pH regulation, was recently held at Strasbourg in conjunction with the International Congress of Physiological Sciences meeting at Paris. Also, two excellent reviews on the subject have recently appeared (Howell and Rahn, 1976; Reeves, 1977).

The consistency of the relationship between blood pH and temperature compel the belief that it is not a fortuitous, inconsequential observation. Indeed, there is a growing body of knowledge which strongly indicates that this effect is of fundamental significance. One observation leading to this conclusion is that the temperature-related changes in acid–base properties of an animal's blood *in vivo* match the behavior of the blood when it is equilibrated in a sealed vessel at various temperatures *in vitro*. From this we learn that the animal's physiological control systems are defending, at each temperature, the acid–base state produced by the effect of temperature on the chemical equilibrium reactions of the body fluids.

Reeves (1972) has examined these reactions and found that the dominant equilibrium reaction contributing to the temperature effect is the dissociation of the histidine–imidazole group. This group has a pK close to 7.0 and an enthalpy of ionization (ΔH^0) close to 7 kcal/mole, both of which are properties the key protein moiety must possess (Albery and Lloyd, 1967). Indeed, Reeves (1972) found that a solution composed simply of 25 mM NaHCO$_3$, 100 mM NaCl, and 20 mM imidazole behaved the same as whole blood, in terms of acid–base properties, when equilibrated at various temperatures. He further pointed out that because pH changes as it does, the fractional dissociation of imidazole, or α-imidazole, remains constant. This led Reeves to hypothesize that perhaps the fractional dissociation of imidazole is the defended variable in the system and that respiratory control is based on a so-called "alphastat."

Recently, Reeves (1976a,b) has established the physiological importance of the pH–temperature relationship. Because the protein ionization state remains unchanged despite changes in temperature (Reeves, 1976a), the distribution of diffusible ions is also unaffected; i.e., the Donnan ratio for these ions stays the same (Reeves, 1976b). This effect was experimentally demonstrated for Cl⁻ (Fig. 10), but it presumably is true for the other diffusible ions as well. This, of course, has great importance for the

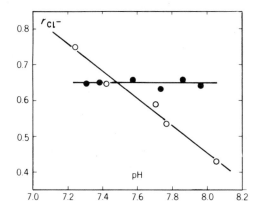

Figure 10.   Effect of pH on the Donnan distribution ratio for chloride ion (r_{Cl^-}). Open symbols represent CO_2 titration at 37.5°C; closed symbols represent changing temperature at constant CO_2 concentration. (From Reeves, 1976b.)

stability of cellular composition and volume. It is not a new idea, however—it was suggested in the pioneering investigation of Austin *et al.* (1927)—but Reeves has provided the experimental verification. It is certain that the integrity of many other intracellular functions related to protein charge is preserved by the observed shift of pH.

It has been noted by Rahn and his colleagues (Rahn, 1966; Howell *et al.*, 1970) that, while pH per se is not constant at different temperatures, the relative alkalinity, or OH^-/H^+ ratio, is held constant. This is true because the slope of the blood pH vs. temperature line is parallel to the line relating the neutral pH of water and temperature. Blood measurements, however, are extracellular measurements, and the intracellular milieu is probably the important site. In the intracellular fluid, pH also varies with temperature, with a slope similar to that of the extracellular fluid (Malan *et al.*, 1976), but the absolute value of pH_i is very close to neutrality (Fig. 11). Rahn and his group (Rahn *et al.*, 1975; Rahn, 1976) drawing upon the analysis of Davis (1958), have postulated that the maintenance of a neutral pH within the cell is essential for keeping the numerous metabolic intermediates within the cell, because at neutrality they are nearly all in the ionized state and cannot easily penetrate through the membrane. The maintenance of a neutral pH within the cells of the ectotherms throughout their temperature range preserves this important property.

Thus, the observed variation of blood and cellular pH of various ectotherms with temperature is a manifestation of a fundamental homeostatic process which preserves essential features of the intra- and extracellu-

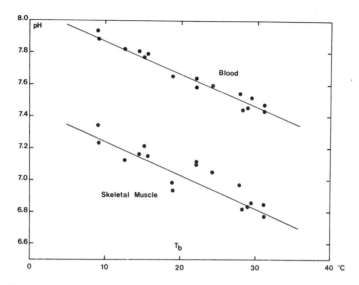

Figure 11. Plasma and intracellular skeletal muscle pH of the turtle, *Pseudemys scripta*, as a function of steady-state body temperature. (From Malan *et al.,* 1976.)

lar fluids. As we have seen, a shift in temperature results in a spontaneous readjustment of the body fluids to the new, correct acid–base state because of the effect of temperature on the chemical equilibria. The preservation of this new state, however, depends upon the proper performance of one or more physiological control mechanisms, for the organism is a metabolizing, open system. There must be a close coupling between the physical system, represented by the blood *in vitro,* and the physiological system, which is exchanging gas and solute molecules with its environment.

B. Respiratory Responses to Temperature in Various Ectothermic Groups

The preceding description is a general one and can be considered to apply to all ectotherms. When we begin to look at individual species, however, or when we compare gill-breathing animals with animals respiring with lungs or skin, we see rather striking differences in the physiological details of the phenomenon. The physiological regulation of acid–base balance is a dual process, involving both the control of P_{CO_2} via the gas exchanger and the control of the strong ion difference via ion transport sites such as the kidney tubules and gill epithelium. Either or both of these mechanisms could adjust its performance to conform to the new requirements imposed by a change in body temperature. In order to decide which mechanism is involved, one must analyze blood from animals equilibrated at different temperatures and observe how P_{CO_2} and the strong ion difference (this is generally approximated by measuring $[HCO_3^-]$) vary with body temperature. I will first consider briefly the response of fish and then discuss in greater detail the responses in lung and skin-breathing ectotherms.

1. Gill Breathers

In their study of the rainbow trout, *Salmo gairdneri,* Randall and Cameron (1973) found that P_{CO_2} was constant between 4.5° and 20°C, while total $[CO_2]$ decreased over this range, leading to the conclusion that an ion transport process, and not ventilatory control of P_{CO_2}, was the control mechanism involved. This failure of fish to conform to the behavior of the *in vitro* system (a constant CO_2 system) is probably related to the tight coupling of fish respiration to its oxygen supply function (Dejours, 1973). Were the fish to follow the pH–temperature line as it ascends to 20°C by elevating its P_{CO_2} the lowered gill ventilation required for this adjustment would undoubtedly jeopardize O_2 supply. The fish is already extracting its O_2 from a relatively O_2-poor medium, and a rise in temperature lowers the available O_2 even further (by reduced O_2 solubility) while the O_2 demand of the fish meanwhile has been increased (Q_{10} effect). The trout is thus obliged to use an ion- transport mechanism which requires at least several hours to readjust to a new temperature.

2. Lung Breathers

Air-breathing ectotherms live in a medium which, compared to water, is abundantly rich in O_2. Consequently, the ventilation of air breathers is not so tightly coupled to O_2 supply, nor is O_2 supply jeopardized by adjusting ventilation within reasonable limits in the interests of acid–base regulation. Thus, we find that arterial blood sampled from the air-breathing ectotherm, acclimated at a series of temperatures, characteristically shows evidence of respiratory adjustment, but no renal adjustment; i.e., P_{CO_2} varies directly with temperature while total $[CO_2]$ is unaffected by temperature. This has been reported to be the case in the bullfrog, *Rana catesbeiana* (Reeves, 1972; Jackson and Mackenzie, 1977); the turtle, *Pseudemys scripta* (Jackson *et al.,* 1974; Jackson and Kagen, 1976); the alligator, *A. mississippiensis* (Davies and Kopetzky, 1976); and the lizard, *Sauromalus obesus* (Crawford and Gatz, 1974). These data are summarized in Table III.

How does the arterial P_{CO_2} correlate with actual measurements of venti-

Table III. Acid–Base Values of Ectotherms at Various Temperatures

Species	Temperature (°C)	pH_a	Pa_{CO_2} (torr)	$[HCO_3^-]$ (mEq/liter)	Reference
Alligator	15	7.64	11.8	16.0	Davies and
(A. mississippiensis)	25	7.48	17.9	15.2	Kopetzky, 1976
(N = 13)	35	7.38	23.2	14.1	
Lizard	16	7.54	11	13.7	Crawford and
(Sauromalus obesus)	27	7.35	26	15.9	Gatz, 1974
(N = 8–14)	40	7.13	40	12.7	
Turtle	10	7.76	14.1	33.1	Jackson et al.,
(Pseudemys scripta)	20	7.67	22.7	34.8	1974
($\dot{N}$ = 11–13)	30	7.56	31.9	31.9	
Bullfrog	5	8.14	7.0	22.6	Reeves, 1972
(Rana catesbeiana)	10	7.99	9.4	22.8	
(N = 5–12)	20	7.83	11.2	21.0	
	34	7.67	23.1	24.1	

lation at different temperatures? In mammals, we can assume that alveolar and arterial P_{CO_2} values are normally quite similar and that steady-state Pa_{CO_2} values will conform closely to the predictions of the alveolar ventilation equation. In reptiles and amphibians, on the other hand, this is not always a safe assumption, because of incomplete separation of the pulmonary and systemic circuits and the potential for significant pulmonary shunting (White, 1976). Nonetheless, the magnitude of the Pa_{CO_2} changes with temperature make a ventilatory adjustment highly likely. Rahn (1966) predicted that because Pa_{CO_2} and metabolic rate of an ectotherm increased with temperature at approximately the same relative rate (i.e., with a similar Q_{10}), the ventilation should increase only slightly, if at all, with temperature. This is based on the alveolar ventilation equation (or gas-law equation):

$$\dot{V}_A = \frac{\dot{M}_{CO_2}}{P_{A_{CO_2}}} \times RT \qquad (1)$$

where $\dot{V}_A$ is alveolar ventilation, $\dot{M}_{CO_2}$ is metabolic CO_2 production, and $P_{A_{CO_2}}$ is alveolar P_{CO_2}.

This prediction was experimentally tested in my laboratory (Jackson, 1971) using the turtle, *Pseudemys scripta*, a reptile which had already been reported to exhibit the typical pH and P_{CO_2} temperature dependence (Robin, 1962). The results verified Rahn's prediction. Respiratory minute volume ($\dot{V}_E$) did not change significantly with temperature, while metabolic rate ($\dot{M}_{O_2}$) increased with a Q_{10} of about 2.0 (Fig. 12). In a subsequent study, these same measurements were made and, in addition,

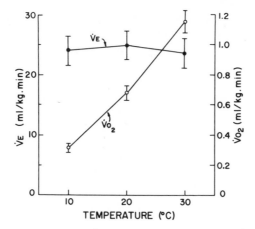

Figure 12. Pulmonary ventilation ($\dot{V}_E$) and oxygen consumption ($\dot{V}_{O_2}$) of turtles, *Pseudemys scripta*. Each is plotted as a function of body temperature. Vertical lines are standard errors. (After Jackson, 1971; Jackson *et al.*, 1974.)

arterial blood samples were taken and the Pa_{CO_2} values determined and correlated with the ventilatory record (Jackson *et al.*, 1974). In this study, the Pa_{CO_2} increased at a slower rate with temperature than did metabolic rate, and ventilation increased moderately with temperature. But the results fit well with the predicted values based on the gas-law equation written in the following terms:

$$\dot{V}_E = \frac{\dot{M}_{O_2}}{Pa_{CO_2}} \times RT \qquad (2)$$

The equation in this form can be used with no correction necessary if the following assumptions are made:

$$P_{A_{CO_2}} = Pa_{CO_2}$$

$$\dot{V}_A = 0.8\dot{V}_E$$

$$\dot{M}_{CO_2} = 0.8\dot{M}_{O_2}$$

Other studies of the temperature–ventilation relationship in reptiles have generally revealed an increase in $\dot{V}_E$ with temperature (Davies, 1975; Giordano and Jackson, 1973; Nielsen, 1961; White and Kinney, 1976). It is important to note that $\dot{V}_E$ by itself does not provide adequate information to assess acid–base status. Measurements of metabolic rate must also be made because, as is clearly seen in Eq. (1) or (2) it is the ratio between ventilation and metabolic rate that determines $P_{A_{CO_2}}$ and Pa_{CO_2}. It is useful, therefore, to assess the respiratory response of ectotherms to changes in body temperature in terms of the ratio, $\dot{V}_E/\dot{M}_{O_2}$. This ratio has been termed the *air convection requirement* (Dejours *et al.*, 1970). For the sake of convenience, this will be designated as ACR.

The ACR has usually been observed to decrease with temperature in the animals (all reptiles) in which it has been measured. These data are presented in Table IV together with data from some reptiles which do not conform to the general pattern. These interesting exceptions will be discussed below. Also included in Table IV are the Pa_{CO_2} values from the same studies, either measured or calculated from Eq. (2). The particular setting for the ACR at each temperature is assumed to be that which is required to regulate arterial (and intracellular) pH at the proper value. For one animal, this may require a higher ACR and lower Pa_{CO_2} than for another animal at the same temperature. If the pH values of the two animals are similar, then the strong ion difference (or $[HCO_3^-]$) of the

Table IV. Air Convection Requirement ($\dot{V}_E/\dot{M}_{O_2}$) Values of Reptiles at Various Temperatures Within Their Normal Range

Species	Temperature (°C)	ACR (liter BTPS/mmole)	Pa_{CO_2} (torr)[a]	Reference
Turtles	10	1.71	(10.3)	Jackson, 1971
Pseudemys scripta	20	0.85	(21.5)	
	30	0.36	(52.5)	
	35	0.24	(80.1)	
Pseudemys scripta	10	1.32	14.1	Jackson *et al.*, 1974
	20	0.71	22.7	
	30	0.44	31.9	
Lizards	10	2.06	(8.6)	Nielsen, 1961
Lacerta	20	1.77	(10.3)	
	30	1.25	(15.1)	
	35	1.24	(15.5)	
Iguana iguana	20	0.94	(19.4)	Giordano and Jackson, 1973
	30	0.68	(27.8)	
	35	0.46	(41.8)	
Sauromalus hispidis	30	2.5	(7.7)	Bennett, 1973a
	40	0.9	(21.7)	
Varanus gouldii	30	0.8	(23.6)	Bennett, 1973a
	40	2.25	(8.7)	
V. exanthematicus	25	0.79	17	Wood *et al.*, 1977
	35	0.73	22	
Alligator	15	0.91	11.8	Davies, 1975
A. mississippiensis	25	0.79	17.9	
	35	0.68	23.2	

[a] Values in parentheses are calculated using measured ACR and Eq. (2).

extracellular fluid (ECF) must be different (Rahn and Garey, 1973). There are too few comprehensive studies available to properly evaluate this effect, but an expected consequence would be that an animal with a low ECF $[HCO_3^-]$ would require a high ACR compared to an animal with a higher ECF $[HCO_3^-]$. Many lizards, snakes, and crocodilians, for example, have low $[HCO_3^-]$ compared to turtles. In the examples cited in Table IV, the alligator's $[HCO_3^-]$ was about 15 mEq/liter, the lizard's, *Sauromalus obesus,* was about 14 mEq/liter, while the turtle's, *Pseudemys scripta,* was about 33 mEq/liter. In the case of these animals, however, the ACR values were not significantly different because of the relatively low pH values of the alligator and the lizard. The lizards *I. iguana* and *Lacerta,* did show high ACR values and, although $[HCO_3^-]$ was not measured, it can be assumed to be much less than in the turtle.

The particular ECF $[HCO_3^-]$ of an ectotherm may be an important constraint on the useful temperature range of the animal. Conversely, the preferred or eccritic temperature range of a particular animal may be a factor influencing the animal's $[HCO_3^-]$ or strong ion difference. My reason for suggesting this is that the $[HCO_3^-]$, in effect, dictates what the P_{CO_2} (and therefore the ACR) must be in order to achieve the proper pH. The factor which severely limits this whole regulatory scheme is the supply of O_2. The ACR can only decrease so far in the interests of acid–base regulation before O_2 supply is impaired. It is therefore to the advantage of an animal with a high eccritic temperature to have a low $[HCO_3^-]$ so that the proper pH at high temperature can be achieved with a low P_{CO_2} and thus a high enough ACR can exist to ensure adequate O_2 supply. On the other hand, a higher $[HCO_3^-]$ would benefit the animal preferring a low-temperature range. It is important to emphasize that these are speculations which lack experimental evidence.

There is evidence for the impairment of O_2 supply at high temperature, however. Calculation of the O_2 extraction coefficient (E) from the ventilation data obtained on *P. scripta* showed that it decreased progressively from about 6% at 10°C to nearly 50% at 35°C (Jackson, 1971). Extrapolation of this relationship to higher temperatures revealed that 100% extraction of inspired O_2 would be required at 42°C to satisfy acid–base requirements, which is clearly an impossibility. The upper lethal temperature of this species is in the range of 40°–42°C (Hutchison *et al.,* 1966). We have studied this turtle at temperatures between 35° and 40°C and found that the ACR increases in this range and metabolic acidosis develops (J. C. Allen and D. C. Jackson, unpublished observations). We believe this result is consistent with a breakdown of the pH–temperature control system because of inadequate O_2 supply.

We may now return to a consideration of the turtle's enhanced respiratory response to hypoxic gas mixtures at increased temperature. Why was the turtle more sensitive at 30°C than at 10°C? One important factor concerns the normal ventilation of the turtle breathing air. At 10°C, the turtle has a high ACR and is, in effect, hyperventilating. This should result in a high $P_{A_{O_2}}$ which, together with high hemoglobin affinity for O_2 and low metabolic need, should make the turtle rather insensitive to large decreases in $P_{I_{O_2}}$, as indeed it was (see Fig. 9). At 30°C, however, the ACR is much lower (relative hypoventilation), hemoglobin affinity is less, and O_2 demand is up; thus, there should be greater vulnerability to hypoxia. Two major questions remain unanswered concerning hypoxic sensitivity in the turtle: first, where are the receptors mediating this response, and second, is there a temperature-dependent difference in O_2 sensitivity at the receptor level?

From this discussion, we see that the respiratory control of the turtle, *P. scripta*, is linked primarily to its acid–base homeostasis over its normal temperature range of 10°–35°C. The ACR decreases as the turtle moves up in temperature in order to effect the appropriate decrease in pH (and to preserve a constant α-imidazole). Throughout this range, O_2 requirements are satisfied. Above 35°C, however, further decreases in the ACR (in the interests of acid–base balance) can no longer be tolerated because O_2 supply is compromised. Thus the ACR stops decreasing, and even increases, to prevent hypoxemia.

In this regard, it is of interest now to consider those reptiles which fail to conform to the general pattern of pH control at different temperatures (see Table IV). The most notable examples are the varanid lizards, *Varanus gouldii* (Bennett, 1973b) and *Varanus exanthematicus* (Wood et al., 1977). Within their normal temperature range (25°–35°C), these animals maintained a relatively constant arterial pH, and ACR either remained unchanged (*V. exanthematicus*) or increased (*V. gouldii*). The varanid lizards are highly aerobic reptiles with cardiopulmonary systems that are mammallike in many respects (Millard and Johansen, 1974). The implication is that the respiratory control of these active lizards is governed by their high O_2 requirements, and that they cannot afford to adhere to the acid–base regulation of other ectotherms. It is of interest here to recall that rainbow trout (Randall and Cameron, 1973) were also considered unable to adhere to the pH–temperature curve by ventilatory means, but they followed it nonetheless by an ionic regulatory adjustment which lowered blood CO_2 concentration as temperature rose. In contrast, Wood et al. (1977) reported that *V. exanthematicus* raised its plasma $[HCO_3^-]$ between 20° and 35°C. Arterial pH remained constant over this range at about 7.55, for Pa_{CO_2} rose somewhat with temperature (Fig. 13). These lizards, therefore, seem to be defending a constant absolute blood pH

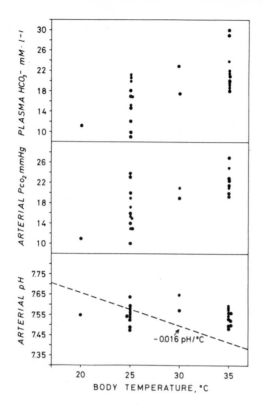

Figure 13. Acid–base variables of monitor lizards, *Varanus exanthematicus*, at different body temperatures. Note the constancy of blood pH in contrast to other ectothermic vertebrates (dashed line). (From Wood *et al.*, 1977.)

value across this temperature range, a form of control which runs counter to the general pattern that has been discussed in this chapter.

3. *Skin Breathers*

Although all vertebrates exchange some respiratory gas through their integuments, this avenue of exchange is most significant and important among the amphibians, where it reaches its zenith in the plethodonts, or lungless salamanders, which lack gills and lungs. Other amphibians rely to varying degrees on cutaneous respiration, although it is usually of greatest importance in smaller individuals (Ultsch, 1976) and in cool environments (Hutchison *et al.*, 1968; Whitford and Hutchison, 1965). Furthermore, in amphibians which respire through both the skin and lungs, the skin is invariably a more important site for CO_2 loss than it is for O_2 uptake

(Krogh, 1941). Hence, even in bimodal breathers, which have an important pulmonary component to their gas exchange, the skin represents a potentially important site for control of CO_2 loss and, therefore, of acid–base balance. The only studies available on the relationship between acid–base balances and gas exchange have been carried out on such bimodal breathers, and we can only speculate from these results about the exclusively skin-breathing forms.

Blood measurements at different temperatures have been made on the anurans *Bufo marinus* (Howell *et al.,* 1970) and *Rana catesbeiana* (Howell *et al.,* 1970; Reeves, 1972; Jackson and Mackenzie, 1977). Both animals displayed the usual decrease of pH and increase of P_{CO_2} with temperature as well as the constancy of plasma CO_2 concentration. Hence, they resemble typical air-breathing ectotherms, but because lung ventilation is an important exchange mode in each species, this is not surprising.

We have recently investigated the skin O_2 exchange of *Rana catesbeiana* at different temperatures in order to determine whether or not the skin conductance is altered by temperature. Skin CO_2 conductance (G_{CO_2}) is defined as follows:

$$G_{CO_2} = \frac{\dot{M}_{S_{CO_2}}}{\Delta P_{CO_2}} \qquad (3)$$

where $\dot{M}_{S_{CO_2}}$ is the net CO_2 flux across the skin and ΔP_{CO_2} is the transcutaneous P_{CO_2} difference. As discussed earlier in this chapter, we found in other investigations of this species that isothermal skin CO_2 exchange is a largely passive, poorly controlled process. Our results in the temperature study were similar: Skin CO_2 conductance was not significantly different at $10°$, $20°$, and $30°C$, and the increased CO_2 loss through the skin which we observed as temperature was increased could be attributed to the rise in arterial P_{CO_2} (Fig. 14). This result may seem surprising in view of the fact that the metabolic rate of the frog increased more than fourfold over this temperature range and cutaneous blood flow would be expected to rise as well. This suggests that cutaneous CO_2 conductance may be insensitive in increases in perfusion. This same conclusion was also reached by Piiper *et al.* (1976) on the basis of their study of inert gas kinetics in the lungless salamander, *Desmognathus fuscus.*

Because the bullfrog has effective respiratory control via its pulmonary system, the absence of effective control over its cutaneous exchange has little effect on its acid–base homeostasis, either at a single temperature, or across a range of temperatures. However, what about an amphibian which respires exclusively through its integument? Our data suggest that, at constant temperature, the internal P_{CO_2} of such an animal would vary directly with the metabolic CO_2 production. A constant skin conductance,

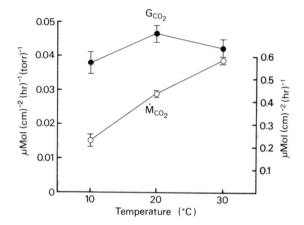

Figure 14. Skin CO_2 conductance and skin CO_2 loss in bullfrogs, *Rana catesbeiana*, at different temperatures. (From Jackson and Mackenzie, 1977.)

therefore, would pose problems for acid–base control at constant temperature. But it may be a valuable adaptation for adjusting acid–base control to a change in body temperature. Consider an increase in body temperature of 10°C in a hypothetical amphibian which breathes exclusively through its skin. The increase in temperature will have two immediate effects on the basic chemical processes of the animal: (a) It will accelerate the rates of reactions and thereby increase the animal's metabolic rate (CO_2 production) by about twofold; and (b) It will alter the chemical equilibria of the body fluids. resulting in a fall in pH of about 0.16 units and a rise in P_{CO_2}. If the new P_{CO_2} is about twice the original P_{CO_2} and the skin conductance is unchanged, then the transcutaneous P_{CO_2} difference will be precisely what is required to excrete the metabolically produced CO_2 and maintain pH with no active physiological adjustment required. If P_{CO_2} does not rise that much, which is probable, then some adjustment in conductance would be required, perhaps by altering convection at the skin surface (Guimond and Hutchison, 1973b). This mechanism would have the further advantage of being a rapid adjustment requiring little or no acclimation time, just as with the adjustment of air breathers (Jackson and Kagen, 1976). To test this model, it will be necessary to measure cutaneous gas exchange and transcutaneous gas pressure differences in a strictly skin-breathing amphibian at various temperatures. As mentioned earlier, this will be difficult technically on the small plethodonts, but the large hellbender, *Cryptobranchus alleghaniensis*, should be an ideal animal for such a study.

V. CONCLUSIONS

What emerges from this discussion is the sense that the basic respiratory control mechanism of the air-breathing ectotherms is not particularly different from the mechanism of mammals. But there are striking differences of detail, and it is these differences that attract our attention to these animals. Because of the diversity of adaptations, there is great diversity in the expression of the basic respiratory pattern. In this chapter particular emphasis has been placed on the adaptation to temperature, because this is what, above all, sets the ectotherms apart from the endotherms. From this we learn that acid–base control occurs along a temperature continuum and that we mammals are specialists residing within a narrow band on the continuum. What we have long regarded as the prime regulated variables of the respiratory control system, [H$^+$] and P_{CO_2}, are revealed by the study of ectotherms to be of secondary importance to some more basic homeostatic variable, such as protein ionization. These specialized adaptations of the ectotherms, to temperature and to other environmental stresses, provide us with valuable experimental models and tools not only for understanding and appreciating how such physiological systems can adapt, but affording insights into mammalian control as well.

ACKNOWLEDGMENT

The support of NSF Grant PCM76-24443 during the writing of this manuscript is gratefully acknowledged.

REFERENCES

Adams, W. E. (1958). "The Comparative Morphology of the Carotid Body and Carotid Sinus," pp. 194–197. Thomas, Springfield, Illinois.

Albery, W. J., and B. B. Lloyd (1967). Variation of chemical potential with temperature. *In* "Development of the Lung" (A. V. A. de Reuck and R. Porter, eds.), pp. 30–33. Churchill, London.

Austin, J. H., F. W. Sunderman, and J. G. Camack (1927). Studies in serum electrolytes. The electrolyte composition and the pH of serum of a poikilothermous animal at different temperatures. *J. Biol. Chem.* **72,** 677–685.

Banzett, R. B., and R. E. Burger (1977). Response of avian intrapulmonary chemoreceptors to venous CO_2 and ventilatory gas flow. *Respir. Physiol.* **29,** 63–72.

Belkin, D. A. (1962). Anaerobiosis in diving turtles. *Physiologist* **5,** 105.

Belkin, D. A. (1963). Anoxia: Tolerance in reptiles. *Science* **139,** 492–493.

Belkin, D. A. (1964). Variations in heart rate during voluntary diving in the turtle, *Pseudemys concinna. Copeia* pp. 321–330.

Belkin, D. A. (1965). Critical oxygen tensions in turtles. *Physiologist* **8**, 109.

Bennett, A. F. (1972). The effect of activity on oxygen consumption, oxygen debt, and heart rate in the lizards *Varanus gouldii* and *Sauromalus hispidus. J. Comp. Physiol.* **79**, 259–280.

Bennett, A. F. (1973a). Ventilation in two species of lizards during rest and activity. *Comp. Biochem. Physiol. A* **46**, 653–671.

Bennett, A. F. (1973b). Blood physiology and oxygen transport during activity in two lizards, *Varanus gouldii* and *Sauromalus hispidus. Comp. Biochem. Physiol. A* **46**, 673–690.

Bennett, A. F., and W. R. Dawson (1976). Metabolism. *Biol. Reptilia* **5**, pp. 127–223.

Berkson, H. (1966). Physiological adjustments to prolonged diving in the Pacific green turtle *(Chelonia mydas agassizii). Comp. Biochem. Physiol.* **18**, 101–119.

Boelaert, R. (1941). Sur la physiologie de la respiration des Lacertiens. *Arch. Intern. Physiol.* **51**, 379–437.

Bouverot, P., and L. -M. Leitner (1972). Arterial chemoreceptors in the domestic fowl. *Respir. Physiol.* **15**, 310–320.

Boyer, D. R. (1966). Comparative effects of hypoxia on respiratory and cardiac function in reptiles. *Physiol. Zool.* **39**, 307–316.

Brattstrom, B. H. (1970). Amphibia. *Comp. Physiol. Thermoregul.* **1**, 135–166.

Bretz, W. L., and K. Schmidt-Nielsen (1971). Bird respiration: Flow patterns in the duck lung. *J. Exp. Biol.* **54**, 103–118.

Burri, P. H., and E. R. Weibel (1971). Morphometric estimation of pulmonary diffusion capacity. II. Effect of P_{O_2} on the growing lung. Adaptation of the growing rat lung to hypoxia and hyperoxia. *Respir. Physiol.* **11**, 247–264.

Chance, B. (1957). Cellular oxygen requirements. *Fed. Proc., Fed. Am. Soc. Exp. Biol.* **16**, 671–680.

Colacino, J. M., D. H. Hector, and K. Schmidt-Nielsen (1977). Respiratory responses of ducks to simulated altitude. *Respir. Physiol.* **29**, 265–281.

Crawford, E. C., Jr., and R. N. Gatz (1974). Carbon dioxide tension and pH of the blood of the lizard *Sauromalus obesus* at different temperatures. *Comp. Biochem. Physiol. A* **47**, 529–534.

Davies, D. G. (1975. The effect of temperature on ventilation and gas exchange in the American alligator. *Fed. Proc., Fed. Am. Soc. Exp. Biol.* **34**, 431.

Davies, D. G., and M. T. Kopetzky (1976). Effect of body temperature on the ventilatory response to hypercapnia in the awake alligator. *Fed. Proc., Fed. Am. Soc. Exp. Biol.* **35**, 840.

Davis, B. D. (1958). On the importance of being ionized. *Arch. Biochem. Biophys.* **78**, 497–509.

Dejours, P. (1973). Problems of control of breathing in fishes. *In* "Comparative Physiology, Locomotion, Respiration, Transport and Blood" (L. Bolis, K. Schmidt-Nielsen and S. H. P. Maddrell, eds.), pp. 117–133, North-Holland Publ., Amsterdam.

Dejours, P. (1975). "Principles of Comparative Respiratory Physiology." North-Holland Publ., Amsterdam.

Dejours, P., W. F. Garey, and H. Rahn (1970). Comparison of ventilatory and circulatory flow rates between animals in various physiological conditions. *Respir. Physiol.* **9**, 108–117.

Fedde, M. R., and D. F. Peterson (1970). Intrapulmonary receptor response to changes in airway-gas composition in *Gallus domesticus. J. Physiol. (London)* **209**, 609–625.

Fedde, M. R., W. D. Kuhlmann, and P. Scheid (1977). Intrapulmonary receptors in the tegu lizard. I. Sensitivity to CO_2. *Respir. Physiol.* **29**, 35–48.

Frankel, H. M., A. Spitzer, J. Blaine, and E. P. Schoener (1969). Respiratory response of turtles *(Pseudemys scripta)* to changes in arterial blood gas composition. *Comp. Biochem. Physiol.* **31**, 535–546.

Gatten, R. E., Jr. (1974). Effects of temperature and activity on aerobic and anaerobic metabolism and heart rate in the turtles *Pseudemys scripta* and *Terrapene ornata*. *Comp. Biochem. Physiol. A* **48**, 610–648.

Gatz, R. N., M. R. Fedde, and E. C. Crawford, Jr. (1975). Lizard lungs: CO_2-sensitive receptors in *Tupinambis nigropunctatus*. *Experientia* **31**, 455–456.

Giordano, R. V., and D. C. Jackson (1973). The effect of temperature on ventilation in the green iguana *(Iguana iguana)*. *Comp. Biochem. Physiol. A* **45**, 235–238.

Gottlieb, G., and D. C. Jackson (1976). Importance of pulmonary ventilation in respiratory control in the bullfrog. *Am. J. Physiol.* **230**, 608–613.

Guimond, R. W., and V. H. Hutchison (1972). Pulmonary, branchial and cutaneous gas exchange in the mud puppy, *Necturus maculosus maculosus (Rafinesque)*. *Comp. Biochem. Physiol. A* **42**, 367–392.

Guimond, R. W., and V. H. Hutchison (1973a). Trimodal gas exchange in the large aquatic salamander, *Siren lacertina (Linnaeus)*. *Comp. Biochem. Physiol. A* **46**, 249–268.

Guimond, R. W., and V. H. Hutchison (1973b). Aquatic respiration: An unusual strategy in the hellbender *Cryptobranchus alleganiensis alleganiensis (Daudin)*. *Science* **182**, 1263–1265.

Hayward, J. S. (1966). Abnormal concentrations of respiratory gases in rabbit burrows. *J. Mammal.* **47**, 723–724.

Hitzig, B. M. (1977). Control of ventilation by central respiratory chemosensors in the unanesthetized turtle, *Pseudemys scripta elegans*. Ph.D. dissertation, Brown University, Providence, Rhode Island.

Hock, R. J. (1964). Animals in high altitudes: Reptiles and amphibians. *Hand. Physiol. Sect. 4: Adapt. Environ.* pp. 841–842.

Howell, B. J., and H. Rahn (1976). Regulation of acid–base balance in reptiles. *Biol. Reptilia.* **5**, 335–363.

Howell, B. J., F. W. Baumgardner, K. Bondi, and H. Rahn (1970). Acid–base balance in cold-blooded vertebrates as a function of body temperature. *Am. J. Physiol.* **218**, 600–606.

Hurtado, A. (1964). Animals in high altitudes: Resident man. *Hand. Physiol. Sect. 4: Adapt. Environ.* pp. 843–860.

Hutchison, V. H., A. Vinegar, and R. J. Kosh (1966). Critical thermal maxima in turtles. *Herpetologica* **22**, 32–41.

Hutchison, V. H., W. G. Whitford, and M. Kohl (1968). Relation of body size and surface area to gas exchange in anurans. *Physiol. Zool.* **41**, 65–85.

Jackson, D. C. (1968). Metabolic depression and oxygen depletion in the diving turtle. *J. Appl. Physiol.* **24**, 503–509.

Jackson, D. C. (1971). The effect of temperature on ventilation in the turtle, *Pseudemys scripta elegans*. *Respir. Physiol.* **12**, 131–140.

Jackson, D. C. (1973). Ventilatory response to hypoxia in turtles at various temperatures. *Respir. Physiol.* **18**, 178–187.

Jackson, D. C., and R. D. Kagen (1976). Effects of temperature transients on gas exchange and acid–base status of turtles. *Am. J. Physiol.* **230**, 1389–1393.

Jackson, D. C., and J. A. Mackenzie (1977). Control of CO_2 exchange in a bimodal breather *(Rana catesbeiana)* at different temperatures. *Proc. Int. Union Physiol. Sci.* **13**, 350.

Jackson, D. C., and H. D. Prange (1977). Respiratory response to inspired CO_2 in the green turtle, *Chelonia mydas*. *Fed. Proc., Fed. Am. Soc. Exp. Biol.* **36**, 478.

Jackson, D. C., and H. Silverblatt (1974). Respiration and acid–base status of turtles following experimental dives. *Am. J. Physiol.* **226**, 903–909.

Jackson, D. C., S. E. Palmer, and W. L. Meadow (1974). The effects of temperature and carbon dioxide breathing on ventilation and acid–base status of turtles. *Respir. Physiol.* **20**, 131–146.

Johansen, K. (1970). Air breathing in fishes. *Fish Physiol.* **4**, 361–411.

Johansen, K., C. Lenfant, and G. C. Grigg (1967). Respiratory control in the lungfish, *Neoceratodus forsteri (Krefft)*. *Comp. Biochem. Physiol.* **20**, 835–854.

Johansen, K., D. Hanson, and C. Lenfant (1970). Respiration in a primitive air breather, *Amia calva*. *Respir. Physiol.* **9**, 162–174.

Jones, D. R., and M. J. Purves (1970). The effect of carotid body denervation upon the respiratory response to hypoxia and hypercapnia in the duck. *J. Physiol. (London)* **211**, 295–309.

Kay, F. R. (1977). Environmental physiology of the banner-tailed kangaroo rat. II. Influences of the burrow environment on metabolism and water loss. *Comp. Biochem. Physiol. A* **57**, 471–477.

Krogh, A. (1941). "The Comparative Physiology of Respiratory Mechanisms," pp. 13–15. Univ. of Pennsylvania Press, Philadelphia.

Lenfant, C., K. Johansen, J. A. Petersen, and K. Schmidt-Nielsen (1970). Respiration in the fresh water turtle, *Chelys fimbriata*. *Respir. Physiol.* **8**, 261–275.

McCutcheon, F. H. (1943). The respiratory mechanism in turtles. *Physiol. Zool.* **16**, 255–269.

Malan, A., R. L. Wilson, and R. B. Reeves (1976). Intracellular pH in cold-blooded vertebrates as a function of body temperature. *Respir. Physiol.* **28**, 29–47.

Millard, R. W., and K. Johansen (1974). Ventricular outflow dynamics in the lizard, *Varanus niloticus:* Responses to hypoxia, hypercarbia and diving. *J. Exp. Biol.* **60**, 871–880.

Millen, J. E., H. V. Murdaugh, Jr., C. B. Bauer, and E. D. Robin (1964). Circulatory adaptation to diving in the freshwater turtle. *Science* **145**, 591–593.

Milsom, W. K., and D. R. Jones (1975). Inhibition by CO_2 of respiratory related, vagal discharge in turtles. *Physiologist* **18**, 322.

Moberly, W. R. (1968a). The metabolic responses of the common iguana, *Iguana iguana*, to activity under restraint. *Comp. Biochem. Physiol.* **27**, 1–20.

Moberly, W. R. (1968b). The metabolic responses of the common iguana, *Iguana iguana*, to walking and diving. *Comp. Biochem. Physiol.* **27**, 21–32.

Nielsen, B. (1961). On the regulation of the respiration in reptiles. I. The effect of temperature and CO_2 on the respiration of lizards *(Lacerta)*. *J. Exp. Biol.* **38**, 301–314.

Nielsen, B. (1962). On the regulation of respiration in reptiles. II. The effect of hypoxia with and without moderate hypercapnia on the respiration and metabolism of lizards. *J. Exp. Biol.* **39**, 107–117.

Ou, L. C., and S. M. Tenney (1970). Properties of mitochondria from hearts of cattle acclimatized to high altitude. *Respir. Physiol.* **8**, 151–159.

Pappenheimer, J. R., V. Fencl, S. R. Heisey, and D. Held (1965). Role of cerebral fluids in control of respiration as studied in unanesthetized goats. *Am. J. Physiol.* **208**, 436–450.

Piiper, J., R. N. Gatz, and E. C. Crawford, Jr. (1975). Gas transport characteristics in an exclusively skin-breathing salamander, *Desmognathus fuscus (Plethodontidae)*. *In* "Respiration of Amphibious Vertebrates" (G. M. Hughes, ed.), 339–356. Academic Press, New York.

Prange, H. D. (1976). Energetics of swimming of a sea turtle. *J. Exp. Biol.* **64**, 1–12.

Prange, H. D., and D. C. Jackson (1976). Ventilation, gas exchange and metabolic scaling of a sea turtle. *Respir. Physiol.* **27**, 369–377.

Prosser, C. L. (1973). Oxygen: Respiration and metabolism. *In* "Comparative Animal Physiology" (C. L. Prosser, ed.), pp. 165–211. Saunders, Philadelphia.

130   Donald C. Jackson

Rahn, H. (1966). Gas transport from the external environment to the cell. *In* "Development of the Lung" (A. V. S. de Reuck and R. Porter, eds.), pp. 3–23. Churchill, London.

Rahn, H. (1976). Why are pH of 7.4 and P_{CO_2} of 40 normal values for man? *Bull. Eur. Physiopath. Respir.* **12**, 5–13.

Rahn, H., and F. W. Baumgardner (1972). Temperature and acid–base regulation in fish. *Respir. Physiol.* **14**, 171–182.

Rahn, H., and W. F. Garey (1973). Arterial CO_2, O_2, pH, and HCO_3^- values of ectotherms living in the Amazon. *Am. J. Physiol.* **225**, 735–738.

Rahn, H., R. B. Reeves, and B. J. Howell (1975). Hydrogen ion regulation, temperature, and evolution. *Am. Rev. Respir. Dis.* **112**, 165–172.

Randall, D. J., and J. N. Cameron (1973). Respiratory control of arterial pH as temperature changes in rainbow trout *Salmo gairdneri. Am. J. Physiol.* **225**, 997–1002.

Reeves, R. B. (1972). An imidazole alphastat hypothesis for vertebrate acid–base regulation: Tissue carbon dioxide content and body temperature in bullfrogs. *Respir. Physiol.* **14**, 219–236.

Reeves, R. B. (1976a). Temperature-induced changes in blood acid–base status: pH and P_{CO_2} in a binary buffer. *J. Appl. Physiol.* **40**, 752–761.

Reeves, R. B. (1976b). Temperature-induced changes in blood acid–base status: Donnan r_{Cl} and red cell volume. *J. Appl. Physiol.* **40**, 762–767.

Reeves, R. B. (1977). The interaction of body temperature and acid–base balance in ectothermic vertebrates. *Annu. Rev. Physiol.* **39**, 559–586.

Robin, E. D. (1962). Relationship between temperature and plasma pH and carbon dioxide tension in the turtle. *Nature, (London)* **195**, 249–251.

Robin, E. D., J. W. Vester, H. V. Murdaugh, Jr., and J. E. Millen (1964). Prolonged anaerobiosis in a vertebrate: Anaerobic metabolism in the freshwater turtle. *J. Cell. Comp. Physiol.* **63**, 287–297.

Scheid, P., and J. Piiper (1972). Cross-current gas exchange in avian lungs: Effects of reversed parabronchial air flow in ducks. *Respir. Physiol.* **16**, 304–312.

Scheid, P., W. D. Kuhlmann, and M. R. Fedde (1977). Intrapulmonary receptors in the tegu lizard. II. Functional characteristics and localization. *Respir. Physiol.* **29**, 49–62.

Shelton, G. (1970). The regulation of breathing. *Fish Physiol.* **4**, 293–359.

Smyth, D. H. (1939). The central and reflex control of respiration in the frog. *J. Physiol. (London)* **95**, 305–327.

Steen, J. B. (1971). "Comparative Physiology of Respiratory Mechanisms," pp. 56–75. Academic Press, New York.

Templeton, J. R. (1970). Reptiles. *Comp. Physiol. Thermoregul.* **1**, 167–221.

Templeton, J. R., and W. R. Dawson (1963). Respiration in the lizard *Crotaphytus collaris. Physiol. Zool.* **36**, 104–121.

Tucker, V. A. (1968). Respiratory physiology of house sparrows in relation to high-altitude flight. *J. Exp. Biol.* **48**, 55–66.

Ultsch, G. R. (1976). Respiratory surface area as a factor controlling the standard rate of O_2 consumption of aquatic salamanders. *Respir. Physiol.* **26**, 357–369.

White, F. N. (1976). Circulation. *Biol. Reptilia* **5**, 275–334.

White, F. N., and J. Kinney (1976). Ventilation–perfusion relationships in the turtle. *Physiologist* **19**, 409.

Whitford, W. G., and V. H. Hutchison (1965). Gas exchange in salamanders. *Physiol. Zool.* **38**, 228–242.

Wood, S. C., M. L. Glass, and K. Johansen (1977). Effects of temperature on respiration and acid–base balance in a monitor lizard, *J. Comp. Physiol.* **116**, 287–296.

CHAPTER 5

Breathing during Sleep

JOHN OREM

I. INTRODUCTION

The influence of sleep on breathing is demonstrated by the occurrence of posthyperventilation apnea. Fink *et al.* (1963) noted that *awake* human subjects rendered hypocapnic by overventilation continue to breathe rhythmically with a minute-volume one-half to two-thirds of normal. This reduced ventilation remains unchanged in the presence of a recovering $P_{A_{CO_2}}$ until the latter rises above the CO_2 response threshold. However, if the subject falls asleep while the $P_{A_{CO_2}}$ is below threshold, he becomes apneic. Fink and colleagues concluded: "The stimulus for the persistent rhythmic respiration is evidently not CO_2 and it has been provisionally designated the wakefulness stimulus."

In bulbar poliomyelitis, periods of hypoventilation during sleep can precede impaired waking respiration and can persist for some months after subsidence of waking symptoms (Plum and Swanson, 1958). Severinghaus and Mitchell (1962) described three patients who became apneic following surgery involving the brainstem or the high cervical cord. Postoperatively, these patients required artificial respiration when

131

Regulation of Ventilation and Gas Exchange
Copyright © 1978 by Academic Press, Inc.
All rights of reproduction in any form reserved.
ISBN 0-12-204650-1

asleep and became apneic when "sleep" was induced with nitrous oxide or with a barbiturate. Animal experiments have also demonstrated that lesions which are asymptomatic in wakefulness may result in respiratory difficulties during sleep. St. John et al. (1972) lesioned the region of the superior cerebellar peduncle, medial parabrachial nucleus, and dorsolateral portions of the reticular formation (pneumotaxic center). Initially, these lesions produced a transient decrease in respiratory rate, but when the animals were anesthetized and vagotomized (after a 1- to 3-month interim), two died and all displayed apneusis. After recovery from anesthesia, the animals displayed inspiratory duration times comparable to those of controls; however, 24 hours after vagotomy the animals were again anesthetized, and all demonstrated apneusis. Hugelin and Bertrand (1973) have shown that sleep has an effect similar to that of anesthesia. These authors observed a progressive recovery from apneusis in unanesthetized, acute preparations after pneumotaxic lesions, but the apneustic tendency reappeared when the electroencephalogram (EEG) showed signs of spontaneous sleep.

There are other cases of sleep-related respiratory failure in neurologically normal awake humans. Gastaut et al. (1965, 1966) described hypoventilation during sleep in obese patients with hypersomnolence (the Pickwickian syndrome) and distinguished this from respiratory insufficiencies which lead to somnolence through CO_2 anesthesia. Their patients dozed off at a time when oxyhemoglobin saturation and alveolar CO_2 concentrations were normal. Since Gastaut's original description, sleep apnea syndromes, possibly including the Sudden Infant Death syndrome (SIDS), have become widely recognized and dramatize the state dependence of respiration (Guilleminault and Dement, 1974; Weitzman and Graziani, 1974; Guilleminault et al., 1974, 1976a,b). The clinical literature on the sleep apnea syndromes is expanding rapidly. Interested readers are referred to reviews by Guilleminault and Dement (1974), Weitzman and Graziani (1974) and Guilleminault et al. (1976b).

Three types of sleep apnea have been distinguished: (a) a diaphragmatic apnea in which the diaphragm may be inactive for up to 3 minutes; (b) an obstructive, upper airway apnea in which persistent diaphragmatic movements fail to achieve ventilation because of an anatomical and/or functional obstruction in the upper airway; and (c) a mixed apnea consisting of short diaphragmatic apneas followed by prolonged obstructive apneas. Obstructive apneas, generally appearing as mixed apneas, represent the most common clinical apneas. These patients may be, but are not necessarily, obese; are predominantly males with a sleep complaint (insomnia or hypersomnia); and are heavy snorers (Lugaresi et al., 1975). The patients are unaware of their apneic episodes (numbering in some cases several hundred per night) which lead to life-threatening pulmonary hypertension and cardiac irregularities (Guilleminault *et al.*, 1976b).

It has been suggested that prolonged sleep apnea may be responsible for some cases of SIDS (Steinschneider, 1972; Guilleminault *et al.*, 1973). Bergman *et al.* (1972) and others (see Weitzman and Graziani, 1974) have noted that essentially every SIDS case was discovered lifeless either when a parent awakened in the morning or at the end of naptime in the afternoon. Steinschneider (1972) studied near-miss cases in which the infant was found not breathing and cyanotic but was able to be revived. These potential SIDS children revealed frequent periods of prolonged apnea during sleep which required resuscitative efforts (see also Guilleminault *et al.*, 1975). Shannon and Kelly (1977) have recently reported that infants who subsequently died of the SIDS showed alveolar hypoventilation during nonrapid eye movement (NREM) sleep and abnormal ventilatory responses to CO_2.

In short, the clinical mandates for the study of breathing during sleep are impressive. Beyond this, the study of respiration during sleep and wakefulness offers the realization that breathing changes result from changing central programs. There have been many studies designed to understand the respiratory system, for example, by eliciting reflex responses to lung inflations and different breathed gases. These responses are of some interest, but the relationships they describe may not pertain to variations in respiration which derive from changes in central programs. For example, in normal breathing during sleep and wakefulness, breath-by-breath tidal volume vs. frequency (V_T–f) plots are distributed crossways to the Hering–Breuer curve (Priban, 1963; Newsom Davis and Stagg, 1975; Orem *et al.*, 1977a). Similarly, variations in V_T and f across states do not fall along the Hering–Breuer curve; rather, the V_T–f configurations in wakefulness (W), NREM, and REM are unique in each state (Orem *et al.*, 1977a).

II. DEFINITION OF SLEEP AND WAKEFULNESS

An entertaining and informative presentation of the phenomenology of sleep can be found in Dement (1972). Sleep researchers recognize three distinct *states* of consciousness: wakefulness; nonrapid eye movement (NREM) sleep, which is sometimes called slow wave sleep, quiet sleep, or synchronized sleep; and rapid eye movement (REM) sleep, which is sometimes named active sleep, paradoxical sleep, or desynchronized sleep. Thirty years ago sleep was considered a homogeneous state. We now know that REM sleep is as different from NREM sleep as it is from wakefulness. There is an early literature on breathing during sleep (see Kleitman, 1963, for a review) which will not be considered because of the confusion of breathing during NREM with breathing during REM.

Human sleep and wakefulness are defined by certain polygraphic criteria which are specified in Rechtschaffen and Kales (1968). NREM sleep is divided into four stages, numbered 1 through 4, according to the state of eye movements and the EEG. Stages 1 and 2 of NREM are considered light sleep, while stages 3 and 4 are deep NREM sleep. There has not been any generally accepted division of NREM sleep into well-defined stages in animals. REM sleep is not divided into stages, but sleep researchers make distinctions between the *tonic* and *phasic* events of REM. The tonic events are those which define the state by their continuous occurrence; phasic events occur episodically throughout the state.

In the laboratory, three criteria are used to define sleep and wakefulness. These are: (a) eye movements or the electrooculogram (EOG), measured by placing surface electrodes at the lateral canthi (the corneoretinal potential acts as a dipole so that rotation of the globes can be detected as a change in potential); (b) the electroencephalogram (EEG), which in humans is generally obtained with surface electrodes placed at C3 and C4 (*The Ten Twenty Electrode System of the International Federation for Electroencephalography and Clinical Neurophysiology*, Jasper, 1958); and (c) the electromyogram (EMG) commonly obtained from submental areas. In animals, electrodes are often implanted chronically to obtain EEGs, EOGs, and EMGs.

NREM sleep is defined by the occurrence of: (a) slow rolling eye movements (light NREM sleep only); (b) varying degrees of slow, large amplitude activity in the EEG until, in deep NREM sleep (stages 3 and 4), the entire EEG consists of 20–50% of waves of 2 cps or slower which have amplitudes of greater than 75 μV peak to peak; and (c) the persistence of tonic EMG activity.

REM sleep is defined by: (a) episodic bursts of rapid eye movements; (b) a desynchronized EEG which is similar to the EEG of wakefulness; and (c) the absence of muscle tone. The desynchronized EEG and the absence of muscle tone are *tonic events* of REM sleep. The rapid eye movement bursts are *phasic events* and are usually accompanied by, for example, myoclonic twitches or episodes of irregular or ataxic breathing.

In animal research, NREM sleep is defined primarily by persisting muscle tone and a synchronized EEG together with the behavioral manifestations of sleep. In REM sleep, the EEG is desynchronized, muscle tone is lost, and rapid eye movements and other phasic events occur episodically. The physiological ubiquity of the states of sleep and wakefulness allows almost any measurable physiological phenomenon to serve as a basis for defining W, NREM, and REM; however, the EOG, EEG, and EMG have become conventional.

III.   A DESCRIPTION OF BREATHING DURING SLEEP

Although breathing is often described in terms of tidal and minute volumes, arterial P_{O_2} and P_{CO_2}, or the pH of the blood or cerebrospinal fluid, these parameters are consequences of (and determinants of) the output of the respiratory muscles. They describe the adequacy of the respiratory pump but fail to indicate the nature of the pumping action itself. Tidal volume is sometimes considered an elemental description of a breath, but from the point of view of the neural and muscular respiratory systems, inspiratory tidal volume is the product of influx of air at varying rates for a certain duration. Fundamentally, the neural and muscular respiratory systems produce influx and efflux of air through airways whose resistance varies under neural control. The influx of air varies as a function of the spatiotemporal interactions onto inspiratory motoneurons and the degree of dilation of the airways. Similarly, efflux is active or passive depending upon the state of the thoracic and abdominal expiratory muscles, and it is resisted or facilitated by the state of dilation of the airways. An understanding of the basis for qualitatively different patterns of influx and efflux of air during each state of sleep and wakefulness is complex.

Characteristics of Breathing during Sleep

1.   Inspiration

Figure 1 illustrates average breaths during sleep and wakefulness in the cat. These have been constructed primarily from the data of Orem et al. (1977a), in which thousands of breaths during W, NREM, and REM sleep were computer analyzed. The modeled breaths show flow rates on the vertical axis and time on the horizontal axis. They are equivalent to airflow tracings obtained with the pneumotachograph.

There are three limbs of the inspiratory curves in Fig. 1: first, from the onset of inspiration (time zero) to the average flow rate (V_T/T_I); second, plotted as a straight line from the point of average flow to the point of peak flow; and third, running from the level of peak flow to zero flow at T_I. Because Remmers et al. (1976) report that the diaphragmatic activation patterns and the slope of the average spirograms are similar during the different states, the slope of the first limb from time zero to the average

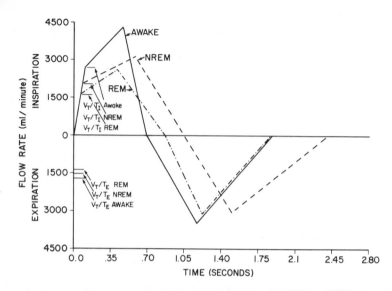

Figure 1. Average flow rate tracing during wakefulness, and NREM and REM sleep in the cat. See text for details.

flow rate is plotted as equivalent during wakefulness, NREM, and REM. These authors note that the mean inspiratory flow rate during REM was sometimes less than in W and NREM; however, they interpret the changes in breathing during sleep as arising primarily from changes in the inspiratory–expiratory phase transition. If this was clearly the case, and if diaphragmatic activation was linearly related to flow rate, a single function would have run from time zero to peak flow in Fig. 1. However, Orem *et al.* (1977a) have shown that there are systematic changes in peak flow during sleep and wakefulness. Peak flow was largest in wakefulness and least in REM, and appeared to derive from a secondary inspiratory effort similar to the sudden increase in inspiratory activity just prior to the termination of inspiration described by Clark and von Euler (1972) in anesthetized cats. Accordingly, the initial pattern of activation of the diaphragm may be similar during sleep and wakefulness, but there is controversy about the similarity of the diaphragmatic activation patterns throughout inspiration during different states.

Factor analysis was employed by Orem *et al.* (1977a) in obtaining correlation matrices of various breathing parameters. From this, a volume and frequency factor consistently emerged. Peak airflow rate was most highly correlated with the volume factor. There was a systematic positive relationship between peak flow and tidal volume within each state when computed on a breath-by-breath basis.

The reduction in peak flow from wakefulness to NREM and to REM (Fig. 1) may signal a diminishing respiratory drive. Peak flow rate would seem to be the isotonic equivalent of the negative pressure developed as the result of occlusion at functional residual capacity (Pomus of Grunstein *et al.*, 1973). A similar interpretation would result from the use of V_T/T_I as an indication of respiratory drive, as this ratio also declines systematically from wakefulness to REM.

The third limb of the inspiratory curve in Fig. 1 is shown as a straight line extending from peak flow to T_I. The time and value of peak flow and T_I were obtained from the data of Orem *et al.* (1977a). The monotonic drop from peak flow to end-inspiration conforms to the pattern generally produced in airflow tracings. The different slopes in sleep and wakefulness indicate that inspiratory efforts are more precipitously ended in wakefulness than sleep. Comparison of the last limb of the inspiratory curve across sleep and wakefulness also shows that T_I is shortest in wakefulness and longest in NREM. This is consistent with several reports of frequency changes across states (Remmers *et al.*, 1976; Phillipson *et al.*, 1976; Aserinsky, 1965; Jouvet *et al.*, 1960; Snyder *et al.*, 1964).

Tidal volume depends on the rate and duration of airflow. In W, airflow rates were high [as judged from peak flow (*Pf*) or V_T/T_I], but the duration was minimal. In NREM, airflow rates decreased, but the duration of the flow was sufficiently long to produce a mean tidal volume which was slightly greater than that during W. In REM, airflow rates were below NREM levels, and the duration was shorter. This combination of reduced airflow rates and short airflow durations in REM produced a tidal volume which was less than those during W and NREM. There is agreement that tidal volume is largest in NREM and smallest in REM in animals (Remmers *et al.*, 1976; Phillipson *et al.*, 1976; Orem *et al.*, 1977a), but there is controversy regarding changes in tidal volume during sleep in humans. Some authors argue that human sleep involves a reduction in tidal volume (Østergard, 1944; Magnussen, 1944; Birchfield *et al.*, 1958), but Duron (1972) reports that tidal volume is large in W, smaller in NREM, and large again in REM. Similarly, there are discrepancies in reported instantaneous minute-volume during sleep and wakefulness. Duron reports an increased minute-volume during NREM sleep, while other authors have reported a decrease (Østergaard, 1944; Magnussen, 1944; Birchfield *et al.*, 1958; Reed and Kellogg, 1958; Robin *et al.*, 1958). Orem *et al.* (1977a) found a decrease in average instantaneous minute-volume during sleep in the cat, with lowest values occurring in REM sleep. In contrast, Phillipson *et al.* (1976) in the dog and Hathorn (1974) and Bolton and Herman (1974) in the human neonate reported increased average instantaneous minute-volumes in REM sleep. The contradiction between these studies derives in part from the hypothetical nature of instantaneous minute-volume. When average minute-volume was calculated as the product of average tidal volume and average frequency (60/mean T_{tot}) in three of the seven cats of Orem et al. (1977a), minute-volume was larger in REM than in NREM, and in all cases, the difference between REM and NREM was smaller. However, the over-all average of the cats of Orem et al. (1977a) shows a minute-volume which is less in REM than in NREM. The average of the data of Phillipson et al. (1976), calculated in the same way, shows a minute-volume which is larger in REM. Actually, the only contradiction between the results of Orem et al. (1977a) and Phillipson et al. (1976) is over the degree of tidal volume and frequency changes during REM and NREM sleep. In the Phillipson study, frequencies were more than twice as high in REM as in NREM, and tidal volume declined only 16% in REM. In the Orem study, frequencies were 1.6 times higher in REM than in NREM, but tidal volume declined 30% in REM.

2. Expiration

In the modeled breaths of Fig. 1, only two limbs of the expiratory curve are depicted. The first limb extends from T_I to peak expiratory flow, the second from peak expiratory flow to T_{tot}. Both limbs are nearly parallel across states. This would be better seen if the limb from peak expiratory flow to T_{tot} in NREM included the expiratory pause which is commonly seen in that state. Although the average expiratory flow rates (V_T/T_E) are essentially similar across states, the order of average flow rates seen in inspiration can still be discriminated.

3. Duration of the Respiratory Cycle

There are minor discrepancies in the fractionation of T_{tot} into T_I and T_E (Orem et al., 1977a; Remmers et al., 1976; Phillipson et al., 1976), but there is general agreement that in animals, breathing rates are rapid in W and REM and slower in NREM. The increases and decreases in the rate of breathing during sleep–wakefulness coincide with elevations and declines in body temperature. In NREM there is a decreased hypothalamic and body temperature (von Euler and Söderberg, 1958; Parmeggiani et al., 1975), and in REM hypothalamic temperature increases to near wakeful-ness levels (Parmeggiani et al., 1975). Incremented frequencies of breath-ing in response to elevated body temperatures are well known (Hal-dane, 1905; Cotes, 1955; Cunningham and O'Riordan, 1957; Hey et al., 1966; von Euler et al., 1970; Bradley et al., 1974), and the changes in the rate of breathing during sleep–wakefulness may derive from changes in body temperature or from changes in central mechanisms common to breathing rate and body temperature.

Several studies have described V_T-f Hering–Breuer curves (Grunstein *et al.*, 1973; Bradley *et al.*, 1974; von Euler *et al.*, 1970; Hey *et al.*, 1966; Clark and von Euler, 1972). These curves show a positive relationship between V_T and f, which indicates a progressive decrease in the threshold of the inspiratory off-switch with time from the onset of inspiration. In an analysis of the relationship between V_T and f within and across states of consciousness, Orem *et al.* (1977a) found a consistent negative rather than a positive V_T-f correlation. The average product moment correlation coefficient between V_T and f across their cats in W was -0.47, in NREM the coefficient was -0.30, and in REM, -0.62. The effect of the negative relationship between f and V_T was a stabilization of minute-volume within each state. A similar relationship in conscious man was described earlier (Priban, 1963), and Bradley *et al.* (1974) have noted that with constant chemical drive the V_T-T_I relationship is mainly distributed in a direction crossways to the volume–threshold curve.

Orem *et al.* (1977a) also failed to obtain a consistent volume–threshold curve by varying chemical drive during sleep and wakefulness. They used a series of added dead spaces and observed ventilation during the sleep–wakefulness cycle. Frequency changes were small and variable until tidal volume increased 300–400% above eupneic values. With this amount of dead space, a reduction in the amplitude of the EEG and a suppression of EMG activity were seen, and there was no indication of sleep. Presumably, when there is a dramatic increase in frequency of breathing, with tidal volume at a maximum, the animals are near the point at which sleep is no longer possible.

Phillipson *et al.* (1976) and Remmers *et al.* (1976) have shown that vagotomy does not alter the frequency changes characteristic of W, NREM, and REM. Both groups have concluded that the frequency changes during sleep derive from central mechanisms rather than vagal reflexes.

IV. RESPIRATORY REFLEXES DURING SLEEP

There have been a number of studies designed to determine the CO_2 sensitivity of the sleeping respiratory system (Bülow, 1963; Magnussen, 1944; Reed and Kellogg, 1958; Robin *et al.*, 1958; Birchfield *et al.*, 1958; Bellville *et al.*, 1959). The majority of these have generated CO_2 response curves during NREM sleep and have found increased alveolar CO_2 concentrations compared to wakefulness and, at times, a reduced slope or a shift in the CO_2 response curve—all of which supposedly indicate a diminished sensitivity of the sleeping brain to CO_2. Recently, Phillipson *et al.* (1977) have demonstrated that, with hyperoxic hypercapnea during NREM, the animals (3 dogs) rebreathe for 0.99 ± 0.05 minutes before arousing with alveolar CO_2 tensions of 54.2 ± 3.4 mm Hg; while during REM, the same animals rebreathe 1.71 ± 0.24 minutes before arousing with alveolar CO_2 tensions of 60.3 ± 4.2 mm Hg. The data of these authors show that minute ventilation, tidal volume, frequency of breathing, V_T/T_I and T_I/T_{tot} when plotted as a function of alveolar CO_2 tension on a breath-by-breath basis during REM describe regressions which were less than those in NREM and which at times did not significantly differ from zero. Their conclusion that there is a marked loss of CO_2 sensitivity during REM sleep can be questioned for several reasons. No data are presented which allow a comparison of ventilation during REM and NREM at various intervals after the onset of rebreathing. Furthermore, the important comparison is between (a) the differences between NREM before and during rebreathing and (b) the differences between REM before and during rebreathing. The reason for this is that the patterns of breathing during these two states of sleep are qualitatively different. Tidal volume is smaller in REM than in NREM; frequency is normally higher and minute-ventilation is normally less in REM than in NREM (Orem *et al.*, 1977a). It is not a matter of how the REM rebreathing compares to NREM; rather, one should investigate how ventilation progresses during both NREM and REM from control to rebreathing and finally to arousal. The regression curves of Phillipson *et al.* (1977) begin with alveolar CO_2 values of 50 mm Hg for dogs 1 and 3 and 40 mm Hg for dog 2; and the levels of tidal volume and minute-volume, frequency of breathing and V_T/T_I at control alveolar CO_2 tensions are not given.

Orem *et al.* (1977a) studied the changes in peak flow, tidal volume, minute-volume, and frequency of breathing with added dead spaces. They did not measure CO_2 tensions. They found that, as in control breathing and regardless of the level of ventilatory demand created by the size of the dead space, frequency increased in REM compared to NREM, peak airflow rate declined in REM compared to NREM, tidal volume decreased in REM compared to NREM, and minute-volume declined slightly in REM compared to NREM (Fig. 2). However, as ventilatory demand increased tidal volume, minute volume, and peak flow all increased proportionately during REM and NREM. The conclusion was that the respiratory system can change to meet increased ventilatory demand in either NREM or REM.

There are major differences between the study of Phillipson *et al.* (1977), in which hyperoxic hypercapnea was used, and the study of Orem *et al.* (1977a), in which added dead spaces were used to increase ventilatory drive. First, tube breathing provides a complex stimulus involving a

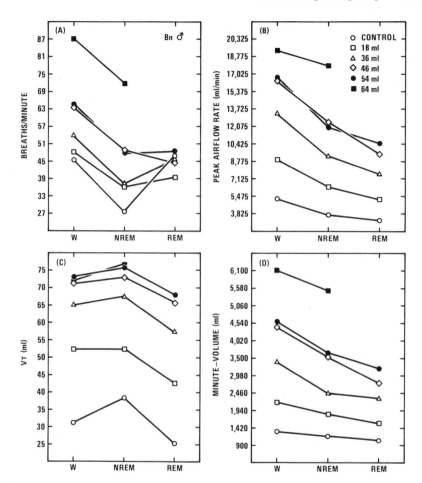

Figure 2.   Means of breaths/minute (A), peak inspiratory airflow rate (B), tidal volume (C), and minute-volume (D) under control conditions and with added dead spaces for one cat.

varying pattern of hypercapnea and hypoxia, and recently Phillipson and Sullivan (1977) have reported that ventilatory responses to hypoxia are intact during REM as well as NREM sleep. Second, in the study of Orem *et al.* (1977a) the added dead spaces were applied during wakefulness, and 15 minutes of breathing were allowed before recordings of breathing during sleep and wakefulness began. The adaptation to the dead space during sleep and wakefulness was compared and not the response to the application of dead space. In the studies of Phillipson *et al.* (1977), it was rather the responses to a suddenly applied respiratory stimuli during NREM and REM that were compared.

The status of pulmonary reflexes during sleep is also nebulous. Farber and Marlow (1976) report that, in the opossum, Hering–Breuer reflexes are as active in REM as in NREM sleep. Henderson-Smart and Read (1976) report that nasal obstruction during REM fails to produce a normal load-compensating reflex with progressive augmentation of inspiratory activity in the intercostal muscles of the lamb. This is not surprising, because the intercostal muscles are known to be inactive during REM sleep (Parmeggiani and Sabattini, 1972; Henderson-Smart and Read, 1976). In their paper, Henderson-Smart and Read (1976) illustrate an example of nasal obstruction in the lamb in which the diaphragm *does* respond to the obstruction, but they note that other recordings from the same animal showed a reduction of diaphragmatic activity and of the negative pleural pressure swings during obstruction. It should be noted that human patients with obstructive sleep apnea show vigorous breathing efforts in an attempt to overcome the obstruction. Similarly, Phillipson *et al.* (1976) report that the responses to elastic loads in W and NREM are similar and independent of vagal influences.

Knill and Bryan (1976) have reported that rapid distortion of the rib cage during sleep in human newborn infants inhibits inspiration. They interpret the inhibitory reflex to arise from the spindles of the intercostal muscles. These authors suggest that this reflex may, at times, pace breathing and produce the irregular breathing pattern of REM sleep. However, Phillipson *et al.* (1977) note that they could not eliminate the irregular breathing patterns of REM by bilateral denervation of the third to seventh intercostal spaces in dogs.

V.   UPPER AIRWAY FUNCTION DURING SLEEP AND WAKEFULNESS

The most common clinical sleep apnea is an obstructive apnea in which, despite diaphragmatic contractions, no air flows through the upper airways. Unusual anatomical features of the upper airways, e.g., enlarged tonsils and adenoids (Menashe *et al.*, 1965; Luke *et al.*, 1966; Levy *et al.*, 1967; Imes *et al.*, 1977) or infiltration of fat into the base of the tongue, have been implicated in some but not all cases of obstructive sleep apnea.

Orem *et al.* (1977b) adapted a technique used by Bartlett *et al.* (1973) for measuring upper airway resistance during sleep and wakefulness in restrained cats (Fig. 3). Mean upper airway resistance levels during NREM were 13.8 ± 2.2 (S.D.) cm H_2O/liter/second greater than during wakefulness. In REM, mean upper airway resistance across cats averaged 17.8 ± 3.6 cm H_2O/liter/second greater than wakefulness. These levels were

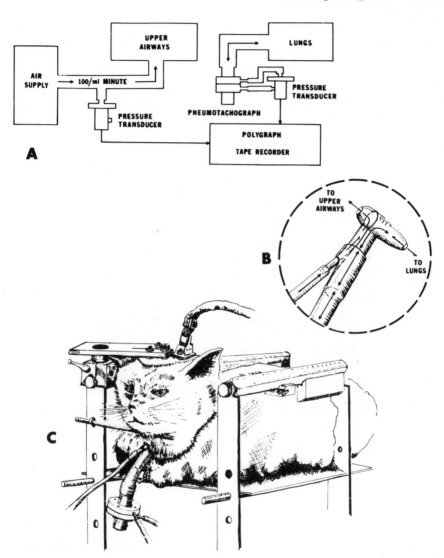

Figure 3. Measurement of upper airway resistance. (A) shows a block diagram of the arrangement for recording breathing and upper airway resistance. In (B) the endotracheal tube which allowed separation of breathing and measurement of upper airway resistance is shown. (C) is a sketch of the apparatus used for chronic recordings with head restraint.

averages of upper airway resistance sampled every 20 milliseconds (ms); they incorporate modulations within the respiratory cycle. In wakefulness, there was a resistance drop during inspiration which averaged about 8 cm H_2O/liter/second; in NREM, cyclic modulation was almost twice that in wakefulness (approximately 15 cm H_2O/liter/second). In REM, cyclic modulation was not significantly different from wakefulness levels (Fig. 4).

This study showed that there is normally an increase in upper airway resistance during sleep. In addition, there is a small resistance drop during inspiration in wakefulness when baseline resistance is low. The drop is

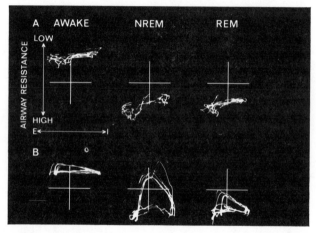

Figure 4. $X-Y$ plots of inspiratory and expiratory airflow rates (horizontal axis) and upper airway resistance (UAR) (vertical axis) during W, NREM, and REM in two cats (A and B). These plots show the coordination between changes in UAR and inspiratory and expiratory airflow rates. On the horizontal axis, points to the right of the intersection of the axes denote inspiratory flow, and the further from the origin, the greater the flow rate. The vertical axis represents UAR. Thus, each point on the curves indicates the level of UAR at a given direction and rate of airflow measured at prelaryngeal levels. In A during wakefulness, UAR was low, and the major changes during each respiratory cycle consisted of a small increase in UAR which occurred as expiratory airflow rates declined. During NREM UAR increased, but the modulations during each cycle were larger. During NREM the coordination pattern is clearest: Following the increase in UAR which occurred as expiratory flow rates declined and near the onset of inspiration, UAR decreased. As inspiratory airflow rates increased, UAR remained low; and as inspiratory flow rates began to drop, UAR increased to a level that was maintained until expiratory flow rates began to decline. Accordingly, this pattern of coordination resulted in a tilted "8" pattern. In REM in part A, the pattern is similar to that in wakefulness, but the level of resistance is higher. In B, another pattern of coordination is shown. In this case, UAR began to decrease as expiratory flow rates decreased. The reduction in UAR was maximal near the onset of inspiration; and as inspiratory airflow increased, UAR increased to reach a maximal level near peak inspiratory airflow. As inspiratory airflow rates declined and as expiratory rates increased, the UAR remained high.

larger in NREM when baseline resistance is high, and in REM it is small again on a high baseline resistance.

Several factors can contribute to upper airway resistance changes. Changes in the head-on-neck angle can influence the patency of the upper airways, but this was held constant in the study of Orem et al. (1977b). Engorgement of the nasal tissues with blood may increase upper airway resistance during sleep. Nasal resistance represents the greater portion of human upper airway resistance with the mouth closed (Ferris et al., 1964), and there is a decrease in blood pressure during sleep (Snyder et al., 1964; Candia et al., 1962; Kanzow et al., 1962). However, blood pressure changes cannot account for respiratory-modulated upper airway resistance changes, and it seems likely that other factors are involved.

Hyperventilation and CO_2 administration produce an increased dilation of the glottis in both humans (Hyatt and Wilcox, 1961) and anesthetized cats (Bartlett et al., 1973). In unanesthetized cats there is a drop in upper airway resistance with CO_2 administration (Bartlett et al., 1973). The similarity of the pressure changes during increasing hypercapnea (see Bartlett et al., 1973, Fig. 3) to those in the progression from sleep to wakefulness is striking. In wakefulness, modulations with each respiratory cycle are as small as those seen during hypercapnia, while in NREM there is a large inspiratory drop in pressure similar to the drop from high expiratory levels seen in normocapnea in the anesthetized cat. The decrease in upper airway resistance during hypercapnia is associated with prolongation of intrinsic laryngeal abductor EMG activity (from the posterior cricoarytenoid muscles) into expiration (Bartlett et al., 1973; Murakami and Kirchner, 1972).

To test the hypothesis that changes in laryngeal function account for the changes in upper airway resistance, Orem et al. (1978) recorded the electromyographic activity of the posterior cricoarytenoid (PCA) muscles in six adult cats (Fig. 5). During wakefulness, the EMG activity from the PCA muscles showed intense bursts of activity beginning about 90 milliseconds before the onset of inspiratory airflow and continuing through inspiration. In addition, there was a substantial activity persisting during expiration. At the end of expiration, PCA activity was minimal. During NREM sleep, there was a decrease in both inspiratory and expiratory PCA activity. The relative decrease in expiratory activity was greater than the decrease in inspiratory activity. In recordings from nine PCA muscle groups in the six cats, the average, integrated wakefulness expiratory activity was 61% of the inspiratory activity. In NREM, the inspiratory PCA activity was 84% of wakefulness levels and the expiratory activity was 34% of wakefulness inspiratory activity. In REM sleep inspiratory activity averaged 66% of wakefulness levels and expiratory

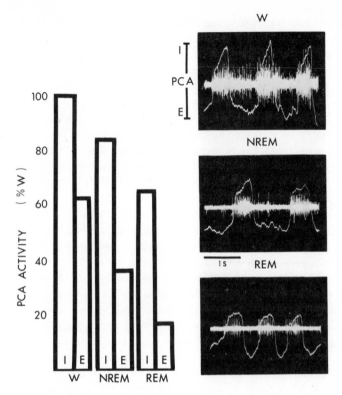

Figure 5. Posterior cricoarytenoid (PCA) muscle activity during sleep and wakefulness. In the histogram, PCA activity occurring during inspiration (I) and expiration (E) in wakefulness, and NREM and REM sleep is expressed as a percentage of wakefulness inspiratory activity levels. The data shown are an average of activity fron nine PCA muscle groups recorded in six cats. Photographs at right show examples of PCA activity during sleep and wakefulness. An upward deflection of the breathing trace signifies inspiration.

activity was 16% of wakefulness inspiratory levels. These results showed a progressive reduction in laryngeal activity from wakefulness to NREM and from NREM to REM. They are consistent with a narrowing of the glottic aperture during sleep.

The relationship of these results on the larynx to the pathophysiology of obstructive sleep apnea is uncertain. A major issue is the source of the upper airway obstruction. There is a recent report on fibroscopic observations of a patient with obstructive apnea (Krieger *et al.*, 1976). The authors report a vocal cord collapse with subsequent complete obstruction of the glottis. This corresponds to the observation that in some patients provision of an oropharyngeal airway down to the level of the larynx does not eliminate obstructive episodes (F. Eldridge and C. Guilleminault, personal communication). On the other hand, at a recent meeting of the Association for the Psychophysiological Study of Sleep (Houston, 1977), Weitzman and his colleagues (1977) presented fibroscopic and fluoroscopic evidence that the obstruction occurs within the pharynx. In their abstract, the authors explain that:

> The superior lateral pharyngeal walls are partially or completely closed at the end of an expiration. If partial, a snore will ensue with the next inspiration; if total, the patient will be silent but obstructed and a respiratory effort produces no airflow. At the end of an apnea (e.g., 40 sec) and after 10–15 respiratory efforts the lateral pharyngeal walls will open partially and a loud snoring noise and deep respiratory movements will occur with a transient arousal.

In clinical obstructive apneas, first the patient falls asleep and breathing ceases. Second, there are efforts to breathe which progressively augment, but no air flows through the upper airway. Upper airway function either fails to resume or is somehow insufficient or out of phase with the pumping action of the diaphragm and chest. In view of recent work (Orem *et al.*, 1977b, 1978; Sauerland and Harper, 1976), it is likely that the central respiratory drive to the dilators of the upper airways is less during sleep than the central respiratory drive to motoneurons of the chest and diaphragm.

Remmers *et al.* (1978) have studied 12 obese patients complaining of daytime somnolence. Ten of the twelve demonstrated obstructive apneic episodes. Nasopharyngeal intubation eliminated the obstructive episodes in four of the patients, and in five patients similar pressure changes were recorded from esophegeal and from supraglottic sites during obstruction. These results are consistent with a patent glottis, and the authors conclude that obstruction occurs within the pharynx. Genioglossal activity was recorded in their patients. The greatest activity occurred coincident with the release of obstruction, and as pharyngeal resistance increased, there was a simultaneous decline in genioglossal activity. However, the correspondence between genioglossal activity and patency of the pharyngeal airway was not exact, for as the authors note, there was some overlap of genioglossal activity levels during obstruction and during ventilation. During obstruction, increases in pharyngeal pressure exceeded increases in genioglossal activity, and release of obstruction was associated with a two- to five-fold increase in genioglossal activity.

From these results, Remmers and his colleagues propose the following sequence of events in the pathogenesis of obstructive apnea. First, they state that because of structural narrowing of the pharyngeal airway, pharyngeal resistance increases, and in association with decreased genioglossal activity at sleep onset, this leads to pharyngeal collapse.

Second, during sleep the increasing chemical drive from the apnea preferentially activates inspiratory efforts. Genioglossal activity is also augmented, but to a lesser extent. Third, asphyxic stimuli produce arousal, and arousal results in an activation of the genioglossus which opens the pharynx.

This chapter affirms the original interpretation of obstructive apnea proposed by Gastaut and his colleagues (1966, 1969) but conflicts with Weitzman's interpretation that although the obstruction occurs at the level of the pharynx, it does not result from a backward movement of the tongue (E. D. Weitzman, personal communication). There is also some controversy concerning the necessity of an anatomical abnormality in the upper airway in the pathogenesis of obstruction. This is a central feature of the interpretation of Remmers and colleagues. The reduction at genioglossal activity during sleep is presumably normal (Sauerland and Harper, 1976) and does not normally lead to obstruction. Guilleminault reports that obstructive apneas also occur in nonobese patients with normal upper airways (personal communication).

VI. NEUROPHYSIOLOGICAL INTERPRETATIONS

A. The Wakefulness Stimulus

The two-way relationship between physiological state and respiration has been demonstrated repeatedly (some of this literature is reviewed in Section I of this chapter). Kumagi et al. (1966) observed changes in the pattern of the electrocorticogram as a function of changes in enforced ventilation in curarized cats. An increase in ventilation subsequent to an accelerated rate or increase of tidal volume in artificial respiration caused a decrease in phrenic activity and slower, higher voltage waves on the cortex. Conversely, a decrease in enforced ventilation increased phrenic nerve volleys and desynchronized the electrocorticogram. Bonvallet et al. (1955) noted earlier that hypercapnea produces an intense cortical activation with intensification of phrenic discharges, and that hypocapnea synchronized cortical activity and reduced phrenic firing. Other studies (Ranson et al., 1935) have demonstrated inspiratory facilitation from hypothalamic stimulation and inspiratory depression from functional and electrolytic hypothalamic lesions (Redgate, 1963). Hugelin and Cohen (1963) and Cohen and Hugelin (1965) have shown in spinal, vagotomized, and artificially respirated cats that stimulation of midbrain and diencephalic regions which elicit patterns of cortical arousal decreased the duration of the expiratory phase (as revealed by phrenic recordings) and increased the slope and amplitude of integrated phrenic activity. To-gether, these results demonstrate a facilitatory effect of arousal upon respiratory activity, and in addition, implicate a significant suprapontine facilitatory action. The latter apparently is not restricted to the hypo-thalamus. Cohen (1964) showed that rostral diencephalic transection de-creased the threshold for apnea as CO_2 concentration was lowered. Simi-larly, Fink et $al.$ (1962) found that the change in ventilation (ΔV) as a function of the change in CO_2 (ΔPa_{CO_2}) expressed as the ratio $\Delta V/\Delta Pa_{CO_2}$ was more than twice the value obtained from animals with intercollicular transections when the transections were made at supracollicular levels. That is, the supracollicular animals were more than twice as responsive to CO_2 as the intercollicular animals.

There is general agreement on the influence of anesthetics on respira-tory neurons. This issue is particularly important in the present context, because anesthesia may be equivalent with sleep to the extent that both involve the loss of the "wakefulness stimulus." It is important to recall the similar findings of St. John et $al.$ (1972) with anesthesia and of Hugelin and Bertrand (1973) in NREM sleep (spinal cats) following pneumotaxic lesions (see Section I). Several studies with varying purposes have dem-onstrated that the population of respiratory neurons fluctuates in response to level of anesthesia and the chemical environment. Sears (1964a) noted the sensitivity of intercostal gamma and alpha motoneurons to the level of anesthesia; Batsel (1965) wrote of a reserve pool of medullary respiratory neurons which are active in conditions requiring deeper breathing—an observation made earlier by Burns and Salmoiraghi (1960). There are also indications that caudal brainstem respiratory neurons are less sensitive to anesthesia than rostral brainstem respiratory neurons. Merrill (1970) ob-served a restriction of the medullary respiratory neuron population under deep barbiturate anesthesia and noted that this restriction limited dis-charge principally to caudal neurons with spinal projections. Eyzaguirre and Taylor (1963) found a loss of expiratory discharges in the recurrent laryngeal nerve with Nembutal anesthesia; similarly, Hugelin and Cohen (1963) found that Nembutal and urethane reduced the slope and amplitude of integrated phrenic nerve activity. Robson et $al.$ (1963) studied the alteration of firing patterns in medullary respiratory neurons under bar-biturates and described a change from discontinuous respiratory firing to continuous discharges under anesthesia. In contrast to results showing recruitment under hypercapnia and decreased populations of respiratory neurons under anesthesia, Nesland et $al.$ (1966) contend that the response to hypercapnia or hyperoxia consists of an increase and decrease, respec-tively, of respiratory discharge frequencies with little or no recruitment or decruitment of neurons. Some of their preparations were anesthetized with sodium pentobarbital, while others were midcollicularly decerebrate. The population of respiratory neurons which they studied in the caudal medulla was, according to other studies, the least sensitive to anesthesia.

These observations suggest certain possible bases for respiratory changes during sleep. The concept of recruitment suggests that during sleep the functioning population of respiratory neurons may decrease. According to the model offered by studies with anesthesia, we might view the restriction of the population of respiratory neurons as progressively increasing from caudal to rostral levels. The issue of the loss of the "wakefulness" stimulus during anesthesia and sleep may be particularly pertinent in understanding the pathophysiology of obstructive sleep apnea and the mechanism behind the dramatic changes in upper airway resistance and laryngeal abductor activity during sleep.

The *upper* motoneurons for the muscles of the upper airways have not been identified. Studies within the central nervous system are almost exclusively concerned with laryngeal motoneurons. Merrill (1970) studied laryngeal EMG activity and laryngeal motoneurons. He noted, reiterating several other authors (Bianconi and Raschi, 1964; Eyzaguirre and Taylor, 1963; Sherrey and Megirian, 1975), that laryngeal respiratory activity decreases with increasing pentobarbital anesthesia and that expiratory laryngeal muscles (thyreoarytenoid and cricothyroid muscles) are more sensitive to anesthesia than the inspiratory posterior cricoarytenoids. The author found that with increasing depth of anesthesia the number of neurons with respiratory activity in nucleus ambiguus decreased. In contrast, nonnucleus ambiguus neurons were relatively insensitive to pentobarbital anesthesia. The mechanism of decruitment of laryngeal motoneurons under anesthesia may be similar to the mechanism of the loss of upper airway control in obstructive sleep apnea cases and, to some extent, during normal sleep.

Bianchi (1971) studied medullary neurons in the chloralose–urethane anesthetized cat. By antidromic stimulation of the vagus, he identified medullary neurons as laryngeal motoneurons. A total of six neurons, all in the vicinity of nucleus ambiguus from 2 mm in front to 1 mm behind the obex, were identified. He noted that it was possible to antidromically invade laryngeal motoneurons which were silent under his experimental conditions. This observation is consistent with the idea that the population of laryngeal motoneurons is under precarious central control which is sensitive to anesthesia and possibly sleep.

In 1974 two independent studies indicated that something similar to barbiturate "decruitment" occurred during natural sleep. Puizillout and Ternaux (1974), utilizing vagoaortic stimulation to induce "sleeplike" behavior in encéphale isolé cats (cords transected at the level of first cervical vertebrae), observed a decrease in integrated medullary multiunit respiratory activity during spontaneous sleep and elimination of this activity during vagoaortic stimulation. The effect was always more dramatic in the latter case than the spontaneously occurring depression. They also noted an accompanying depression in phrenic nerve activity. The multiunit activity was recorded from the region of nucleus ambiguus, around the solitary tract, along the medullary midline and into the hypoglossal nucleus. Orem *et al.* (1974) recorded single respiratory neurons in restrained but intact cats during sleep and wakefulness. They reported a class of respiratory neurons which were decruited during sleep (Fig. 6). Their neurons were situated in the ventrolateral brain stem in regions corresponding to the area of the retrofacial nucleus. Taber (1961) describes the feline nucleus ambiguus as extending from just caudal to the inferior olive up to the caudal pole of the facial nucleus. Rostrally, according to Taber, the nucleus is composed of a dorsal and ventral group. The ventral group which appears continuous with the facial nucleus is commonly called the retrofacial nucleus. It is then likely that the decruited respiratory neurons of Orem *et al.* (1974) were related to the control of the upper airways.

The respiratory muscles of the larynx are thought to be controlled by an oscillating system also common to muscles of the respiratory pump (diaphragm and intercostal muscles) (Cohen, 1975). However, both from experimental studies showing an unusual sensitivity of laryngeal motoneurons to anesthesia and from the occurrence of clinical sleep apneas, it seems that the central control of the upper airways is more precarious than the control of the diaphragm. The mechanism underlying this difference between laryngeal motoneurons and phrenic motoneurons is unknown, nor has it been strictly proven in the case of sleep. For example, peak flow and V_T/T_I decrease in sleep, and phrenic activity may decline as much as laryngeal activity. It seems paradoxical that the threshold for activation of laryngeal motoneurons by the common respiratory oscillator should be lower than for activation of neurons driving phrenic motoneurons (Cohen, 1975), while at the same time these laryngeal elements are preferentially depressed by anesthesia (Merrill, 1970).

Moruzzi (1972) has hypothesized that reticular deactivation is a prerequisite for the appearance of active sleep mechanisms. Reticular deactivation may be equivalent to what is called here "the loss of the wakefulness stimulus"—that common element between NREM sleep and anesthesia. There are several aspects of breathing during sleep which may result from reticular deactivation, e.g., the slow frequency of breathing and the reduction in peak airflow rate during NREM. Cohen and Hugelin (1965) have shown that stimulation of midbrain and diencephalic regions which

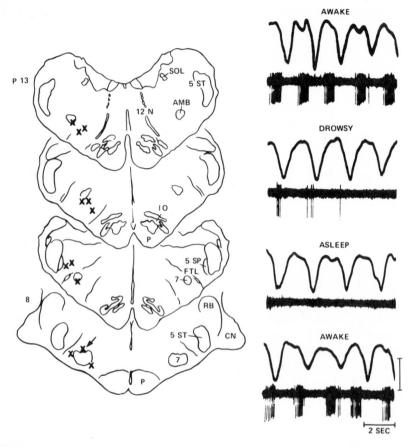

Figure 6. Locations of 12 sleep-sensitive respiratory neurons. Arrow marks the location of the cell whose activity is illustrated on the right. AMB, nucleus ambiguus; CN, cochlear nucleus; FTL, lateral tegmental field; IO, inferior olive; P, pyramidal tract; RB, restiform body; SOL, solitary tract; 5SP, nucleus of the spinal tract of V; 5ST, spinal tract of V; 7, facial nucleus; 12N, hypoglossal nerve.

elicit patterns of cortical arousal decreased the duration of expiration and increased the slope and amplitude of integrated phrenic activity. However, the correspondence between Cohen and Hugelin's work in acute animals and changes in breathing rates during sleep and wakefulness is not exact. Orem *et al.* (1977a) note that the ratio T_I/T_{tot} increases from wakefulness to NREM and REM, while the shortening of T_E in Cohen and Hugelin's animals would produce a larger T_I/T_{tot} ratio in stimulated arousal than in the unstimulated condition.

Reticular deactivation may largely explain the changes which occur in upper airway resistance and laryngeal abductor activity during sleep. Orem and Lydic (1978) have shown that Nembutal anesthesia can be used to replicate the depression in tonic and phasic posterior cricoarytenoid activity which occurs during sleep. Stimulation in the reticular activating system (Moruzzi and Magoun, 1949) converts the laryngeal activity from patterns characteristic of sleep to patterns equivalent to those seen in wakefulness.

The details of the mode of action of the reticular activating system on respiration are unknown. Their elucidation will explain much about the mechanisms of breathing during sleep and wakefulness.

B. Respiratory Influences Arising from Sleep Processes

1. The Atonia of REM Sleep

Parmeggiani and Sabattini (1972) were first to point out that intercostal EMG was lost during REM sleep while diaphragmatic efforts persisted. Knill and Bryan (1976) and Henderson-Smart and Read (1976) have confirmed this by noting paradoxical rib cage movements in REM in newborn humans and from electromyographic recordings in lambs. In 1918, Coombs (cited in Newsom Davis, 1974) noted that thoracic dorsal root section in the cat was associated with decreased costal respiratory, and it is now known that this decrease results from an interruption of excitatory influences on alpha motoneurons from the muscle spindle loop (Critchlow and von Euler, 1963; Sears, 1964a,b,c; Corda et al., 1965; Eklund et al., 1964). In contrast to the intercostals, the diaphragm appears to be primarily controlled by central influences and intercostal-to-phrenic reflexes (see Newsom Davis, 1974). The diaphragm is essentially devoid of muscle spindles (Corda et al., 1965) and fusimotor fibers (Gasser and Grundfest, 1939). Corda et al. (1965) found that more than one-half the spindles encountered in the diaphragm showed no evidence of rhythmic fusimotor driving. Rhythmic fusimotor bias of diaphragmatic muscle spindles in inspiration, in a few cases, increased firing rates of the alpha motoneurons.

The contrasting behavior of the intercostal and diaphragmatic neuromuscular systems in response to stretch and during REM may be a significant factor in the interpretation of REM atonia as well as sleep-associated respiratory changes. The paralysis of REM sleep has been noted often, and there will be no attempt here to review all the related literature. A number of studies have shown a depression of various brainstem and spinal reflexes (Giaquinto et al., 1964; Hodes and Dement,

1964; Kubota *et al.*, 1965; Chase, 1970), and a series of studies in 1964 and 1965 from Pisa were designed to explain the nature and neural basis of atonia and reflex depression of REM (Giaquinto *et al.*, 1964; Morrison and Pompeiano, 1965a,b,c; Gassel *et al.*, 1964a,b,c). Pompeiano (1966, 1967, 1973) has reviewed this work, and two aspects are emphasized: (a) that there is a tonic inhibition throughout REM sleep which derives from a hyperpolarization of alpha motoneurons; and (b) that during the bursts of eye movements in REM, a phasic inhibition is superimposed upon the tonic inhibition. The phasic inhibition derives from a presynaptic inhibition of Ia terminals (PAD) determined by Wall's method (Wall, 1958). However, hyperpolarizations have actually not been recorded from alpha motoneurons in REM but inferred from reflex changes, an analysis of the recurrent discharge, and direct stimulation of the ventral horns. None of these can differentiate hyperpolarizations from disfacilitation.

There is evidence that the loss of fusimotor activity may be at least a partial cause of the REM paralysis. Parallel reticular influences on muscle spindles and state of consciousness can be inferred from the work of Granit and Kaada (1953) and Moruzzi and Magoun (1949). Von Euler and Söderberg (1956, 1957) showed that activated EEG patterns were accompanied by increased discharges from muscle spindles; Buchwald and Eldred (1961) found a general positive correlation between fusimotor discharges and the level of cortical activity—whether the latter was spontaneous or induced by drugs or by stimulation. In von Euler and Söderberg's studies and in the study by Buchwald and Eldred, the activated patterns were presumably those of wakefulness, not REM. Gassel and Pompeiano (1965), using a technique developed by Paillard (1955), demonstrated that gamma motoneurons as well as alpha motoneurons were depressed in REM sleep. Kubota and Tanaka (1966) confirmed a REM depression of fusimotor activity by direct recordings of gamma efferent fibers from cats recovering from barbiturate anesthesia. Some fusimotor fibers fired in frequencies varying from 0 to 50 cps during NREM, but the majority were silent. Spontaneously active units during NREM reduced their firing rate or ceased altogether during REM. Occasional discharges were observed during intense eye movement bursts in REM sleep.

It seems, therefore, that the REM paralysis involves, at least in part, a loss of fusimotor tone. The loss of intercostal EMG activity during REM with a perseverance of diaphragmatic activity is consistent with this interpretation because autogenic facilitation is of differing importance to the two muscle systems.

The contribution of costal breathing to the airflow patterns of wakefulness and NREM sleep is not known. Knill and Bryan (1976) contend that the loss of intercostal activity allows rapid rib cage distortion and pacing of breathing (and ataxic or irregular breathing) during REM, but, as mentioned above, the importance of the intercostal inspiratory inhibitory reflex is uncertain. The significance of REM paralysis in other aspects of breathing during REM sleep is also unknown. Although laryngeal myotactic reflexes have been reported (Abo-el-Enein and Wyke, 1966), it is not clear that the atonia of REM is involved in the reduction of tonic and phasic laryngeal abductor activity, as this latter event begins in NREM sleep. Similarly, the paralysis of REM sleep appears to have little relationship to the central and obstructive sleep apnea syndromes in which apneas appear in both NREM and REM sleep.

2. REM-Specific Neurons

Moruzzi (1972) distinguished between the loss of wakefulness or reticular deactivation and the presence of processes peculiar to sleep. There are aspects of breathing during sleep which cannot be accounted for by a reticular deactivation. In particular, the increased rate of breathing in REM and the ubiquitous irregularities during that state of sleep seem to derive from processes peculiar to REM. Opinion as to the nature of these processes is not unanimous: Knill and Bryan (1976) have stressed the role of an intercostal inspiratory inhibitory reflex in the rapid rate and irregularity of breathing during REM, but Phillipson et al. (1977) doubt the importance of this reflex. Recently, Netick et al. (1977) have reported REM-specific tonic neurons whose rate of discharge was positively correlated with the rate of breathing during that state. While several authors have suggested that such neurons may exist (Andersen and Sears, 1970; Cohen, 1970; Pitts et al., 1939), these cells are the first demonstration of possible tonic respiratory neurons. The regions from which the neurons were recorded correspond to the regions from which Andersen and Sears (1970) obtained inspiratory apneuses. These tonic respiratory neurons are characterized in the following ways: First, they were observed while recording respiratory neurons between the caudal pole of the facial nucleus and nucleus ambiguus. They were in regions medial and dorsal to the retrofacial nucleus which correspond to the medullary region of the lateral and gigantocellular tegmental field. Their action potentials were larger than those of the respiratory neurons. Second, they were silent or intermittently active during the deep NREM periods preceding REM. At the onset of REM, they began discharging at a gradually accelerating rate for the first few seconds of the REM period. They then reached a level of tonic activity which continued, with modulation, throughout the REM period (Fig. 7). Third, they began discharging tonically from 7 seconds prior to 6.5 seconds after the onset of REM as judged from cortical desynchronization. Fourth, variations of the individual interspike intervals from the

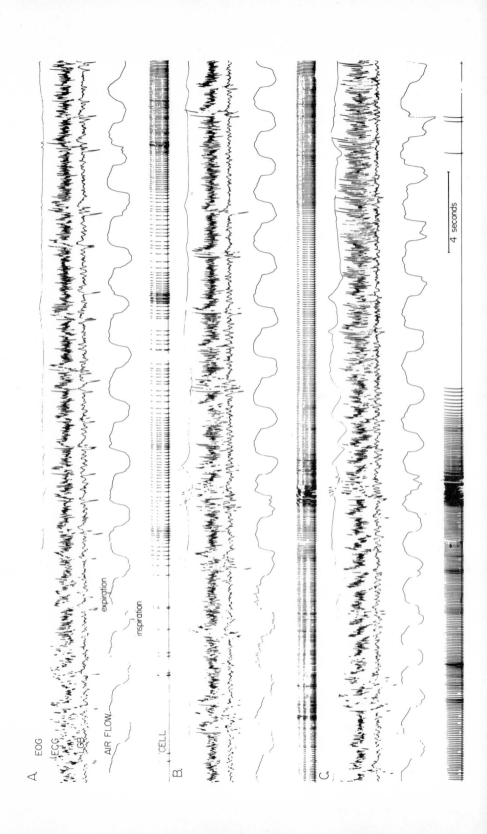

A. EOG

ECG

LGB

AIR FLOW

expiration

inspiration

B. CELL

C.

4 seconds

mean interspike interval were sufficiently small to conclude that the discharges were more evenly spaced in time than if they occurred at random; i.e., they showed a pacemakerlike activity. Fifth, the rhythmic activity of the cells was modulated throughout the REM periods. Discharge frequencies during each respiratory cycle were positively correlated with frequencies of the cycles (Fig. 8). Finally, the highest discharge rates were associated with bursts of eye movements and the irregular respirations associated with these. This irregular respiration at times consisted of rapid swings of small amplitude around zero airflow which, during intense firing of the neurons, contributed in part to the positive correlations between rate of respiration and rate of discharge of the neurons.

The characteristics of these REM-specific neurons pose an interpretative dilemma: There is reason to believe either that they are generators of REM sleep and/or that they represent a REM-specific influence on breathing. Hobson and McCarley (Hobson, 1974; Hobson *et al.*, 1974, 1975; McCarley and Hobson, 1971, 1975a,b) have reported two classes of pontine reticular units with higher discharge rates during REM than during W or NREM. Cells located in the gigantocellular tegmental field have high selectivity ratios (discharge frequency in REM/discharge frequency in W and NREM) and phasic discharge bursts which correlate with eye movement bursts. In contrast, cells in the central tegmental field have lower selectivity ratios and are relatively tonic in their discharge pattern.

The Hobson–McCarley theory of REM generation is not without its difficulties. First, recent work (Jones *et al.*, 1977) has shown that lesions of locus coeruleus do not prevent the occurrence of REM sleep, but may be involved in certain phasic REM events and the muscle atonia of REM sleep. (Hobson and McCarley have proposed that REM sleep arises from reciprocal interactions between REM-specific neurons of the gigantocellular tegmental field and neurons within the locus coeruleus.) Second, Siegel and McGinty (1976, 1977) and Vertes (1977) have shown that

Figure 7. A polygraphic recording of REM-specific tonic activity. In parts A–C, the top trace is the EOG; the second trace down is the electrocorticogram (ECoG) recorded from the occipital cortex; the third trace down is pontogeniculooccipital activity recorded from the dorsal lateral geniculate body; the fourth trace is airflow recorded at prelaryngeal levels with a pneumotachograph. The bottom trace is the output to the polygraph of a pulse height discriminator which was adjusted to give a pulse for each action potential of the neuron. A: The onset of REM. At the beginning of A, the animal was in deep NREM sleep. As the ECoG desynchronized, the neuron began discharging, at first falteringly, but after a few seconds activity was established. B: An episode within the REM period. Note the coninuing tonic activity with modulation. Near the middle of B, there is an episode of intense discharges which coinicdes with a burst of eye movements. C: The end of REM. Note the progressively decelerating pattern of discharge coinciding with REM termination.

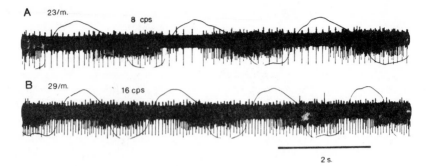

Figure 8. Relationship between the discharge frequency of a REM-specific neuron and rate of respiration. In A, the respiration rate is approximately 23 per minute, and the neuron discharged at a rate of 8 cps. In B, the neuronal discharge rate was 16 cps, and respiration was approximately 29 per minute. The REM-specific neuron appeared at the onset of REM while recording the phase spanning expiratory–inspiratory show in the figure. Downward deflections of the respiration tracings signify inspiration.

pontine, presumably gigantocellular tegmental field neurons, demonstrate a high REM selectivity only when the animals are restrained. If spontaneous waking movements are allowed, the neurons discharge at rates equivalent to or exceeding those in REM. These important studies dispute the REM specificity of the gigantocellular tegmental field neurons of Hobson and McCarley.

The discharge patterns of the medullary cells reported by Netick *et al.* (1977) are fundamentally different from the pontine cells of Hobson and McCarley. Their cells were as REM-selective as the pontine cells, and the discharge patterns were also highly regular but sufficiently modulated to allow correlations with breathing rate and eye movement bursts. The cells reported by Netick *et al.* combined REM selectivity with tonicity and phasic modulation. McCarley and Hobson have concluded that the lack of regularity in their pontine cells ". . . weakens the hypothesis that pacemaker cells become active in desynchronized sleep, and thus generate the signs of this state" (Hobson *et al.*, 1974, p. 762). In view of the cells of Netick *et al.* (1977) which were highly selective to REM with regular, pacemakerlike discharge patterns, this conclusion and the later elaboration of a mechanism for REM generation, based in part upon the nonexistence of such cells (Hobson *et al.*, 1975), seems premature.

In terms of breathing, some theories of respiratory rhythmicity require tonic influences (Cohen, 1970). However, these have never been directly demonstrated. In view of the strong influence of state on respiration, it would not be surprising if such tonic elements were also state specific.

VII. SUMMARY

Experimental and clinical evidence concurs that breathing efforts are reduced during sleep. Although the incidence of sleep apnea is unknown, it constitutes a significant sleep disorder which has become increasingly recognized. Apnea during sleep may account for many cases of Sudden Infant Death syndrome. Animal studies indicate reductions during sleep in peak flow, V_T/T_I, and perhaps in the ventilatory response to CO_2.

Although a central or diaphragmatic apnea has been described as a type of sleep apnea, it is clear that this type of apnea is rare in adult patients. The obstructive apneas are much more prevalent, and in these cases, it is clear that diaphragmatic efforts are vigorous at a time when upper airway function is lost. Both human and animal electromyographic studies show dramatic reductions in some of the dilator muscles of the upper airways during sleep in normal subjects. However, it has never been directly demonstrated that the percentage reduction in activity of, e.g., the posterior cricoarytenoids, exceeds the reduction in the diaphragm. It may be that tolerances in the upper airways are less, so that a 30% reduction in an upper airway dilator will result in complete obstruction (particularly in association with an anatomical irregularity), whereas a 30% reduction in diaphragmatic activity produces only a 30% reduction in airflow rates.

The central fact is that breathing during sleep is different from breathing during wakefulness. The differences derive from changes in central programs. The mechanisms are largely unknown, but breathing changes partly result from sleep processes and partly from the loss of the wakefulness stimulus. The differentiation of sleep processes from the loss of wakefulness involves a structure–function central nervous system distinction. The loss of wakefulness implies a reticular deactivation which may be the physiological substance common to coma, anesthesia, and quiet sleep. Respiratory influences arising from sleep processes, e.g., the atonia of REM sleep with intercostal muscle flaccidity and possibly the phasic events of REM sleep (with episodes of ataxic breathing included as one of these), presumably depend on sleep-mediating structures and can be considered as active influences on respiration. In contrast, the respiratory effects of reticular deactivation may be passive and may represent the unactivated respiratory system.

REFERENCES

Abo-el-Enein, M. A., and B. Wyke (1966). Laryngeal myotatic reflexes. *Nature* (*London*) **209**, 682–686.

Andersen, P., and T. A. Sears (1970). Medullary activation of intercostal fusimotor and alpha motoneurones. *J. Physiol. (London)* **209**, 739–755.

Aserinsky, E. (1965). Periodic respiratory pattern occurring in conjunction with eye movements during sleep. *Science* **150**, 763–766.

Bartlett, D., Jr., J. E. Remmers, and H. Gautier (1973). Laryngeal regulation of respiratory airflow. *Respir. Physiol.* **18**, 194–204.

Batsel, H. L. (1965). Some functional properties of bulbar respiratory units. *Exp. Neurol.* **11**, 341–366.

Bellville, J. W., W. S. Howland, J. C. Seed, and R. W. Houde (1959). The effect of sleep on the respiratory response to carbon dioxide. *Anaesthesia* **20**, 628–634.

Bergman, A. B., C. G. Ray, M. A. Pomeroy, P. W. Wahl, and J. B. Beckwith (1972). Studies of the sudden infant death syndrome in King County, Washington. III. Epidemiology. *Pediatrics* **49**, 860–870.

Bianchi, A. L. (1971). Localisation et étude des neurones respiratoires bulbaires. Mise en jeu antidromique par stimulation spinal ou vagale. *J. Physiol. (Paris)* **63**, 5–40.

Bianconi, R., and F. Raschi (1964). Respiratory control of motoneurones of the recurrent laryngeal nerve and hypocapnic apnoea. *Arch. Ital. Biol.* **102**, 56–73.

Birchfield, R. I., H. O. Sieker, and A. Heyman (1958). Alterations in blood gases during natural sleep and narcolepsy. *Neurology* **8**, 107–112.

Bolton, D. P. G., and S. Herman (1974). Ventilation and sleep state in the new-born. *J. Physiol. (London)* **240**, 67–77.

Bonvallet, M., A. Hugelin, and P. Dell (1955). Sensibilité compare du système reticule activateur ascendant et du centre respiratoire aux gaz du sang et à l'adrenaline. *J. Physiol. (Paris)* **47**, 651–654.

Bradley, G. W., C. von Euler, I. Marttila, and B. Roos (1974). Steady state effects of CO_2 and temperature on the relationship between lung volume and inspiratory duration (Hering–Breuer threshold curve). *Acta Physiol. Scand.* **92**, 351–363.

Buchwald, J. S., and E. Eldred (1961). Relations between gamma efferent discharge and cortical activity. *Electroencephalogr. Clin. Neurophysiol.* **13**, 243–247.

Bülow, K. (1963). Respiration and wakefulness in man. *Acta Physiol. Scand.* **59**,Suppl. 209, 1–110.

Burns, B. D., and G. C. Salmoiraghi (1960). Repetitive firing of respiratory neurones during their burst activity. *J. Neurophysiol.* **23**, 27–46.

Candia, O., E. Favale, A. Guissani, and G. F. Rossi (1962). Blood pressure during natural sleep and during sleep induced by electrical stimulation of the brain stem reticular formation. *Arch. Ital. Biol.* **100**, 216–233.

Chase, M. H. (1970). The digastric reflex in the kitten and adult cat: Paradoxical amplitude fluctuations during sleep and wakefulness. *Arch. Ital. Biol.* **108**, 403–422.

Clark, F. J., and C. von Euler (1972). On the regulation of depth and rate of breathing. *J. Physiol. (London)* **222**, 267–295.

Cohen, M. I. (1964). Respiratory periodicity in the paralyzed, vagotomized cat: Hypocapnic polypnea. *Am. J. Physiol.* **206**, 845–854.

Cohen, M. I. (1975). Phrenic and recurrent laryngeal discharge patterns and the Hering–Breuer reflex. *Am. J. Physiol.* **228**, 1489–1496.

Cohen, M. I. (1970). How respiratory rhythm originates: Evidence from discharge patterns of brainstem respiratory neurons. *In* "Breathing: Hering–Breuer Centenary Symposium" (R. Porter, ed.), pp. 125–157. Churchill, London.

Cohen, M. I., and A. Hugelin (1965). Suprapontine reticular control of intrinsic respiratory mechanisms. *Arch. Ital. Biol.* **103**, 317–334.

Corda, M., C. von Euler, and G. Lennerstrand (1965). Proprioceptive innervation of the diaphragm. *J. Physiol. (London)* **178**, 161–177.

Cotes, J. E. (1955). The role of body temperature in controlling ventilation during exercise in one normal subject breathing oxygen. *J. Physiol. (London)* **129**, 554–563.

Critchlow, V., and C. von Euler (1963). Intercostal muscle spindle activity and its gamma motor control. *J. Physiol. (London)* **168**, 820–847.

Cunningham, D. J. C., and J. L. H. O'Riordan (1957). The effect of a rise in the temperature of the body on the respiratory response to carbon dioxide at rest. *Q. J. Exp. Physiol. Cogn. Med. Sci.* **42**, 329–345.

Dement, W. C. (1972). "Some Must Watch While Some Must Sleep." Stanford Alumni Assoc., Stanford, California.

Duron, B. (1972). Le fonction respiratoire pendant le sommeil physiologique. *Bull. Physiopathol.* **8**, 1277–1288.

Eklund, G., C. von Euler, and S. Rutkowski (1964). Spontaneous and reflex activity of intercostal gamma motoneurons. *J. Physiol. (London)* **171**, 139–163.

Eyzaguirre, C., and J. R. Taylor (1963). Respiratory discharge of some vagal motoneurons. *J. Neurophysiol.* **26**, 61–78.

Farber, J. P., and T. A. Marlow (1976). Pulmonary reflexes and breathing pattern during sleep in the opossum. *Respir. Physiol.* **27**, 73–86.

Ferris, B. G., Jr., J. Mead, and L. H. Opie (1964). Partitioning of respiratory flow resistance in man. *J. Appl. Physiol.* **19**, 653–658.

Fink, B. R., R. Katz, H. Reinhold, and A. Schoolman (1962). Suprapontine mechanisms in regulation of respiration. *Am. J. Physiol.* **202**, 217–220.

Fink, B. R., E. C. Hanks, S. H. Ngai, and E. M. Papper (1963). Central regulation of respiration during anesthesia and wakefulness. *Ann. N.Y. Acad. Sci.* **109**, 892–900.

Gassel, M. M., and O. Pompeiano (1965). Fusimotor function during sleep in unrestrained cats. An account of the modulation of the mechanically and electrically evoked monosynaptic reflexes. *Arch. Ital. Biol.* **103**, 347–368.

Gassel, M. M., P. L. Marchiafava, and O. Pompeiano (1964a). Phasic changes in muscular activity during desynchronized sleep in unrestrained cats. An analysis of the pattern and organization of myoclonic twitches. *Arch. Ital. Biol.* **102**, 449–470.

Gassel, M. M., P. L. Marchiafava, and O. Pompeiano (1964b). Tonic and phasic inhibition of spinal reflexes during deep, desynchronized sleep in unrestrained cats. *Arch. Ital. Biol.* **102**, 471–499.

Gassel, M. M., P. Marchiafava, and O. Pompeiano (1964c). An analysis of the supraspinal influences acting on motoneurons during sleep in the unrestrained cat. *Arch. Ital. Biol.* **103**, 25–44.

Gasser, H. S., and H. Grundfest (1939). Axon diameters in relation to the spike dimensions and the conduction velocity in mammalian A fibers. *Am. J. Physiol.* **127**, 393–414.

Gastaut, H., C. Tassinari, and B. Duron (1965). Etude polygraphic des manifestations épisodiques (hypniques et respiratoires) diurnes et nocturnes de syndrome de Pickwick. *Rev. Neurol.* **112**, 568–578.

Gastaut, H., C. A. Tassinari, and B. Duron (1966). Polygraphic studies of the episodic and nocturnal (hypnic and respiratory) manifestations of the Pickwick syndrome. *Brain Res.* **2**, 167–186.

Gastaut, H., B. Duron, C. A. Tassinari, S. Luagoubi, and J. Saier (1969). Mechanism of the respiratory pauses accompanying slumber in the Pickwickian syndrome. *Act.Nerv. Super.* **11**, 209–215.

Giaquinto, S., O. Pompeiano, and I. Somogyi (1964). Supraspinal modulation of heteronymous monosynaptic and of polysynaptic reflexes during natural sleep and wakefulness. *Arch. Ital. Biol.* **102**, 245–281.

Granit, R., and B. R. Kaada (1953). Influence of stimulation of central nervous structures on muscle spindles in cat. *Acta Physiol. Scand.* **27**, 130–160.

Grunstein, M. M., M. Younes, and J. Milic-Emili (1973). Control of tidal volume and respiratory frequency in anesthetized cats. *J. Appl. Physiol.* **25**, 463–476.

Guilleminault, C., and W. Dement (1974). Pathologies of excessive sleep. *Adv. Sleep Res.* **1**, 345–390.

Guilleminault, C., W. Dement, and N. Monod (1973). Syndrome "mort subite du nourrisson": apnées au cours du sommeil. Nouvelle hypothèse. *Nouv. Presse Med.* **2**, 1355–1358.

Guilleminault, C., R. Peraita, M. Souquet, and W. C. Dement (1975). Apneas during sleep in infants: Possible relationship with sudden infant death syndrome. *Science* **190**, 677–679.

Guilleminault, C., F. L. Eldridge, F. B. Simmons, and W. C. Dement (1976a). Sleep apnea in eight children. *Pediatrics* **58**, 23–30.

Guilleminault, C., A. Tilkian, and W. C. Dement (1976b). The sleep apnea syndromes. *Annu. Rev. Med.* **27**, 465–484.

Haldane, J. S. (1905). The influence of high air temperature. *I. J. Hyg.* **5**, 494–513.

Hathorn, M. K. S. (1974). The rate and depth of breathing in new-born infants in different sleep states. *J. Physiol. (London)* **243**, 101–113.

Henderson-Smart, D. J., and D. J. C. Read (1976). Depression of respiratory muscles and defective responses to nasal obstruction during active sleep in the newborn. *Aust. Pediatr. J.* **12**, 261–266.

Hey, E. N., B. B. Lloyd, D. J. C. Cunningham, M. G. M. Jukes, and D. P. G. Bolton (1966). Effects of various respiratory stimuli on the depth and frequency of breathing in man. *Respir. Physiol.* **1**, 193–205.

Hobson, J. A. (1974). The cellular basis of sleep cycle control. *Adv. Sleep Res.* **1**, 217–250.

Hobson, J. A., R. W. McCarley, R. T. Pivik, and R. Freedman (1974). Selective firing by cat pontine brain stem neurons in desynchronized sleep. *J. Neurophysiol.* **37**, 497–511.

Hobson, J. A., R. W. McCarley, and P. W. Wyzinski (1975). Sleep cycle oscillation: Reciprocal discharge by two brainstem neuronal groups. *Science* **189**, 55–58.

Hodes, R., and W. C. Dement (1964). Depression of electrically induced reflexes ("H-reflexes") in man during low voltage EEG "sleep." *Electroencephalogr. Clin. Neurophysiol.* **17**, 617–629.

Hugelin, A., and F. Bertrand (1973). Le système pneumotaxique. *Arch. Ital. Biol.* **111**, 527–545.

Hugelin, A., and M. I. Cohen (1963). The reticular activating system and respiratory regulation in the cat. *Ann. N.Y. Acad. Sci.* **109**, 586–603.

Hyatt, R. E., and R. E. Wilcox (1961). Extrathoracic airway resistance in man. *J. Appl. Physiol.* **16**, 326–330.

Imes, N. K., W. C. Orr, R. O. Smith, and R. M. Rogers (1977). Refrognathia and sleep apnea. A life-threatening condition masquerading as narcolepsy. *J. Am. Med. Assoc.* **237**, 1596–1597.

Jasper, H. H. (1958). Report of the committee on methods of clinical examination in electroencephalography. *Electroencephalogr. Clin. Neurophysiol.* **10**, 370–375.

Jones, B. E., S. T. Harper, and A. E. Halavis (1977). Effects of locus coeruleus lesions upon cerebral monoamine content, sleep–wakefulness states and the response to amphetamine in the cat. *Brain Res.* **124**, 473–496.

Jouvet, M. F., F. Michel, and D. Mounier (1960). Analyse electroencephalographique comparée du sommeil physiologique chez le chat et chez l'homme. *Rev. Neurol.* **103**, 189–205.

Kanzow, E., D. Krause, and H. Kuhnel (1962). Die Vasomotorik der Hirnrinde in den Phasen desynchronisierter EEG-Aktivitat im naturlichen Schlaf der Katze. *Pfluegers Arch.* **274**, 593–607.

Kleitman, N. (1963). "Sleep and Wakefulness." Univ. of Chicago Press, Chicago, Illinois.

Knill, R., and A. C. Bryan (1976). An intercostal–phrenic inhibitory reflex in human newborn infants. *J. Appl. Physiol.* **40**, 352–356.

Krieger, J., D. Kurtz, and N. Roeslin (1976). Observation fibroscopique directé au cours de apnées hypniques chez un sujet pickwickien. *Nouv. Presse Med.* **5**, 2890.

Kubota, K., and R. Tanaka (1966). The fusimotor activity and natural sleep in the cat. *Brain Res.* **3**, 198–201.

Kubota, K., Y. Iwamura, and Y. Niimi (1965). Monosynaptic reflex and natural sleep in the cat. *J. Neurophysiol.* **28**, 125–138.

Kumagi, H., F. Sakai, A. Sukuma, and T. Hukuhara (1966). Relationship between activity of respiratory center and EEG. *Progr. Brain. Res.* **21A**, 98–111.

Levy, A. M., B. S. Tabakin, J. S. Hanson, and R. M. Narkewicz (1967). Hypertrophied adenoids causing pulmonary hypertension and severe congestive heart failure. *N. Engl. J. Med.* **277**, 506–511.

Lugaresi, E., P. Coccagna, P. Farneti, M. Mantovani, and F. Cirignotta (1975). Snoring. *Electroencephalogr. Clin. Neurophysiol.* **39**, 59–64.

Luke, M. J., A. Mehrizi, G. M. Folger, Jr., and R. D. Rowe (1966). Chronic nasopharyngeal obstruction as a cause of cardiomegaly, cor pulmonale, and pulmonary edema. *Pediatrics* **37**, 762–768.

McCarley, R. W., and J. A. Hobson (1971). Single neuron activity in cat gigantocellular tegmental field: Selectivity of discharge in desynchronized sleep. *Science* **174**, 1250–1252.

McCarley, R. W., and J. A. Hobson (1975a). Discharge patterns of cat pontine brain stem neurons during desynchronized sleep. *J. Neurophysiol.* **38**, 751–766.

McCarley, R. W., and J. A. Hobson (1975b). Neuronal excitability modulation over the sleep cycle: A structural and mathematical model. *Science* **189**, 58–60.

Magnussen, G. (1944). "Studies of the Respiration during Sleep: A Contribution to the Physiology of Sleep Function." Lewis, London.

Menashe, V. D., C. Farrehi, and M. Miller (1965). Hypoventilation and cor pulmonale due to chronic upper airway obstruction. *J. Pediatr.* **67**, 198–203.

Merrill, E. G. (1970). The lateral respiratory neurones of the medulla: Their associations with nucleus ambiguus, nucleus retroambigualis, the spinal accessory nucleus and the spinal cord. *Brain Res.* **24**, 11–28.

Morrison, A. R., and O. Pompeiano (1965a). An analysis of the supraspinal influences acting on motoneurons during sleep in the unrestrained cat. Responses of the alpha motoneurons to direct electrical stimulation during sleep. *Arch. Ital. Biol.* **103**, 497–516.

Morrison, A. R., and O. Pompeiano (1965b). Central depolarization of group Ia afferent fibers during desynchronized sleep. *Arch. Ital. Biol.* **103**, 517–537.

Morrison, A. R., and O. Pompeiano (1965c). Pyramidal discharge from somatosensory cortex and cortical control of primary afferents during sleep. *Arch. Ital. Biol.* **103**, 538–568.

Moruzzi, G. (1972). The sleep-waking cycle. *Ergeb. Physiol., Biol. Chem. Exp. Pharmakol.* **64**, 1–165.

Moruzzi, G., and H. W. Magoun (1949). Brain stem reticular formation and activation of the EEG. *Electroencephalogr. Clin. Neurophysiol.* **1**, 455–473.

Murakami, Y., and J. A. Kirchner (1972). Respiratory movements of the vocal cords, an electromyographic study in the cat. *Laryngoscope* **82**, 454–467.

Nesland, R. S., F. Plum, J. R. Nelson, and H. D. Siedler (1966). The graded response to stimulation of medullary respiratory neurons. *Exp. Neurol.* **14**, 57–76.

Netick, A., J. Orem, and W. Dement (1977). Neuronal activity specific to REM sleep and its relationship to breathing. *Brain Res.* **120**, 197–207.

Newsom Davis, J. (1974). Control of the muscles of breathing. *In* "Respiratory Physiology" (J. G. Widdicombe, ed.), pp. 221–245, University Park Press, Baltimore, Maryland.

Newsom Davis, J., and D. Stagg (1975). Interrelationships of the volume and time components of individual breaths in resting man. *J. Physiol. (London)* **245**, 481–498.

Orem, J. and R. Lydic (1978). Upper airway function during sleep and wakefulness: Experimental studies on normal and anesthetized cats. *Sleep* **1** (in press).

Orem, J., J. Montplaisir, and W. C. Dement (1974). Changes in the activity of respiratory neurons during sleep. *Brain Res.* **82**, 309–315.

Orem, J., A. Netick, and W. C. Dement (1977a). Breathing during sleep and wakefulness in the cat. *Respir. Physiol.* **30**, 265–289.

Orem, J., A. Netick and W. C. Dement (1977b). Increased upper airway resistance to breathing during sleep in the cat. *Electroencephalogr. Clin. Neurophysiol.* **43**, 14–22.

Orem, J., P. Norris, and R. Lydic (1978). Laryngeal abductor activity during sleep. *Chest* **73**, 300–301.

Østergaard, T. (1944). The excitability of the respiratory centre during sleep and during evipan anaesthesia. *Acta Physiol. Scand.* **8**, 1–15.

Paillard, J. (1955). "Reflexes et regulations d'origine proprioceptive chez l'homme. Etude neurophysiologique et psychophysiologique." Libraire Arnette, Paris.

Parmeggiani, P. L., and L. Sabattini (1972). Electromyographic aspects of postural, respiratory and thermoregulatory mechanisms in sleeping cats. *Electroencephalogr. Clin. Neurophysiol.* **33**, 1–13.

Parmeggiani, P. L., L. F. Agnati, G. Zamboni, and T. Cianci (1975). Hypothalamic temperature during the sleep cycle at different ambient temperatures. *Electroencephalogr. Clin. Neurophysiol.* **38**, 589–596.

Phillipson, E. A., and C. E. Sullivan (1977). Ventilatory and waking responses to hypercapnia and hypoxia during sleep. *Assoc. Psychophysiol. Study Sleep, 17th Annu. Meet.* Abstract.

Phillipson, E. A., E. Murphy, and L. F. Kozar (1976). Regulation of respiration in sleeping dogs. *J. Appl. Physiol.* **40**, 688–693.

Phillipson, E. A., L. F. Kozar, A. S. Rebuck, and E. Murphy (1977). Ventilatory and waking responses to CO_2 in sleeping dogs. *Am. Rev. Respir. Dis.* **115**, 251–259.

Pitts, R. F., H. W. Magoun, and S. W. Ranson (1939). Localization of the medullary respiratory centers in the cat. *Am. J. Physiol.* **126**, 673–688.

Plum, F., and A. G. Swanson (1958). Abnormalities in central regulation of respiration in acute and convalescent poliomyelitis. *Arch. Neurol. Psychiatry.* **80**, 267–285.

Pompeiano, O. (1966). Muscular afferents and motor control during sleep. *Muscular Afferents Motor Control. Proc. Nobel Symp., 1st, 1965* pp. 415–436.

Pompeiano, O. (1967). Sensory inhibition during motor activity in sleep. In "Neurophysiological Basis of Normal and Abnormal Motor Activities" (M. D. Yahr and D. P. Purpura, eds.), pp. 323–375. Raven Press, New York.

Pompeiano, O. (1973). Mechanisms of sensorimotor integration during sleep. *Prog. Physiol. Psychiatry* **3**, 1–179.

Priban, I. P. (1963). An analysis of some short-term patterns of breathing in man at rest. *J. Physiol. (London)* **166**, 425–434.

Puizillout, J.-J., and J.-P. Ternaux (1974). Variations d'activités toniques, phasiques et respiratoires, au niveau bulbaire pendant l'endormement de la préparation "encephale isolé." *Brain Res.* **66**, 67–83.

Ranson, S. W., H. Kabat, and H. W. Magoun (1935). Autonomic responses to electrical stimulation of hypothalamus, preoptic region and septum. *Arch. Neurol. Psychiatry* **33**, 467–477.

Rechtschaffen, A., and A. Kales (1968). "A Manual of Standardized Terminology, Techniques and Scoring System for Sleep Stages of Human Subjects," pp. 1–62. Public Health Serv., US Gov. Printing Office, Washington, D.C.

Redgate, E. S. (1963). Hypothalamic influence on respiration. *Ann. N.Y. Acad. Sci.* **109**, 606–618.

Reed, D. J., and R. H. Kellogg (1958). Changes in respiratory response to CO_2 during natural sleep at sea level and at altitude. *J. Appl. Physiol.* **13**, 325–330.

Remmers, J. E., D. Bartlett, Jr., and M. D. Putnam (1976). Changes in the respiratory cycle associated with sleep. *Respir. Physiol.* **28**, 227–238.

Remmers, J. E., W. J. deGroot, E. K. Sauerland, and A. M. Anch (1978). Pathogenesis of upper airway occlusion during sleep. *J. Appl. Physiol.* (in press).

Robin, E. D., R. D. Whaley, C. H. Crump, and D. M. Travis (1958). Alveolar gas tensions, pulmonary ventilation and blood pH during physiologic sleep in normal subjects. *J. Clin. Invest.* **37**, 981–989.

Robson, J. G., M. A. Houseley, and O. H. Solis-Quiroga (1963). The mechanism of respiratory arrest with sodium pentobarbital and sodium thiopental. *Ann. N.Y. Acad. Sci.* **109**, 494–502.

St. John, W. M., R. L. Glasser, and R. A. King (1972). Rhythmic respiration in awake vagotomized cats with chronic pneumotaxic area lesions. *Respir. Physiol.* **15**, 233–244.

Sauerland, E. K., and R. M. Harper (1976). The human tongue during sleep: Electromyographic activity of the genioglossus muscle. *Exp. Neurol.* **51**, 160–170.

Sears, T. A. (1963). Activity of fusimotor fibres innervating muscle spindles in the intercostal muscles of the cat. *Nature (London)* **197**, 1013–1014.

Sears, T. A. (1964a). Efferent discharges in alpha and fusimotor fibres of intercostal nerves of the cat. *J. Physiol. (London)* **174**, 295–315.

Sears, T. A. (1964b). Some properties and reflex connections of respiratory motoneurons of the cat's thoracic spinal cord. *J. Physiol. (London)* **175**, 386–403.

Sears, T. A. (1964c). The slow potentials of thoracic respiratory motoneurones and their relationship to breathing. *J. Physiol. (London)* **175**, 404–424.

Severinghaus, J. W., and R. A. Mitchell (1962). Ondine's curse—Failure of respiratory center automaticity while awake. *Clin. Res.* **10**, 122.

Shannon, D. C., and D. Kelly (1977). Impaired regulation of alveolar ventilation and the sudden infant death syndrome. *Science* **197**, 367–368.

Sherrey, J. H., and D. Megirian (1975). Analysis of the respiratory role of intrinsic laryngeal motoneurons of cat. *Exp. Neurol.* **49**, 456–465.

Siegel, J. M., and D. J. McGinty (1976). Brainstem neurons without spontaneous unit discharge. *Science* **193**, 240–242.

Siegel, J. M., and D. J. McGinty (1977). Pontine reticular formation neurons: Relationship of discharge to motoractivity. *Science* **196**, 678–680.

Snyder, F., J. A. Hobson, D. F. Morrison, and F. Goldfrank (1964). Changes in respiration, heartrate, and systolic blood pressure in human sleep. *J. Appl. Physiol.* **19**, 417–422.

Steinschneider, A. (1972). Prolonged apnea and the sudden infant death syndrome: Clinical and laboratory observations. *Pediatrics* **50**, 646–654.

Taber, E. (1961). The cytoarchitecture of the brain stem of the cat. I. Brain stem nuclei of cat. *J. Comp. Neurol.* **116**, 27–69.

Vertes, R. P. (1977). Selective firing of rat pontine gigantocellular neurons during movement and REM sleep. *Brain Res.* **128**, 146–152.

von Euler, C., and U. Söderberg (1956). The relation between gamma motor activity and the electroencephalogram. *Experientia* **12**, 278–279.

von Euler, C., and U. Söderberg (1957). The influence of hypothalamic thermoceptive structures on the electroencephalogram and gamma motor activity. *Electroencephalogr. Clin. Neurophysiol.* **9**, 391–408.

von Euler, C., and U. Söderberg (1958). Co-ordinated changes in temperature thresholds for thermoregulatory reflexes. *Acta Physiol. Scand.* **42**, 112–129.

von Euler, C., F. Herrero, and I. Wexler (1970). Control mechanisms determining rate and depth of respiratory movements. *Respir. Physiol.* **10,** 93–108.

Wall, P. D. (1958). Excitability changes in afferent fibre terminations and their relation to slow potentials. *J. Physiol. (London)* **142,** 1–21.

Weitzman, E. D., and L. Graziani (1974). Sleep and the sudden infant death syndrome. *Adv. Sleep Res.* **1,** 327–344.

Weitzman, E. D., C. Pollak, B. Borowiecki, B. Burack, R. Shprintzen, and S. Rakogg (1977). The hypersomnia sleep-apnea syndrome (CHSA): Site and mechanism of upper airway obstruction. Assoc. Psychophysiol. Study Sleep, *17th Annu. Meet.* Abstract.

CHAPTER 6

Hydrogen Ion Homeostasis
of the Cerebral
Extracellular Fluid

DONALD G. DAVIES

I. INTRODUCTION

The hydrogen ion homeostasis of the brain extracellular fluid (ECF) and its role in the regulation of pulmonary ventilation and cerebral blood flow

Regulation of Ventilation and Gas Exchange
Copyright © 1978 by Academic Press, Inc.
All rights of reproduction in any form reserved.
ISBN 0-12-204650-1

have been critically evaluated in several books, monographs, and review articles (Cunningham and Lloyd, 1963; Kellogg, 1964; Semple, 1965; Brooks *et al.*, 1965; Mitchell, 1966; Ingvar *et al.*, 1968; Cameron, 1969; Siesjö and Kjällquist, 1969; Siesjö and Sørensen, 1971; Siesjö, 1972; Leusen, 1972; Loeschcke, 1976). Cerebrospinal fluid (CSF) acid–base balance and its role in the regulation of ventilation was comprehensively reviewed by Leusen in 1972. Since then, there has been a prodigious increase in the number of investigations concerned with the regulation of CSF and ECF pH in chronic acid–base abnormalities. In the course of these investigations, several conflicting hypotheses dealing with the regulation of the CSF and ECF P_{CO_2} and bicarbonate concentration ($[HCO_3^-]$) have emerged, including: active transport of H^+ and/or HCO_3^-; active buffering of H^+ by brain tissue; passive distribution of H^+ and HCO_3^- between CSF and blood along electrochemical gradients; changes in cerebral metabolism; the Wien effect; carbonic anhydrase-mediated production of HCO_3^- by the central nervous system (CNS). In this chapter, I will discuss the research which led to the formulation of these hypotheses.

II.   REGULATION OF CSF P_{CO_2}

A.   Normal Values

1.   *Humans*

The majority of CSF acid–base measurements in humans have been made on lumbar samples and indicate that the CSF P_{CO_2} is 8–11 mm Hg higher than simultaneously measured arterial P_{CO_2} (Severinghaus *et al.*, 1963; Mitchell and Singer, 1965; van Heijst *et al.*, 1966; Siesjö, 1972; Dempsey *et al.*, 1974, 1975). The bicarbonate concentrations are approximately equal; lumbar pH is 0.7–0.8 units less than arterial.

Many of the deductions of cerebral acid–base homeostasis have been made on the assumption that the composition of lumbar CSF is representative of the ECF of the brain, based on the original observation of Bradley and Semple (1962) that cisternal and lumbar CSF were identical in the human. However, several recent investigations have demonstrated the existence of steady-state differences in the acid–base composition of lumbar and cisternal CSF, which become even more pronounced during acute respiratory alterations of arterial blood gases. Van Heijst *et al.* (1966) found that lumbar P_{CO_2} was 2.6 mm Hg higher than simultaneously measured cisternal P_{CO_2}. The bicarbonate concentrations were identical, and lumbar pH was 0.021 units less than cisternal. Plum and Posner (1968) compared lumbar and cisternal pH in ten acutely ill patients and found differences of up to 0.08 units, the cisternal being higher. Plum and Price (1973) observed a mean P_{CO_2} differences of 3.8 mm Hg between lumbar and cisternal CSF in 47 hospitalized patients. Similar measurements were recorded by Blayo et al. (1975). They found a mean lumbar–cisternal P_{CO_2} difference of 6.7 mm Hg in 20 healthy Andes natives at 3800 m altitude. Although Ganshirt (1968) noted qualitatively similar differences in hospitalized patients (7.6 mm Hg), he did not demonstrate that they were in a steady state.

Differences between lumbar and cisternal pH and P_{CO_2} have been observed in a variety of other animals. Plum and Posner (1968) measured a mean difference between cisternal and lumbar pH of 0.04 pH units in three tranquilized apes. Pavlin and Hornbein (1975a) found a mean difference in P_{CO_2} of 1.5 mm Hg between lumbar and cisternal CSF in control measurements in 29 anesthetized dogs. No differences were observed between the two values after 6 hours of either metabolic acidosis (Pavlin and Hornbein, 1975a) or metabolic alkalosis (Pavlin and Hornbein, 1975b); whereas, lumbar P_{CO_2} was 1.0 mm Hg higher after 6 hours of respiratory alkalosis (Hornbein and Pavlin, 1975) and 6.8 mm Hg higher after 6 hours of respiratory acidosis (Pavlin and Hornbein, 1975c).

The inhomogeneity of lumbar and cisternal CSF is magnified during acute respiratory changes in acid–base balance. Fisher and Christianson (1963) studied 12 patients and observed alterations in cisternal P_{CO_2} after 10 minutes of hyperventilation, but practically none in lumbar. Bradley et al. (1965) found that at least 20–30 minutes were required for cisternal P_{CO_2} to reach a steady state during CO_2 breathing. Also, Bradley and Semple (1962) demonstrated that lumbar CSF is not constantly related to cisternal until at least 4 hours after any large change in arterial acid–base status has occurred. In tranquilized apes, Plum and Posner (1968) found during induced respiratory acidosis or alkalosis that the cisternal–lumbar pH difference widened from a normal value of 0.04 pH units to a value of 0.06 pH units (0.108 pH units–the maximum difference). This difference was maintained for up to 5 hours.

In view of the discrepancies between lumbar and cisternal CSF, caution must be exercised when lumbar acid–base values are used to make inferences about the acid–base composition of the ECF of the brain, for the recorded changes in lumbar CSF may bear an uncertain relationship to those occurring in the brain.

A limited number of cisternal CSF acid–base measurements have been made in humans (Schwab, 1962; van Heijst et al., 1966; Plum and Price, 1973). The data indicate that cisternal P_{CO_2} is 5–8 mm Hg higher than arterial, that the bicarbonate concentrations are similar, and that the cisternal pH is 0.05–0.10 pH units less than arterial.

2. *Other Species*

The majority of CSF acid–base measurements in other species have been made in the dog, although some data have been reported for other animals, including the cat, goat, pony, and rat. Table I contains a list of the control acid–base values for cisternal CSF and arterial blood for a variety of animals.

In the dog, the P_{CO_2} differences between CSF and arterial blood range from 5 to 14 mm Hg, whereas, the pH differences range from -0.004 to -0.089 pH units. The extreme variability in reported CSF acid–base values is probably the result of at least two things: experimental error, and lack of a steady state. It is well recognized that it is difficult to make accurate measurements of CSF pH and P_{CO_2} because it is so poorly buffered (Mitchell, 1965; Leusen, 1965; Pappenheimer *et al.*, 1965; Fencl *et al.*, 1966, 1969; van Heijst *et al.*, 1966; Davies, 1976, 1977). Assuming that the low CSF P_{CO_2} and high pH CSF pH values are probably the result of experimental error, most investigators would agree that the normal CSF–arterial P_{CO_2} difference is between 10 and 14 mm Hg and the normal pH difference is between -0.07 and -0.08 pH units.

B. Relationship between CSF and Cerebral Venous P_{CO_2}

A great deal of controversy exists concerning whether CSF P_{CO_2} is less, equal to, or greater than cerebral venous P_{CO_2}. Lambertsen (1960) predicted on theoretical grounds that CSF P_{CO_2} should be equal to cerebral venous P_{CO_2}. Bradley and Semple (1962) found in humans that lumbar CSF and internal jugular venous P_{CO_2} values were equal, whereas Pappenheimer *et al.* (1965) concluded that CSF and cerebral venous P_{CO_2} were equal based on similarities between CSF/arterial and arterial/cerebral venous P_{CO_2} values.

Pontén and Siesjö (1966), on the other hand, believe that CSF P_{CO_2} is less than cerebral venous P_{CO_2}. From simultaneous measurements in cats of Pa_{CO_2} from the femoral artery, cerebral venous P_{CO_2} from the superior sagittal sinus, and cisternal CSF P_{CO_2}, they found that CSF P_{CO_2} was significantly lower than cerebral venous and was close to 1 mm Hg above the arithmetic mean of arterial and cerebral venous P_{CO_2} values. They concluded from their study that CSF and brain tissue P_{CO_2} could be calculated either from arterial and cerebral venous P_{CO_2} values or from the arterial P_{CO_2} when the normal arterial–venous P_{CO_2} difference is known.

These relationships among cisternal CSF, arterial and cerebral venous P_{CO_2} values have been confirmed by Plum and Price (1973) in 47 patients and by Blayo *et al.* (1975) in 20 healthy Andes natives. Similar observations have been noted by Caronna *et al.* (1974) in unanesthetized rats in

Table I. Normal Control Acid–Base Values for Cisternal CSF

Species	n	P_{CO_2}			[HCO$_3^-$]			pH			Source
		Art	CSF	Δ	Art	CSF	Δ	Art	CSF	Δ	
Cat	9	26.6	31.6	5.0	14.7	16.4	1.7	7.370	7.350	−0.020	Swanson and Rosengren (1962)
Sheep	4	39.2	44.0	4.8	28.1	22.8	5.3	7.480	7.320	−0.016	Hodson et al. (1968)
Goat	4	37.6	47.6	10.0	27.4	20.7	−6.7	7.487	7.283	−0.204	Fencl et al. (1966)
Rat	16	38.1	45.0	6.9	28.9	27.6	−1.3	7.499	7.417	−0.082	Pontén and Siesjö (1967)
Calf	8	38.7	48.6	9.9	10.6	21.3	0.7	7.340	7.280	−0.060	Bisgard et al. (1973)
Pony	4	38.7	47.6	8.9	24.5	24.7	0.2	7.424	7.334	−0.090	Orr et al. (1975)
Pony	10	39.6	46.0	6.4	25.6	22.9	−2.7	7.429	7.339	−0.090	Forster et al. (1976)
Pony	9	41.5	50.4	9.0	25.8	24.8	−1.0	7.415	7.327	−0.088	Bisgard et al. (1976)
Dog	10	40.0	46.0	6.0	21.8	22.6	0.8	7.370	7.320	−0.050	Robin et al. (1958)
Dog	35	36.0	45.0	9.0	24.2	23.5	−0.7	7.420	7.357	−0.063	Bleich et al. (1964)
Dog	30	39.4	46.8	7.4	22.9	24.1	1.2	7.352	7.348	−0.004	Adaro et al. (1969)
Dog	20	40	47	7.0	25	24.7	−0.3	7.386	7.351	−0.035	Chazan et al. (1969)
Dog	6	36.5	41.4	4.9	21.5	20.5	−1.0	7.408	7.349	−0.059	Kazemi et al. (1969)
Dog	19	41.8	50.7	8.9	24.0	24.5	0.5	7.400	7.322	−0.078	Mines et al. (1971)
Dog	15	42.7	50.7	8.0	24.4	24.4	0	7.398	7.316	−0.082	Mines and Sørensen (1971)
Dog	6	40	47	7.0	22.8	21.0	−1.8	7.371	7.282	−0.089	Kazemi et al. (1973)
Dog	4	34.6	44.4	9.8	22.3	23.9	1.6	7.392	7.334	−0.058	Bureau and Bouverot (1975)
Dog	29	33.5	48.0	14.5	22.4	24.9	2.5	7.401	7.347	−0.054	Pavlin and Hornbein (1975a)
Dog	4	39.4	48.9	9.5	24.3	23.8	−0.5	7.401	7.320	−0.081	Bledsoe and Mines (1975)
Dog	54	40.7	46.3	5.6	21.9	22.8	0.9	7.350	7.328	−0.022	Pelligrino and Dempsey (1976)
Dog	6	38.8	48.1	9.3	22.3	23.0	0.7	7.382	7.324	−0.058	Choma and Kazemi (1976)
Dog	10	36.2	46.8	10.6	22.9	22.7	−0.2	7.393	7.307	−0.086	Davies (1978)
Man	15	37.5	45.2	7.7	24.9	23.6	−1.3	7.424	7.349	−0.075	Schwab (1962)
Man	13	40.5	46.5	6.0	24.3	24.9	0.6	7.397	7.346	−0.051	van Heijst et al. (1966)
Man	6	38.1	42.9	4.8	24.7	22.1	−2.6	7.428	7.328	−0.100	Plum and Price (1973)

acute respiratory acidosis and alkalosis and in chronic metabolic acidosis. These relationships were also validated during carbonic anhydrase inhibition in the cat and rat (Brzezinski *et al.*, 1967).

Davies, Gurtner, and colleagues (Davies *et al.*, 1973; Davies and Gurtner, 1973; Gurtner *et al.*, 1972, 1974; Razavi *et al.*, 1977), have reported experimental results which do not conform to the predictions of Pontén and Siesjö (1966). They demonstrated that cisternal CSF P_{CO_2} was higher than simultaneously measured cerebral venous P_{CO_2} (Gurtner *et al.*, 1972, 1974; Razavi *et al.*, 1977). The CSF P_{CO_2} also exceeded the value that would have been calculated by Pontén and Siesjö (1966) from arterial and venous P_{CO_2} values (Davies *et al.*, 1973; Davies and Gurtner, 1973). Similar observations have been made by other investigators. Kazemi *et al.* (1973) and Wichser and Kazemi (1975) reported cisternal CSF P_{CO_2} values which exceeded superior sagittal sinus P_{CO_2}; whereas, larger than predicted CSF–arterial P_{CO_2} differences have been reported in goat (Fencl *et al.*, 1966), calf (Bisgard *et al.*, 1973), pony (Orr *et al.*, 1975; Bisgard *et al.*, 1976), and dog (Bleich *et al.*, 1964; Mines *et al.*, 1971; Mines and Sørensen, 1971; Bureau and Bouverot, 1975; Pavlin and Hornbein, 1975a; Bledsoe and Mines, 1975; Choma and Kazemi, 1976; Davies, 1978).

The "charged membrane hypothesis" (Wien effect) was proposed (Davies and Gurtner, 1973, 1975; Davies *et al.*, 1973) to account for these observations. According to the hypothesis, when blood enters a capillary there is a rapid movement of H^+ away from blood proteins toward the negatively charged capillary wall and a slower repulsion of HCO_3^- away from the wall, resulting in the formation of H_2CO_3 which immediately dissociates to form $CO_2 + H_2O$. This CO_2 increases the P_{CO_2} at the capillary wall and acts as a barrier to the diffusion of CO_2 out of the CSF and thereby increases the CSF P_{CO_2}. The most important aspect of this nonequilibrium is that H^+ must move toward the wall at a faster rate than the HCO_3^- can diffuse away in order for the reaction to proceed to the right and form CO_2. This is hypothesized to be due to the increased H^+ dissociation of blood proteins when they are exposed to the electrical field in the capillary caused by the fixed negative charges on the wall (Wien effect). The hypothesis predicts that the magnitude of the P_{CO_2} difference should vary inversely with arterial pH and capillary transit time. A decrease in cerebral blood flow rate (increase in transit time) will cause the P_{CO_2} gradient to diminish because there will be enough time for the increased $[H^+]$ at the capillary wall to be balanced by a decrease in $[HCO_3^-]$ as a result of electrostatic repulsion by the fixed negative charges. An increase in acidity will increase the P_{CO_2} difference, because there is more H^+ available to diffuse toward the capillary wall.

C. Relationship between CSF–Arterial P_{CO_2} Difference and Cerebral Blood Flow

1. Humans

The P_{CO_2} difference between CSF and arterial blood depends on the rate of CO_2 production by brain tissue, the diffusion coefficient for CO_2, the distance for diffusion, and the cerebral blood flow rate (CBF). At a given metabolic rate, provided all other factors are assumed to be constant, the P_{CO_2} difference should be inversely related to the CBF if no other mechanism is acting, e.g., the charged membrane effect. Because the CBF varies directly with arterial P_{CO_2} (Kety and Schmidt, 1948; Reivich, 1964), the CSF–arterial P_{CO_2} difference should decrease in respiratory acidosis and increase in respiratory alkalosis.

Inverse relationships between the CSF–arterial P_{CO_2} gradient and arterial P_{CO_2} have been observed in humans during chronic respiratory acidosis and alkalosis (Fisher and Christianson, 1963; Posner et al., 1965; Alroy and Flenley, 1967; Sørensen and Milledge, 1971; Plum and Price, 1973; Pontén, 1977) and during chronic metabolic acidosis and alkalosis (Plum and Price, 1973; Marks et al., 1973). However, the majority of human measurements indicates that the P_{CO_2} difference increases with arterial P_{CO_2} in both chronic respiratory acidosis (Merwarth et al., 1961; Pauli et al., 1962; Severinghaus et al., 1963; Severinghaus and Carcelén B., 1964; Mitchell et al., 1965; Mitchell, 1966; Huang and Lyons, 1966; Bulger et al., 1966; Dempsey et al., 1974; Blayo et al., 1975) and metabolic acidosis (Pauli et al., 1962; Cowie et al., 1962; Bradley and Semple, 1962; Pauli and Reubi, 1963; Posner et al., 1965; Mitchell and Singer, 1965; Mitchell et al., 1965; Mitchell, 1966; Posner and Plum, 1967; Pierce et al., 1971).

Both Siesjö (1972) and Caronna et al. (1974) stressed that the physiological significance of these observations with regard to brain ECF acid–base regulation must be interpreted with caution; in many instances, patients with chronic acid–base abnormalities also have accompanying hypoxia and heart failure. Also, the majority of values reported here were obtained from lumbar samples and, as mentioned previously, lumbar CSF measurements are usually not adequate for estimating the acid–base status of the brain ECF, especially during nonsteady-state conditions. The problem of cerebral ECF acid–base regulation in humans will not be understood fully until more cisternal CSF measurements have been made.

2. Experimental Animals

Several studies in various experimental animals have demonstrated an inverse relationship between the cisternal CSF–arterial P_{CO_2} difference and arterial P_{CO_2}. Leusen and Demeester (1964) observed an increase in the P_{CO_2} difference from 6 to 12 mm Hg in anesthetized dogs after 7–8 hours of hypocapnia. Pappenheimer *et al.* (1965) and Fencl *et al.* (1966), in six awake goats, noted a decrease from 11.0 to 7.5 mm Hg as arterial P_{CO_2} increased from 25 to 55 mm Hg during perfusion of the ventricular–cisternal system with artificial CSF. Pontén and Siesjö (1966) observed a decrease with increased arterial P_{CO_2} over the range of 30–90 mm Hg in anesthetized cats. Caronna *et al.* (1974) made the same observation in rats.

However, there have been a number of instances in which a direct relationship between the CSF–arterial P_{CO_2} gradient and arterial P_{CO_2} was found. Bleich *et al.* (1964) studied chronic respiratory acidosis (12% CO_2 for 5 days) in 35 unanesthetized dogs and observed an increase from 9 to 16 mm Hg as the arterial P_{CO_2} increased from 36 to 75 mm Hg. Chazan *et al.* (1969) made measurements of CSF and arterial blood in six dogs during chronic respiratory acidosis (8.8% CO_2 for 5 days) and noted an increase from 7 to 10 mm Hg as arterial P_{CO_2} increased from 40 to 63 mm Hg. Adaro *et al.* (1969), in ten anesthetized dogs, observed an increase from 8.1 to 16.4 mm Hg as the arterial P_{CO_2} was increased from 38.3 to 81.3 mm Hg for 4 hours.

Plum and Posner (1967) studied respiratory alkalosis in six anesthetized dogs for 6 hours. A decrease in the difference from 10.1 to 7.0 mm Hg was noted as arterial P_{CO_2} was reduced from 45.5 to 7.9 mm Hg. Similarly, Plum *et al.* (1968) demonstrated a decrease from 10.1 to 7.6 mm Hg in five anesthetized dogs after 5 hours of hyperventilation when arterial P_{CO_2} was reduced from 45.5 to 8.0 mm Hg.

Davies and Gurtner (1973) measured CSF and arterial acid–base balance during respiratory acidosis and respiratory alkalosis and found a gradient in four anesthetized dogs of 17.9 mm Hg when the arterial P_{CO_2} was increased from 31.8 to 49.1 mm Hg for 5 hours, and a gradient in four other dogs of 4.2 mm Hg when the P_{CO_2} was decreased from 31.1 to 12.6 mm Hg for 5 hours. Similar observations were recorded by Pavlin and Hornbein (1975c), who found a difference of 24.4 mm Hg after 6 hours of hypercapnia (arterial P_{CO_2} increased from 33.6 to 56.8 mm Hg) in six anesthetized dogs and a difference of 13.4 mm Hg after 6 hours of hyperventilation (arterial P_{CO_2} decreased from 31.8 to 19.5 mm Hg) in six dogs (Hornbein and Pavlin, 1975).

Although these studies demonstrate that the magnitude of the CSF–arterial P_{CO_2} difference increases in respiratory acidosis and decreases in respiratory alkalosis, they do not prove that there is a direct relationship between the P_{CO_2} difference and the cerebral blood flow rate, because cerebral blood flow was not measured. Siesjö and Zwentnow (1970), observed a slight increase in rats in the difference (from 10 to 12 mm Hg) with hypovolemic hypotension, but they did not measure cerebral blood flow. MacMillan and Siesjö (1971) demonstrated an inverse relationship between the difference and arterial P_{O_2} when it was less than 40 mm Hg. Cerebral blood flow was also not measured in this study.

There are two reports in the literature which include both cerebral blood flow and CSF–arterial P_{CO_2} measurements. However, the results are contradictory. Shannon et al. (1970), in eight anesthetized dogs, observed an increase when cerebral blood flow was reduced to 42% of its control value, whereas Razavi et al. (1977) demonstrated a direct relationship between both the CSF–sagittal sinus and the CSF–arterial P_{CO_2} difference and cerebral blood flow rate over a range of 10–160 ml min^{-1} 100 gm^{-1} in 20 healthy, anesthetized dogs. Because there is experimental evidence both for and against a direct relationship between the CSF–arterial P_{CO_2} difference and cerebral blood flow rate, additional studies which include simultaneous measurements of cerebral blood flow and CSF and blood P_{CO_2} values will have to be performed if this question is to be resolved.

D. Relationship between CSF–Arterial P_{CO_2} Difference and Arterial Acidity ([H$^+$]a)

Under normal circumstances, changes in the CSF–arterial P_{CO_2} difference with arterial acidity would not be expected unless there were accompanying alterations in the cerebral blood flow rate. In this case, an inverse relationship should pertain. Leusen and Demeester (1964) demonstrated an increase in the difference, with decreases in acidity induced by respiratory alkalosis; Pappenheimer et al. (1965) and Fencl et al. (1966) observed a decrease with increased acidity during respiratory acidosis in six awake goats. Inverse relationships between the P_{CO_2} gradient and acidity have also been noted by Pontén and Siesjö (1966) in the cat and by Caronna et al. (1974) in the rat during respiratory acidosis and respiratory alkalosis. Pontén (1977) made measurements during metabolic alterations in acid–base balance in 12 dogs but was unable to demonstrate any correlation between the P_{CO_2} difference and acidity.

There are several studies in the literature which are in contrast to these observations. Bleich et al. (1964), in 35 dogs, observed an increase in the P_{CO_2} difference from 9 to 16 mm Hg during chronic respiratory acidosis when [H$^+$]a increased from 38 to 52 nM/liter. Chazan et al. (1969) noted an increase from 7 to 10 mm Hg in six dogs during chronic respiratory acidosis as [H$^+$]a was increased from 44.6 to 53.0 nM/liter. Furthermore,

Adaro *et al.* (1969) demonstrated in ten dogs an increase from 9.0 to 16.4 mm Hg after 4 hours of respiratory acidosis superimposed on metabolic alkalosis when [H^+]a increased from 22 to 47 nM/liter.

During respiratory alkalosis in six anesthetized dogs, Plum and Posner (1967) observed a decrease in the P_{CO_2} difference from 10.1 to 7.0 mm Hg after 6 hours of hyperventilation when [H^+]a decreased from 54.5 to 16.7 nM/liter. Plum *et al.* (1968) noted a similar decrease (from 10.1 to 7.6 mm Hg) in five dogs after 5 hours of hyperventilation when [H^+]a decreased from 54.5 to 17.3 nM/liter.

More recently, Davies and Gurtner (1973) observed a CSF–arterial P_{CO_2} difference of 17.9 mm Hg in four anesthetized dogs after 5 hours of respiratory acidosis when [H^+] was increased from 42.8 to 62.3 nM/liter, and a difference of 4.2 mm Hg in four dogs during 5 hours of respiratory alkalosis when [H^+]a was decreased from 46.6 to 27.4 nM/liter. In addition, Pavlin and Hornbein (1975c) noted differences of 24.4 mm Hg in six anesthetized dogs after 6 hours of hypercapnia ([H^+]a increased from 19.3 to 59.6 nM/liter) and 13.4 mm Hg in six anesthetized dogs after 6 hours of hypocapnia ([H^+]a decreased from 39.6 to 26.3 nM/liter) (Hornbein and Pavlin, 1975).

Direct relationships between the P_{CO_2} gradient and [H^+]a have also been demonstrated several times during metabolic alterations in acid–base balance. Alexander *et al.* (1962) observed an increase from 11.5 to 17.4 mm Hg in three anesthetized dogs during hyperthermia and lactic acidosis when [H^+]a increased from 47.9 to 66.4 nM/liter. Fencl *et al.* (1966), in the awake goat, noted differences of 11.2 mm Hg in chronic metabolic acidosis ([H^+]a = 59.9 nM/liter) and 7.9 mm Hg in chronic metabolic alkalosis ([H^+]a = 28.5 nM/liter). In nine anesthetized dogs, Mines *et al.* (1971) observed an increase in the difference from 9.0 to 11.0 mm Hg during 6 hours of metabolic acidosis when [H^+]a increased from 39.6 to 50.6 nM/liter. Davies and Gurtner (1973) observed differences of 24.7 mm Hg in five anesthetized dogs after 6 hours of metabolic acidosis ([H^+]a increased from 35.9 to 66.1 nM/liter) and 14.5 mm Hg in four anesthetized dogs after 5 hours of metabolic alkalosis ([H^+]a decreased from 50.5 to 27.3 nM/liter). Pavlin and Hornbein (1975a) noted a difference of 19.2 mm Hg in six anesthetized dogs after 6 hours of metabolic acidosis when [H^+]a was increased from 40.4 to 64.9 nM/liter. Recently, Razavi *et al.* (1977) studied 20 healthy, anesthetized dogs during 6 hours of compensated metabolic acidosis and observed a CSF–arterial P_{CO_2} gradient of 13.4 mm Hg and a CSF–superior sagittal sinus P_{CO_2} gradient of 7.2 mm Hg. These values were intermediate to those found by Davies and Gurtner (1973) during metabolic acidosis and respiratory alkalosis in the anesthetized dog.

E. Conclusions

It is evident from the preceding discussion that there is a great deal of controversy concerning the normal values for the CSF–arterial and CSF–cerebral venous P_{CO_2} differences as well as relationships between the magnitude of these differences and both arterial acidity and cerebral blood flow rate. At least part of the discrepancy must be attributed to the technical difficulties associated with making accurate measurements of CSF acid–base composition. Another factor to be considered is that many conclusions concerning CSF acid–base balance have been made utilizing measurements of lumbar CSF; lumbar CSF is not necessarily representative of cerebral extracellular fluid, especially during nonsteady state conditions.

There is experimental evidence which indicates that CSF P_{CO_2} can be either greater than, less than, or equal to cerebral venous P_{CO_2}; it therefore appears that any definitive conclusions regarding these relationships must await further investigation. Similar conclusions must be drawn regarding the relationships between the CSF–arterial P_{CO_2} difference and both cerebral blood flow and arterial acidity.

III. REGULATION OF CSF BICARBONATE CONCENTRATION

The relative stability of the CSF pH in chronic metabolic acid–base disturbances has been known since the early work of Collip and Backus (1920), and numerous reports have subsequently demonstrated that CSF pH is close to its normal value in chronic metabolic acidosis (Bradley and Semple, 1962; Cowie et al., 1962; Manfredi, 1962; Pauli et al., 1962; Schwab, 1962; Agrest and Roehr, 1963; Buhlmann et al., 1963; Pauli and Reubi, 1963; Mitchell et al., 1965; Posner et al., 1965; Albert et al., 1966; Fencl et al., 1966; Chazan et al., 1969) and chronic metabolic alkalosis (Bradley and Semple, 1962; Manfredi, 1962; Schwab and Dammaschke, 1962; Agrest and Roehr, 1963; Mitchell et al., 1965; Posner et al., 1965; Fencl et al., 1966; Pontén and Siesjö, 1967).

CSF pH is similarly regulated, although to a lesser degree, in chronic respiratory acidosis (Merwarth et al., 1961; Swanson and Rosengren, 1962; Schwab, 1962; Buhlmann et al., 1963; Fisher and Christianson, 1963; Bleich et al., 1964; Mitchell et al., 1965; Huang and Lyons, 1966; Pontén, 1966; Alroy and Flenley, 1967; Kazemi et al., 1967; Adaro et al., 1969; Lee et al., 1969) and respiratory alkalosis (Pauli et al., 1962; Severinghaus et al., 1963; Leusen and Demeester, 1964; Mitchell et al., 1965; van Vaerenbergh et al., 1965; Kazemi et al., 1967; Plum et al., 1968).

Several mechanisms have been proposed to account for the relative stability of the CSF pH including: (a) active transport of HCO_3^- between CSF and blood by a pump located at the blood–brain barrier; (b) passive distribution of H^+ and HCO_3^- between CSF and blood along electrochemical potential gradients; (c) carbonic anhydrase-mediated formation of CSF HCO_3^- from cells in the CNS; (d) HCO_3^- generation via active H^+ buffering by the brain tissue due to the selective increase in brain ammonia levels; (e) metabolic alteration of the $[HCO_3^-]$ in the choroid plexus secretion by variable brain lactic acid production; (f) Wien effect.

A.   Active Transport of HCO_3^- between CSF and Blood

Severinghaus *et al.* (1963), in studies of ventilatory acclimatization to high altitude in man, observed that the hypoxia-induced respiratory alkalosis resulted in a fall in CSF $[HCO_3^-]$ which was sufficient to restore the CSF pH back to a normal value. They found after acclimatization that CSF $[H^+]$ and $[HCO_3^-]$ were not in electrochemical equilibrium with blood, and postulated that the restoration of the CSF pH during respiratory alkalosis was due to the active transport of HCO_3^- out of the CSF by a pump located at the blood–brain barrier. Active transport has also been proposed for the relative stability of CSF pH observed in a variety of other chronic acid–base abnormalities (Pappenheimer *et al.*, 1965; Pappenheimer, 1967; Fencl *et al.*, 1966; Mitchell, 1965; Mitchell *et al.*, 1965). Severinghaus (1965) obtained experimental evidence in favor of the active transport hypothesis by demonstrating significant increases in the electrochemical potentials for H^+ and HCO_3^- during both metabolic and respiratory alkalosis. During metabolic alkalosis, the final electrochemical potentials for H^+ and HCO_3^- were at twice the normal disequilibrium. However, the electrochemical potential values were calculated on the assumption that the electrical potential difference between CSF and blood (E) returned to normal during sustained alterations in blood acid–base balance; and subsequent measurements of E have shown that this is not the case. Goodrich (1965) found in rats, that the potential difference slope $(\Delta E/\Delta pH)$ and intercept remained constant after 3 days of either metabolic acidosis or metabolic alkalosis, indicating that the transient responses observed in acute changes in arterial pH are upheld in the chronic state of acid–base imbalance. This observation has been substantiated by several other investigators (Kjällquist and Siesjö, 1967; Kjällquist, 1970; Messeter and Siesjö, 1971a; Pavlin and Hornbein, 1975a,b,c; Hornbein and Pavlin, 1975). In addition, Bledsoe and Mines (1975) have shown that the potential difference remains elevated during sustained elevations of plasma K^+ concentration.

**B. Passive Distribution of H^+ and HCO_3^- between CSF
and Blood along Electrochemical Potential
Gradients**

Siesjö and Kjällquist (1969) proposed that the distribution of H^+ and HCO_3^- between CSF and blood might be explained by a passive ion distribution according to E. They also suggested that the electrochemical disequilibrium which exists under normal conditions was due to metabolic production of H^+ by the brain cells in conjunction with a low permeability of the blood–brain barrier to H^+ and HCO_3^-. According to the hypothesis, the CSF pH would be set by a balance between the rate of influx of acid from the cerebral tissue and the rat outflux of H^+ from the CSF along the electrochemical potential gradient. During chronic acid–base derangements, the CSF and ECF $[H^+]$ and $[HCO_3^-]$ would be regulated by alterations in the CSF–blood potential difference and by the factors which readjust plasma pH, i.e., changes in pulmonary ventilation and plasma $[HCO_3^-]$. In addition, under certain circumstances, e.g., during hypoxia or hyperventilation, the outflux of lactic acid from cells would become important.

Before considering any further the experimental evidence which supports or refutes the concept of passive regulation of the CSF and ECF $[H^+]$ and $[HCO_3^-]$, I would first like to discuss what is presently known about the CSF–blood potential difference.

1. CSF–Blood Potential Difference

The existence of a dc potential difference between CSF and blood was first reported by Lehmann and Meesman (1924), who found a difference of 6–15 mV in anesthetized cats and rabbits. Numerous CSF–blood potential difference measurements have been reported since then (Tschirgi and Taylor, 1958; Severinghaus et al., 1963; Held et al., 1964; Goodrich, 1965; Severinghaus, 1965; Kjällquist and Siesjö, 1967; Bradbury and Kleeman, 1967; Kjällquist, 1970; Cameron and Kleeman, 1970; Sørensen and Severinghaus, 1970; Messeter and Siesjö, 1971a; Hornbein and Sørensen, 1972; Davies and Dutton, 1972; Cameron et al., 1973; Cameron and Miller, 1973; Bledsoe and Mines, 1975; Pavlin and Hornbein, 1975a,b,c; Hornbein and Pavlin, 1975).

Tschirgi and Taylor (1958) demonstrated that E was sensitive to changes in the pH of the arterial blood, the CSF potential becoming more positive with increasing acidity. This relationship was quantified in anesthetized dogs by Held et al. (1964). They found that E, measured between the cisterna magna and the jugular vein, was 4–6 mV at an arterial pH of 7.4 and that it varied linearly with changes in pH with a slope of

-31.7 mV/pH unit during respiratory acidosis and alkalosis and -42.6 mV/pH unit during metabolic acidosis and alkalosis. The potential is not sensitive to changes in the acidity of the ECF of the brain, induced either by ventriculocisternal perfusion (Held *et al.*, 1964) or by cerebral hypoxia (Sørensen and Severinghaus, 1970).

Neither the origin of the potential difference nor the cause of its sensitivity to changes in the pH of the arterial blood is known. Held *et al.* (1964) found that decreasing the CSF $[K^+]$ increased the potential difference, but that changes in plasma $[K^+]$ had no effect. However, several other investigators have shown that acutely increasing the K^+ concentration of the plasma does cause an increase in the magnitude of the potential difference (Tschirgi and Taylor, 1958; Bradbury and Kleeman, 1967; Cameron and Kleeman, 1970; Cameron and Miller, 1973; Cameron *et al.*, 1973; Bledsoe and Mines, 1975). The potential difference is at least partially related to the active transport of Na^+ into the CSF, for Held *et al.* (1964) demonstrated that perfusion of the ventriculocisternal system for 2 hours with 10^{-5} M ouabain reduced $\Delta E/\Delta pH$ by about 50%. The effect of ouabain on the potential difference led Woodbury (1971) to postulate that the pH sensitivity might be the result of pH-related changes in the permeability of the blood–brain barrier to Na^+, i.e., that a decrease in plasma pH causes an increase in Na^+ permeability. However, he thinks it more probable that the pH sensitivity is related to a decrease in Cl^- permeability which occurs as the pH decreases. The decrease in permeability would increase the drag on Cl^-, necessitating an increase in the rate of Na^+ pumping into the CSF. This hypothesis is supported by measurements in frog skeletal muscle, in which a decrease in pH caused a decrease in Cl^- permeability (Hutter and Warner, 1967).

Davies and Dutton (1972) administered acetazolamide both intracisternally (50 mg) and intravenously (50 mg/kg) in anesthetized dogs, and found that $\Delta E/\Delta pH$ was reduced by approximately 50%. On the basis of this observaton, they postulated that part of the potential difference was a HCO_3^- diffusion potential, which was abolished by carbonic anhydrase inhibition because of the reduction in CSF $[HCO_3^-]$. This hypothesis is supported by several studies which have shown that acetazolamide decreases CSF HCO_3^- formation when given intravenously (Maren and Broder, 1970; Maren, 1971, 1972; Vogh and Maren, 1975) or intraventricularly (Wichser and Kazemi, 1975; Hasan and Kazemi, 1976; Kazemi and Choma, 1977). The pH sensitivity of the potential difference could also be accounted for on the basis of a HCO_3^- diffusion potential, because the CSF/blood $[HCO_3^-]$ ratio changes in the required direction during both respiratory and metabolic alterations of acid–base balance.

Messeter (1972) measured the potential difference before and after the administration of acetazolamide and found no difference in $\Delta E/\Delta pH$. However, the drug was only administered intravenously, and Davies and Dutton (1972) found that the potential difference was reduced only when the acetazolamide was given both intravenously and intracisternally.

Hornbein and Sørensen (1972) attempted to establish the site of formation of the CSF–blood potential. They made potential difference measurements in anesthetized dogs between blood and (a) lateral ventricle; (b) cisterna magna; and (c) lumbar subarachnoid space, before and after cervical spinal cord transection. Before transection, the respective slopes were -35.9, -26.2, and -5.2 mV/pH unit. The observation of a decreasing slope with distance from the lateral ventricle indicated a role of the choroid plexus in the generation of the potential difference. However, the pH sensitivity was still present when the spinal subarachnoid space was isolated from the rest of the brain, indicating that whatever role the choroid plexus may play, it is not the sole source of the pH-sensitive potential. The authors postulated that the entire blood–brain barrier in both the brain and spinal cord is a major source of the potential difference.

2. Observations Consistent with Passive Distribution of H^+ and HCO_3^- between CSF and Blood According to Changes in E

If H^+ and HCO_3^- were passively distributed between CSF and blood during sustained acid–base abnormalities, assuming the rate of production of H^+ by the tissue and the permeability of the blood–brain barrier to H^+ and HCO_3^- remained constant, the electrochemical potential differences should not be significantly different from the control values once a new steady state has been reached. This hypothesis was tested in the elegant experiments of Pavlin and Hornbein (1975a,b,c; Hornbein and Pavlin, 1975), in which they made simultaneous measurements of the CSF–blood potential difference and CSF and arterial $[H^+]$ and $[HCO_3^-]$ in anesthetized dogs and calculated the changes in the electrochemical potential difference for H^+ ($\Delta\mu H^+$) and HCO_3^- ($\Delta\mu HCO_3^-$) during 6 hours of either metabolic or respiratory acidosis and alkalosis. They found after 6 hours of isocapnic metabolic acidosis (Pavlin and Hornbein, 1975a), isocapnic metabolic alkalosis (Pavlin and Hornbein, 1975b), respiratory acidosis (Pavlin and Hornbein, 1975c), and respiratory alkalosis that both $\Delta\mu H^+$ and $\Delta\mu HCO_3^-$ had returned to within 1 mV of the control values. According to the hypothesis, the return of $\Delta\mu$ to the control values can be explained by passive distribution of H^+ and HCO_3^- across the blood–brain barrier.

Several other experiments provide data consistent with the passive distribution concept. Electrochemical potential difference values for H^+

and HCO_3^-, calculated from data obtained during sustained metabolic acidosis of either 5–6 hours (Adaro et al., 1969; Kjällquist, 1970; Mines et al., 1971) or 4–8 days (Fencl et al., 1966; Chazan et al., 1969) duration, were relatively close to the control values. Similar results were obtained for sustained metabolic alkalosis lasting either 5 hours (Adaro et al., 1969) or 5–9 days (Fencl et al., 1966; Chazan et al., 1969); respiratory acidosis lasting either 4–5 hours (Kazemi et al., 1967; Adaro et al., 1969) or 3–5 days (Bleich et al., 1964; Chazan et al., 1969; Messeter and Siesjö, 1971b); and respiratory alkalosis lasting 6 hours (Kazemi et al., 1967).

Hornbein and Pavlin (1975) have suggested that if H^+ and HCO_3^- are distributed passively between CSF and blood according to changes in E, it should be possible to predict the acid–base status of CSF from that in blood. They also suggested that the greater protection of the CSF pH observed during metabolic acid–base derangements than during those of respiratory origin might be the result of the greater potential difference slope found in metabolic changes in acid–base balance (-42.6 vs. -31.7 mV/pH unit) Held et al., 1964).

3. Observations Inconsistent with Passive Distribution of H^+ and HCO_3^- between CSF and Blood According to Changes in E

Bledsoe and Mines (1975) elevated the CSF–blood potential difference for 6 hours by increasing the plasma K^+ concentration from 3.3 to 8.0 mEq/liter, keeping the arterial acid–base composition at its normal value. This procedure did not result in the redistribution of either H^+ or HCO_3^- in the four dogs studied. Similar results were obtained by Cameron et al. (1973) in dogs in experiments of 2 hours duration. Although these results suggest that the potential difference may not play a role in determining the distributions of H^+ and HCO_3^- during chronic acid–base abnormalities, they do suggest that passive changes in CSF $[HSO_3^-]$ may be dependent on changes in plasma $[HCO_3^-]$, as will be discussed in the next section.

C. Dependence of Changes in CSF $[HCO_3^-]$ on Changes in Plasma $[HCO_3^-]$

Several recent experiments support the concept that CSF $[HCO_3^-]$ regulation during hypocapnia and hypoxemic hypocapnia is passive and primarily dependent on concurrent changes in plasma $[HCO_3^-]$. The role of changes in plasma $[HCO_3^-]$ in CSF $[HCO_3^-]$ regulation in these conditions has been investigated most extensively by Dempsey, Forster, and colleagues. During studies of ventilatory acclimatization to hypoxemia (26 hours to 5 weeks sojourn at 3100, 3400, or 4300 m altitude) in man and pony, they observed that pH compensation was similar in CSF and blood, and postulated that the compensatory reduction in CSF [HCO_3^-] was dependent on corresponding changes in arterial [HCO_3^-] (Dempsey *et al.*, 1974, 1975; Forster *et al.*, 1975; Orr *et al.*, 1975). Pelligrino and Dempsey (1976) tested this hypothesis in anesthetized paralyzed dogs by determining the effects of prolonged hypocapnia, hypoxemia, or hypoxemic hypocapnia (7 or 14 hours) on CSF acid–base status. Arterial [HCO_3^-] was either allowed to decrease normally or maintained at its control level by the infusion of $NaHCO_3$. The decrease in CSF [HCO_3^-] and % pH compensation were always less than or equal to those in arterial blood. The magnitude of the decrease in CSF [HCO_3^-] was reduced by more than 50% in both normoxic hypocapnia and hypoxemic hypocapnia when the arterial [HCO_3^-] was maintained at the control value. In addition, the dependence of the CSF [HCO_3^-] regulation on the reduction in plasma [HCO_3^-] was greater in moderate hypocapnia (89%) than in more severe, prolonged hypocapnia (51%). This is undoubtedly due to the increase in CSF lactate which occurs during severe hypocapnia (Leusen, 1965; van Vaerenbergh *et al.*, 1965; Leusen and Demeester, 1966; Leusen *et al.*, 1967; Plum and Posner, 1967; Plum *et al.*, 1968; Granholm and Siesjö, 1968, 1969; Kazemi *et al.*, 1969; Miller *et al.*, 1970; Weyne *et al.*, 1970; Leusen and Weyne, 1976). The increase in lactate could be due either to hypoxia secondary to decreased cerebral blood flow or to the direct effect of the alkalosis itself on intracellular metabolism (Plum *et al.*, 1968). Cohen (1972) has demonstrated that alkalosis increases lactate production through increased glycolysis related to stimulation of phosphofructokinase.

During normocapnic hypoxemia, CSF [HCO_3^-] was reduced independently of any corresponding changes in plasma [HCO_3^-]; the degree of reduction was increased significantly when the arterial P_{O_2} fell below 40 mm Hg. This observation is consistent with those of Kogure *et al.* (1970) and MacMillan and Siesjö (1971), made during progressive, acute hypoxemia in the anesthetized rat and dog. This "CSF-specific" reduction in [HCO_3^-] can be attributed at least partially to a selective increase in cerebral tissue lactacidosis (Cotev and Severinghaus, 1968; Sørensen and Mines, 1970; Sørensen, 1971; Mines and Sørensen, 1971; Plum and Posner, 1967).

Pelligrino and Dempsey (1976) concluded that CSF [HCO_3^-] regulation in hypocapnia and hypoxemic hypocapnia is primarily dependent on, and therefore limited by, the concomitant decrease in plasma [HCO_3^-]. However, there was a "CSF-specific" mechanism, associated with an increase in the CSF lactic acid concentration, which accounted for approximately one-third of the decrease in CSF [HCO_3^-]. However, they feel that the "CSF-specific" mechanisms participating in the regulation of CSF [HCO_3^-] might be time dependent and are important only in the first stages of chronic hypoxemic hypocapnia. The authors believe that the compensatory movement of HCO_3^- out of the CSF is unrelated to the plasma pH and is not attributable to the independent effects of a reduced plasma [HCO_3^-] or CSF P_{CO_2}, but that it requires a concomitant reduction in both plasma [HCO_3^-] and CSF P_{CO_2}.

Similar observations have been made by other investigators. Experiments that were almost identical to those of Pelligrino and Dempsey (1976) were being carried out simultaneously by Choma and Kazemi (1976). They too demonstrated that the changes in plasma [HCO_3^-] in respiratory alkalosis have a dominant and significant effect on the changes in CSF [HCO_3^-] and therefore, on H^+ homeostasis of the brain. When the fall in plasma [HCO_3^-] in hypocapnia was prevented, the CSF [HCO_3^-] decreased by an amount that was equal to the rise in CSF lactate. When the plasma [HCO_3^-] decrease was accentuated, the decrease in CSF [HCO_3^-] did not follow the plasma blindly but reached a lower limit, which was similar to that reached in pure respiratory alkalosis. They concluded that changes in plasma [HCO_3^-] are of critical importance in CSF [HCO_3^-] regulation in hypocapnia, and that the increase in brain and CSF lactate (the local mechanism) is of limited value. However, the fall in plasma [HCO_3^-] is not followed indefinitely by the CSF [HCO_3^-], because the CSF [HCO_3^-] will not decrease below a lower limit despite further falls in plasma [HCO_3^-]. The authors suggested that this limit is set by the CSF [H^+].

Davies (1978) measured ventilation and CSF and blood acid–base balance in anesthetized dogs during 3 hours of severe hypoxia (Pa_{O_2} = 40 mm Hg), and found that the changes in CSF [HCO_3^-] were dependent on corresponding changes in plasma [HCO_3^-]. A significant amount of CSF [HCO_3^-] reduction was also attributed to increased lactic acid formation by the cerebral tissue as a result of the severe degree of hypoxia that was present. Similar observations have been made by Bureau and Bouverot (1975).

Nattie and Tenney (1976) studied the effect of plasma K^+ depletion on CSF HCO_3^- homeostasis, and observed that the changes in CSF [HCO_3^-] in hypokalemia were also dependent on simultaneous changes in plasma [HCO_3^-]. However, they found that CSF [HCO_3^-] was only related to CSF P_{CO_2} when arterial [HCO_3^-] was less than the normal CSF [HCO_3^-]. When the plasma [HCO_3^-] was above this level, the CSF [HCO_3^-] was related to both CSF P_{CO_2} and plasma $[HCO_3^-]$, which was similar to the observation made by Pelligrino and Dempsey (1976).

D. CSF HCO_3^- Formation in Respiratory Acidosis: Roles of Carbonic Anhydrase and Active Buffering by Brain Tissue

1. Carbonic Anhydrase

The role of carbonic anhydrase-mediated formation of CSF HCO_3^- by cells in the CNS, i.e., choroid plexus and glia cells, as well as the role of active buffering by brain tissue in the regulation of CSF and ECF $[HCO_3^-]$ in respiratory acidosis, have been investigated by Kazemi and colleagues (Kazemi *et al.*, 1973, 1976; Kelley and Kazemi, 1974; Wichser and Kazemi, 1975; Hasan and Kazemi, 1976; Kazemi and Choma, 1977). CSF pH compensation is better than blood in respiratory acidosis because of the greater increase in CSF $[HCO_3^-]$ (Kazemi *et al.*, 1967, 1969, 1973; Kjällquist *et al.*, 1969; Adaro *et al.*, 1969; Lee *et al.*, 1969; Weyne and Leusen, 1971; Maren, 1972; Davies and Gurtner, 1973; Monroe and Kazemi, 1973; Wichser and Kazemi, 1975). Kazemi and co-workers (Wichser and Kazemi, 1975; Hasan and Kazemi, 1976; Kazemi *et al.*, 1976; Kazemi and Choma, 1977) measured the changes in CSF $[HCO_3^-]$ during respiratory acidosis before and after repeated intraventricular injections of acetazolamide and/or ouabain. When acetazolamide and ouabain were administered intraventricularly, either separately or together, the increase in CSF $[HCO_3^-]$ during respiratory acidosis was limited and became of the same magnitude as that which occurred in the arterial blood. They concluded that the increase in CSF $[HCO_3^-]$ is due to two factors ("dual contribution theory"): one factor is related to the simultaneous increase in plasma bicarbonate, probably diffusion, and the other is the bicarbonate formed within the CNS. The HCO_3^- derived from the CNS is formed by the choroid plexus and glia cells by the hydration of CO_2, a reaction catalyzed by carbonic anhydrase and inhibited by acetazolamide. The importance of carbonic anhydrase in the generation of CSF HCO_3^- has been stressed by Maren and associates (Maren and Broder, 1970; Maren, 1971, 1972; Vogh and Maren, 1975). According to Kazemi and Choma (1977) and Maren (1972), the H^+ that is formed by this reaction is actively removed from the choroid plexus and glia cells in exchange for plasma Na^+, utilizing the Na–K ATPase pump. Kazemi and Choma (1977) attributed the decrease in CSF $[HCO_3^-]$ formation they observed following the intraventricular injection of ouabain alone to the fact that Na^+ was not available for exchange with H^+, preventing the reaction ($CO_2 \times H_2O \leftrightarrows H_2CO_3 \leftrightarrows HCO_3^- + H^+$) from proceeding to the right.

2. Brain Tissue Buffering

Kazemi *et al.* (1973) determined the role of organic buffers in the brain and CSF in the formation of CSF HCO_3^- during respiratory acidosis by measuring the changes which occurred in $[HCO_3^-]$, glutamic acid, glutamine, and ammonia concentrations in CSF and blood before and after 6 hours of hypercapnia in anesthetized dogs. They observed a decrease in brain glutamic acid concentration and an increase in brain and CSF ammonia concentrations, and suggested that these changes could account for some of the observed increase in CSF $[HCO_3^-]$ and brain buffering capacity in respiratory acidosis. Kelley and Kazemi (1974) tested the role of increases in brain ammonia levels on the generation of CSF HCO_3^- in anesthetized dogs by measuring the changes in brain and CSF ammonia and CSF $[HCO_3^-]$ induced by intravenous administration of ammonium chloride while normal acid–base balance was maintained. They observed that the increase in CSF $[HCO_3^-]$ was linearly related to the increase in CSF ammonia content and concluded that the brain can regulate its ammonia content through its glutamine–glutamic acid pathway and thereby act as an important buffer mechanism for controlling the CSF pH. The relationships between CSF and brain ammonia, glutamic acid, glutamine, and CSF $[HCO_3^-]$ in respiratory acidosis were confirmed by Kazemi *et al.* (1976) in the anesthetized rat.

The observation that the increase in CSF $[HCO_3^-]$ in respiratory acidosis is greater than the increase in arterial $[HCO_3^-]$ might only apply to relatively short-term periods, for some investigators have observed similar increases in CSF and arterial blood $[HCO_3^-]$ in long-term hypercapnia. Bouverot and Bureau (1975) made measurements of CSF and blood acid–base balance for up to 5 weeks in carotid-denervated dogs at 3550 m altitude and observed parallel changes in acid–base composition of CSF and blood; i.e., the pH compensation in both fluids was equal. Similar observations have been reported by Bouverot and Bureau (1975) in the dog and by Forster *et al.* (1976) and Bisgard *et al.* (1976) in the awake pony. Bisgard *et al.* (1976) concluded that the changes in CSF $[HCO_3^-]$ in chronic respiratory acidosis also are primarily dependent on simultaneous changes in plasma $[HCO_3^-]$ as previously shown to be the case for hypocapnia and hypoxemic hypocapnia.

E. The Charged Membrane Hypothesis (Wien Effect)

As mentioned previously, Davies and Gurtner (1973) observed a direct relationship between the CSF–arterial P_{CO_2} difference and arterial $[H^+]$ in both respiratory and metabolic acidosis and alkalosis. This relationship was explained by the charged membrane hypothesis (Davies *et al.*, 1973;

Davies and Gurtner, 1973). They also observed that the ratio of CSF/ blood [H$^+$] was close to unity at high levels of arterial [H$^+$], and that the ratio of CSF/blood [HCO$_3^-$] was close to unity at low levels of arterial [H$^+$]. Based on these observations, Davies and Gurtner (1973) proposed that CSF acid–base regulation could be explained by changes in the CSF–blood P_{CO_2} difference caused by the Wien effect and on pH-sensitive changes in the permeability of the blood–brain barrier to H$^+$ and HCO$_3^-$.

Changes in the CSF–blood P_{CO_2} difference which occurred with changes in acid–base balance of the blood could be important in the regulation of CSF [HCO$_3^-$], because the generation of CSF [HCO$_3^-$] appears to be related to the CSF or choroid plexus P_{CO_2} in both respiratory alkalosis (Pelligrino and Dempsey, 1976) and respiratory acidosis (Wichser and Kazemi, 1975; Hasan and Kazemi, 1976; Kazemi *et al.*, 1976; Kazemi and Choma, 1977). A change in the CSF–blood P_{CO_2} difference could also account, in part, for the rightward shift of the brain CO$_2$ dissociation observed in respiratory alkalosis and the leftward shift observed in respiratory acidosis (Kazemi *et al.*, 1967, 1969).

F. Conclusions

The overwhelming majority of CSF and blood acid–base data obtained during chronic acid–base derangements is consistent with the concept of passive regulation of the CSF and ECF [H$^+$] and [HCO$_3^-$], and almost all the observed changes in CSF [HCO$_3^-$] in these conditions can be accounted for either by variations in the dc potential difference between CSF and blood or by simultaneous changes in plasma [HCO$_3^-$]. "CSF-specific" mechanisms such as lactic acid production by brain cells, active buffering by the brain tissue itself via the formation of ammonia, and carbonic anhydrase-mediated formation of CSF HCO$_3^-$ by glia and choroid plexus cells become important in certain conditions of hypercapnia, hypocapnia, and hypoxia. Alterations in the CSF–arterial P_{CO_2} difference caused by the Wien effect and pH-sensitive changes in the permeability of the blood–brain barrier to H$^+$ and HCO$_3^-$ may also be important in the regulation of the CSF pH.

IV. CEREBRAL ECF ACIDITY AND THE REGULATION OF CEREBRAL BLOOD FLOW AND VENTILATION

A. Cerebral Blood Flow

Several investigators have suggested that cerebral ECF [H$^+$] is important in the regulation of cerebral blood flow (Severinghaus *et al.*, 1966;

Donald G. Davies

Severinghaus and Lassen, 1967; Skinhøj, 1966; Betz and Heuser, 1967; Lassen, 1968; Fencl *et al.*, 1969; Wahl *et al.*, 1970; Pannier *et al.*, 1972). Severinghaus *et al.* (1966) hypothesized that the return of CBF to normal in man during acclimatization to high altitude was due to the return of the CSF and ECF pH to normal. Betz and Heuser (1967) observed in anesthetized cats that changes in cortical blood flow were correlated to changes in cortical pH during metabolic and respiratory acidosis and alkalosis and hypoxemia; Wahl *et al.* (1970) demonstrated alterations in the diameter of cortical arterioles induced by local injections of acidic and alkalotic artificial CSF. Fencl *et al.* (1969) made measurements of CSF acid–base composition and CBF in man and concluded that the changes in CBF were correlated to changes in the calculated pH of cerebral ECF.

    Pannier *et al.* (1972) investigated the effects on CBF of changes in the acid–base composition of the ventriculocisternal system in the anesthetized cat. They found that perfusion with artificial CSF containing a reduced HCO_3^- concentration caused an increase in blood flow to the caudate nucleus, whereas, perfusion with increased $[HCO_3^-]$ caused the opposite effect. No changes in blood flow were elicited in the cerebral hemispheres. Britton *et al.* (1977) performed similar experiments in the anesthetized dog and obtained different results. They perfused the ventriculocisternal system with artificial CSF equilibrated with 7% CO_2 and containing either 10, 25, or 35 mEq/liter $[HCO_3^-]$. Arterial P_{CO_2} was maintained constant at the control level during the 60 minutes of perfusion. In contrast to the results of Pannier *et al.* (1972), they observed a direct relationship between CSF $[H^+]$ and the total CBF. They also found that the greatest change in flow occurred in tissue that was in close proximity to the ventricular system, which suggests that the perfusion had created a HCO_3^- concentration gradient across the cerebral ECF space.

B. Ventilation

    The importance of the cerebral $[H^+]$ in the regulation of ventilation has been demonstrated by Pappenheimer, Fencl, and colleagues (Pappenheimer *et al.*, 1965; Pappenheimer, 1967; Fencl *et al.*, 1966). They found, in awake goats during perfusion of the ventriculocisternal system with artificial CSF containing different HCO_3^- concentrations, that ventilation was correlated to changes in a calculated interstitial fluid pH and not CSF pH. Pierce *et al.* (1971) measured the acid–base status of CSF and arterial blood and ventilation in cholera patients, and observed that the changes in ventilation which occurred during the development and correction of the disease were also not correlated to CSF pH. However, the ventilatory response was negatively correlated to arterial and CSF

[HCO₃⁻], which suggested to them that ventilation was responding to changes in the acidity of the ECF.

Davies (1978) made similar observations in anesthetized dogs exposed to 10% O_2 for 3 hours. The hypoxia caused an initial increase in ventilation in the first 30 minutes, as a result of stimulation of the peripheral chemoreceptors. Following the initial ventilatory response, there was a secondary increase in ventilation which was not correlated to CSF [H⁺]. However, during the hypoxic exposure, there was a gradual and continuous decrease in arterial and CSF [HCO₃⁻]. Similar results have been reported by Dempsey, Forster, and colleagues from their studies of ventilatory acclimatization to high altitude in humans and pony (Dempsey et al., 1974, 1975; Forster et al., 1975; Orr et al., 1975). Davies (1978) calculated the cerebral ECF [H⁺], assuming the ventilatory chemosensitive area was located three-fourths of the distance along a HCO₃⁻ concentration gradient between CSF and blood and that CSF and ECF P_{CO_2} were equal. The changes in ventilation were highly correlated to the changes in the calculated ECF [H⁺], which suggested to the author that alterations in ECF [H⁺] might be playing a role in ventilatory acclimatization to hypoxia.

ACKNOWLEDGMENTS

I am indebted to Ms. Ellen Wendlandt, Technical Reports Editor, for invaluable assistance in the preparation of this chapter.

The author's research described in this chapter was supported by grants HLB 10342, 12564 and 5433 from the National Institutes of Health and by the American Heart Association, Texas Affiliate, Inc.

REFERENCES

Adaro, F. V. M., E. E. Roehr, A. R. Viola, and C. Wymerszberg de Obrutzky (1969). Acid–base equilibrium between blood and cerebrospinal fluid in acute hypercapnia. *J. Appl. Physiol.* **27**, 271–275.

Agrest, A., and E. E. Roehr (1963). Relacion electrolitica y acido–basica entre sangre arterial y liquido cefalorraquiedo en trastornos del equilibrio acido–base. *Medicina (Buenos Aires)* **23**, 173–187.

Albert, M. S., W. J. Rahill, L. Vega, and R. W. Winters (1966). Acid–base changes in cerebrospinal fluid of infants with metabolic acidosis. *N. Engl. J. Med.* **274**, 719–721.

Alexander, S. C., R. D. Workman, and C. J. Lambertsen (1962). Hyperthermia, lactic acid infusion, and the composition of arterial blood and cerebrospinal fluid. *Am. J. Physiol.* **202**, 1049–1054.

Alroy, G. G., and D. C. Flenley (1967). The acidity of the cerebrospinal fluid in man with particular reference to chronic ventilatory failure. *Clin. Sci.* **33**, 335–343.

Betz, E., and D. Heuser (1967). Cerebral cortical blood flow during changes of acid–base equilibrium of the brain. *J. Appl. Physiol.* **23**, 726–733.

Bisgard, G. E., A. V. Ruiz, R. F. Grover, and J. A. Will (1973). Ventilatory control in the Hereford calf. *J. Appl. Physiol.* **35**, 220–226.

Bisgard, G. E., H. V. Forster, J. A. Orr, D. D. Buss, C. A. Rawlings, and B. Rasmussen (1976). Hypoventilation in ponies after carotid body denervation. *J. Appl. Physiol.* **40**, 184–190.

Blayo, M. C., J. Coudert, and J. J. Pocidalo (1975). Comparison of cisternal and lumbar cerebrospinal fluid pH in high altitude natives. *Pfluegers Arch.* **356**, 159–167.

Bledsoe, S. W., and A. H. Mines (1975). Effect of plasma [K$^+$] on the DC potential and on ion distributions between CSF and blood. *J. Appl. Physiol.* **39**, 1012–1016.

Bleich, H. L., P. M. Berkman, and W. B. Schwartz (1964). The response of cerebrospinal fluid composition to sustained hypercapnia. *J. Clin. Invest.* **43**, 11–16.

Bouverot, P., and M. Bureau (1975). Ventilatory acclimatization and CSF acid–base balance in carotid chemodenervated dogs at 3550 m. *Pfluegers Arch.* **361**, 17–23.

Bradbury, M. W. B., and C. R. Kleeman (1967). Stability of the potassium content of cerebrospinal fluid and brain. *Am. J. Physiol.* **213**, 519–528.

Bradley, R. D., and S. J. G. Semple (1962). A comparison of certain acid–base characteristics of arterial blood, jugular venous blood and cerebrospinal fluid in man, and the effect on them of some acute and chronic acid–base disturbances. *J. Physiol. (London)* **160**, 381–391.

Bradley, R. D., S. J. G. Semple, and G. T. Spencer (1965). Rate of change of carbon dioxide tension in arterial blood, jugular venous blood and cisternal cerebrospinal fluid on carbon dioxide administration. *J. Physiol. (London)* **179**, 442–455.

Britton, S., C. Nuñez, and D. G. Davies (1977). Cerebral extracellular fluid acidity and cerebral blood flow. *Physiologist* **20**, 12.

Brooks, C. McC., F. F. Kao, and B. B. Lloyd, eds. (1965). "Cerebrospinal Fluid and the Regulation of Ventilation." Blackwell, Oxford.

Brzezinski, J., Å. Kjällquist, and B. K. Siesjö (1967). Mean carbon dioxide tension in the brain after carbonic anhydrase inhibition. *J. Physiol. (London)* **188**, 13–23.

Buhlmann, A., W. Scheitlin, and P. H. Rossier (1963). Die Beziehungen zwischen Blut und Liquor Cerebrospinalis bei Störungen des Säure Basen-Gleichgewichtes. *Schweiz. Med. Wochenschr.* **93**, 427–432.

Bulger, R. J., R. W. Schrier, W. P. Arend, and A. G. Swanson (1966). Spinal-fluid acidosis and the diagnosis of pulmonary encephalopathy. *N. Engl. J. Med.* **274**, 433–437.

Bureau, M., and P. Bouverot (1975). Blood and CSF acid–base changes, and rate of ventilatory acclimatization of awake dogs to 3,550 m. *Respir. Physiol.* **24**, 203–216.

Cameron, I. R. (1969). Acid–base changes in cerebrospinal fluid. *Br. J. Anaesth.* **41**, 213–221.

Cameron, I. R., and C. R. Kleeman (1970). The effect of acute hyperkalaemia on the blood–CSF potential difference. *J. Physiol. (London)* **207**, 68p–69p.

Cameron, I. R., and R. Miller (1973). The effect of plasma potassium concentration and arterial pH on the CSF–blood potential difference. *Bull. Physio-Pathol. Respir.* **9**, 796–800.

Cameron, I. R., J. Caronna, and R. Miller (1973). The effect of acute hyperkalaemia on the CSF–blood potential difference and the control of CSF pH. *J. Physiol. (London)* **232**, 102p–103p.

Caronna, J. J., F. Plum, and B. K. Siesjö (1974). P_{CO_2} gradients between blood and CSF in rat during alterations of acid–base balance. *Am. J. Physiol.* **227**, 1173–1177.

Chazan, J. A., F. M. Appleton, A. M. London, and W. B. Schwartz (1969). Effects of chronic metabolic acid–base disturbances on the composition of cerebrospinal fluid in the dog. *Clin. Sci.* **36**, 345–358.

Choma, L., and H. Kazemi (1976). Importance of changes in plasma HCO_3^- on regulation of CSF HCO_3^- in respiratory alkalosis. *Respir. Physiol.* **26**, 265–278.

Cohen, P. J. (1972). The metabolic functions of oxygen and biochemical lesions of hypoxia. *Anesthesiology.* **37**, 148–177.

Collip, J. B., and P. L. Backus (1920). The alkali reserve of the blood plasma, spinal fluid and lymph. *Am. J. Physiol.* **51**, 551–567.

Cotev, S., and J. W. Severinghaus (1968). Cerebral ECF acidosis induced by hypoxia at normal and reduced Pa_{CO_2}. *Scand. J. Lab. Clin. Invest., Suppl.* **102**, III-E.

Cowie, J., A. T. Lambie, and J. S. Robson (1962). The influence of extracorporeal dialysis on the acid–base composition of blood and cerebrospinal fluid. *Clin. Sci.* **23**, 397–404.

Cunningham, D. J. C., and B. B. Lloyd, eds. (1963). "The Regulation of Human Respiration." Blackwell, Oxford.

Davies, D. G. (1976). CSF sampling technique and astrup pH and P_{CO_2} values. *J. Appl. Physiol.* **40**, 123–125.

Davies, D. G. (1977). CSF pH and P_{CO_2} measurement. *J. Appl. Physiol.* **43**, 566–567.

Davies, D. G. (1978). Evidence for cerebral extracellular fluid $[H^+]$ as a stimulus during acclimatization to hypoxia. *Respir. Physiol.* **32**, 167–182.

Davies, D. G., and R. E. Dutton (1972). The effect of acetazolamide and ouabain on the D-C potential difference between CSF and blood. *Physiologist* **15**, 114.

Davies, D. G., and G. H. Gurtner (1973). CSF acid–base balance and the Wien effect. *J. Appl. Physiol.* **34**, 249–254.

Davies, D. G., and G. H. Gurtner (1975). The physiological significance of the Wien effect. *Am. J. Physiol.* **229**, 1725–1726.

Davies, D. G., R. S. Fitzgerald, and G. H. Gurtner (1973). Acid–base relationships between CSF and blood during acute metabolic acidosis. *J. Appl. Physiol.* **34**, 243–248.

Dempsey, J. A., H. V. Forster, and G. A. doPico (1974). Ventilatory acclimatization to moderate hypoxemia im man. The role of spinal fluid $[H^+]$. *J. Clin. Invest.* **53**, 1091–1100.

Dempsey, J. A., H. V. Forster, N. Gledhill, and G. A. doPico (1975). Effects of moderate hypoxemia and hypocapnia on CSF $[H^+]$ and ventilation in man. *J. Appl. Physiol.* **38**, 665–674.

Fencl, V., T. B. Miller, and J. R. Pappenheimer (1966). Studies on the respiratory response to disturbances of acid–base balance, with deductions concerning the ionic composition of cerebral interstitial fluid. *Am. J. Physiol.* **210**, 459–472.

Fencl, V., J. R. Vale, and J. A. Broch (1969). Respiration and cerebral blood flow in metabolic acidosis and alkalosis in humans. *J. Appl. Physiol.* **27**, 67–76.

Fisher, V. J., and L. C. Christianson (1963). Cerebrospinal fluid acid–base balance during a changing ventilatory state in man. *J. Appl. Physiol.* **18**, 712–716.

Forster, H. V., J. A. Dempsey, and L. W. Chosy (1975). Incomplete compensation of CSF $[H^+]$ in man during acclimatization to high altitude (4300 m). *J. Appl. Physiol.* **38**, 1067–1072.

Forster, H. V., G. E. Bisgard, B. Rasmussen, J. A. Orr, D. D. Buss, and M. Manohar (1976). Ventilatory control in peripheral chemorecptor-denervated ponies during chronic hypoxemia. *J. Appl. Physiol.* **41**, 878–885.

Ganshirt, H. (1968). Der Sauerstoffdruck der Cerebrospinalflüssigkeit des Menscher. Seine physiologische und klinische Bedeutung. *Klin Wochenschr.* **46**, 771–778.

Goodrich, C. (1965). Effect of chronic acidosis and alkalosis on rat CSF–blood potential. *Physiologist* **8**, 178.

Granholm, L. and B. K. Siesjö (1968). Signs of cerebral hypoxia in hyperventilation. *Experientia* **24**, 337–338.

Granholm, L., and B. K. Siesjö (1969). The effects of hypercapnia and hypocapnia upon the cerebrospinal fluid lactate and pyruvate concentrations and upon the lactate, pyruvate, ATP, ADP, phosphocreatine and creatine concentrations of cat brain tissue. *Acta Physiol. Scand.* **75**, 257–266.

Gurtner, G. H., B. Burns, and D. G. Davies (1972). Steady state differences in P_{CO_2}, [HCO_3^-] and [H^+] between blood and extravascular tissue. Results for lung, CSF and brain. *Chest* **61**, 31s–39s.

Gurtner, G. H., B. Burns, M. Sciuto, and D. G. Davies (1974). Interrelationships between blood and extravascular pH, P_{CO_2} and [HCO_3^-]. *In* "CO_2 and Metabolic Regulations" (G. Nahas and K. Schaeffer, eds.), pp. 35–45. Springer-Verlag, Berlin and New York.

Hasan, F. M., and H. Kazemi (1976). Dual contribution theory of regulation of CSF HCO_3^- in respiratory acidosis. *J. Appl. Physiol.* **40**, 559–567.

Held, D., V. Fencl, and J. R. Pappenheimer (1964). Electrical potential of cerebrospinal fluid. *J. Neurophysiol.* **27**, 942–959.

Hodson, W. A., A. Fenner, G. Brumley, V. Chernick, and M. E. Avery (1968). Cerebrospinal fluid and blood acid–base relationships in fetal and neonatal lambs and pregnant ewes. *Respir. Physiol.* **4**, 322–332.

Hornbein, T. F., and E. G. Pavlin (1975). Distribution of H^+ and HCO_3^- between CSF and blood during respiratory alkalosis in dogs. *Am. J. Physiol.* **228**, 1149–1154.

Hornbein, T. F., and S. C. Sørensen (1972). D-C potential difference between different cerebrospinal fluid sites and blood in dogs. *Am. J. Physiol.* **223**, 415–418.

Huang, C. T., and H. A. Lyons (1966). The maintenance of acid–base balance between cerebrospinal fluid and arterial blood in patients with chronic respiratory disorders. *Clin. Sci.* **31**, 273–284.

Hutter, O. F., and A. E. Warner (1967). The pH sensitivity of the chloride conductance of frog skeletal muscle. *J. Physiol. (London)* **189**, 403–425.

Ingvar, D. H., N. A. Lassen, B. K. Siesjö, and E. Skinhøj (1968). Cerebral blood flow and cerebrospinal fluid. *Scand. J. Lab. Clin. Invest.* **22**, Suppl. 102.

Kazemi, H., and L. Choma (1977). H^+ transport from CNS in hypercapnia and regulation of CSF [HCO_3^-]. *J. Appl. Physiol.* **42**, 667–672.

Kazemi, H., D. C. Shannon, and E. Carvalo-Gil (1967). Brain CO_2 buffering capacity in respiratory acidosis and alkalosis. *J. Appl. Physiol.* **22**, 241–246.

Kazemi, H., M. Valenca, and D. C. Shannon (1969). Brain and cerebrospinal fluid lactate concentration in respiratory acidosis and alkalosis. *Respir. Physiol.* **6**, 178–186.

Kazemi, H., N. S. Shore, V. E. Shih, and D. C. Shannon (1973). Brain organic buffers in respiratory acidosis and alkalosis. *J. Appl. Physiol.* **34**, 478–482.

Kazemi, H., J. Weyne, F. Van Leusen, and I. Leusen (1976). The CSF HCO_3^- increase in hypercapnia. Relationship to HCO_3^-, glutamate, glutamine and NH_3 in brain. *Respir. Physiol.* **28**, 387–401.

Kelley, M. A., and H. Kazemi (1974). Role of ammonia as a buffer in the central nervous system. *Respir. Physiol.* **22**, 345–359.

Kellogg, R. H. (1964). Central chemical regulation of respiration. *Hand. Physio. Sect. 3: Respir.* 507–534.

Kety, S. S., and C. F. Schmidt (1948). The effects of altered arterial tensions of carbon dioxide and oxygen on cerebral blood flow and cerebral oxygen consumption of normal young men. *J. Clin. Invest.* **27**, 484–492.

Kjällquist, Å. (1970). The CSF/blood potential in sustained acid–base changes in the rat with calculations of electrochemical potential differences for H^+ and HCO_3^-. *Acta Physiol. Scand.* **78**, 85–93.

Kjällquist, Å., and B. K. Siesjö (1967). The CSF/blood potential in sustained acidosis and alkalosis in the rat. *Acta Physiol. Scand.* **71**, 255–256.

Kjällquist, Å., M. Nardini, and B. K. Siesjö (1969). The effect of acetazolamide upon tissue concentrations of bicarbonate, lactate, and pyruvate in the rat brain. *Acta Physiol. Scand.* **77**, 241–251.

Kogure, K., P. Scheinberg, O. M. Reinmuth, J. Fujishima, and R. Busto (1970). Mechanisms of cerebral vasodilation in hypoxia. *J. Appl. Physiol.* **34**, 478–482.

Lambertsen, C. J. (1960). Carbon dioxide and respiration in acid–base homeostasis. *Anesthesiology* **21**, 642–651.

Lassen, N. A. (1968). Brain extracellular fluid pH: Main factor controlling cerebral blood flow. *Scand. J. Clin. Lab. Invest.* **22**, 247–251 (editorial).

Lee, J. E., F. Chu, J. B. Posner, and F. Plum (1969). Buffering capacity of cerebrospinal fluid in acute respiratory acidosis in dogs. *Am. J. Physiol.* **217**, 1035–1038.

Lehmann, G., and A. Meesman (1924). Über das Bestehen eines Donnangleichgewichtes zwischen Blut und Kammerwasser bzw. Liquor Cerebrospinalis. *Pfluegers Arch.* **205**, 210–232.

Leusen, I. (1965). Aspects of the acid–base balance between blood and cerebrospinal fluid. *In* "Cerebrospinal Fluid and the Regulation of Ventilation" (C. McC. Brooks, F. F. Kao, and B. B. Lloyd, eds.), pp. 55–89. Blackwell, Oxford.

Leusen, I. (1972). Regulation of cerebrospinal fluid composition with reference to breathing. *Physiol. Rev.* **52**, 1–56.

Leusen, I., and G. Demeester (1964). Acid–base balance in cerebrospinal fluid during prolonged artificial hyperventilation. *Arch. Int. Physiol. Biochim.* **72**, 721–724.

Leusen, I., and G. Demeester (1966). Lactate and pyruvate in the brain of rat during hyperventilation. *Arch. Int. Physiol. Biochim.* **74**, 25–34.

Leusen, I., and J. Weyne (1976). Metabolic processes in the brain during respiratory and non-respiratory alkalosis and acidosis. *In* "Acid–Base Homeostasis of the Brain Extracellular Fluid and the Respiratory Control System" (H. H. Loeschcke, ed.), pp. 27–42. Publishing Sciences Group, Inc., Littleton, Massachusetts.

Leusen, I., E. Lacroix, and G. Demeester (1967). Lactate and pyruvate in the brain of rats during changes in acid–base balance. *Arch. Int. Physiol. Biochim.* **75**, 310–324.

Loeschcke, H. H., ed. (1976). "Acid–Base Homeostasis of the Brain Extracellular Fluid and the Respiratory Control System. Publishing Sciences Group, Inc., Littleton, Massachusetts.

MacMillan, V., and B. K. Siesjö (1971). The effect of arterial hypoxemia upon acid–base parameters in arterial blood and cisternal cerebrospinal fluid of the rat. *Acta Physiol. Scand.* **83**, 454–462.

Manfredi, F. (1962). Acid–base relations between serum and cerebrospinal fluid in man under normal and abnormal conditions. *J. Lab. Clin. Med.* **59**, 128–136.

Maren, T. H. (1971). The effect of acetazolamide on HCO_3^- and Cl^- uptake into cerebrospinal fluid of cat and dogfish. *In* "Ion Homeostasis of the Brain" (B. K. Siesjö and S. C. Sørensen, eds.), pp. 290–311. Academic Press, New York.

Maren, T. H. (1972). Bicarbonate formation in cerebrospinal fluid: Role in sodium transport and pH regulation. *Am. J. Physiol.* **222**, 885–899.

Maren, T. H., and L. E. Broder (1970). The role of carbonic anhydrase in anion secretion into cerebrospinal fluid. *J. Pharmacol. Exp. Ther.* **172**, 197–202.

Marks, C. E., Jr., R. M. Goldring, J. J. Vecchione, and E. E. Gordon (1973). Cerebrospinal fluid acid–base relationships in ketoacidosis and lactic acidosis. *J. Appl. Physiol.* **35**, 813–819.

Merwarth, C. R., H. O. Sieker, and F. Manfredi (1961). Acid–base relations between blood and cerebrospinal fluid in normal subjects and patients with respiratory insufficiency. *N. Engl. J. Med.* **265**, 310–313.

Messeter, K. (1972). The effect of acetazolamide upon the regulation of the cerebrospinal fluid pH in the rat. *Acta Physiol. Scand.* **85**, 58–70.

Messeter, K., and B. K. Siesjö (1971a). The DC potential between CSF and plasma in respiratory acidosis. *Acta Physiol. Scand.* **83**, 13–20.

Messeter, K., and B. K. Siesjö (1971b). Regulation of the CSF pH in acute and sustained respiratory acidosis. *Acta Physiol. Scand.* **83**, 21–30.

Miller, A. I., Jr., K. E. Curtin, A. L. Shen, and C. K. Suiter (1970). Brain oxygenation in the rat during hyperventilation with air and with low O_2 mixtures. *Am. J. Physiol.* **219**, 798–801.

Mines, A. H., and S. C. Sørensen (1971). Changes in the electrochemical potential difference for HCO_3^- between blood and cerebrospinal fluid and in cerebrospinal fluid lactate concentration during isocarbic hypoxia. *Acta Physiol. Scand.* **81**, 225–233.

Mines, A. H., C. G. Morril, and S. C. Sørensen (1971). The effect of isocarbic metabolic acidosis in blood on $[H^+]$ and $[HCO_3^-]$ in CSF with deductions about the regulation of an active transport of H^+/HCO_3^- between blood and CSF. *Acta Physiol. Scand.* **81**, 234–245.

Mitchell, R. A. (1965). The regulation of respiration in metabolic acidosis and alkalosis. *In* "Cerebrospinal Fluid and the Regulation of Ventilation" (C. McC. Brooks, F. F. Kao, and B. B. Lloyd, eds.) pp. 109–131. Blackwell, Oxford.

Mitchell, R. A. (1966). Cerebrospinal fluid and the regulation of respiration. *In* "Advances in Respiratory Physiology" (C. G. Caro, ed.), pp. 1–47. Arnold, London.

Mitchell, R. A., and M. M. Singer (1965). Respiration and cerebrospinal fluid pH in metabolic acidosis and alkalosis. *J. Appl. Physiol.* **20**, 905–911.

Mitchell, R. A., C. T. Carman, J. W. Severinghaus, B. W. Richardson, M. M. Singer, and S. Shnider (1965). Stability of cerebrospinal fluid pH in chronic acid–base disturbances in blood. *J. Appl. Physiol.* **20**, 443–452.

Monroe, C. B., and H. Kazemi (1973). Effect of changes in plasma bicarbonate level on CSF bicarbonate in respiratory acidosis. *Respir. Physiol.* **17**, 386–393.

Nattie, E. E., and S. M. Tenney (1976). Effect of potassium depletion on cerebrospinal fluid bicarbonate homeostasis. *Am. J. Physiol.* **231**, 579–587.

Orr, J. A., G. E. Bisgard, H. V. Forster, D. D. Buss, J. A. Dempsey, and J. A. Will (1975). Cerebrospinal fluid alkalosis during high-altitude sojourn in unanesthetized ponies. *Respir. Physiol.* **25**, 23–37.

Pannier, J. L., J. Weyne, G. Demeester, and I. Leusen (1972). Influence of changes in the acid–base composition of the ventricular system on cerebral blood flow in cats. *Pfluegers Arch.* **333**, 337–351.

Pappenheimer, J. R. (1967). The ionic composition of cerebral extracellular fluid and its relation to the control of breathing. *Harvey Lect.* **61**, 71–94.

Pappenheimer, J. R., V. Fencl, S. R. Heisey, and D. Held (1965). Role of cerebral fluids in control of respiration as studied in unanesthetized goats. *Am. J. Physiol.* **208**, 436–450.

Pauli, H. G., and F. Reubi (1963). Respiratory control in uremic acidosis. *J. Appl. Physiol.* **18**, 717–721.

Pauli, H. G., C. Vorburger, and F. Reubi (1962). Chronic derangements of cerebrospinal fluid acid–base components in man. *J. Appl. Physiol.* **17**, 993–998.

Pavlin, E. G., and T. F. Hornbein (1975a). Distribution of H^+ and HCO_3^- between CSF and blood during metabolic acidosis in dogs. *Am. J. Physiol.* **228**, 1134–1140.

Pavlin, E. G., and T. F. Hornbein (1975b). Distribution of H^+ and HCO_3^- between CSF and blood during metabolic alkalosis in dogs. *Am. J. Physiol.* **228**, 1141–1144.

Pavlin, E. G., and T. F. Hornbein (1975c). Distribution of H^+ and HCO_3^- between CSF and blood during respiratory acidosis in dogs. *Am. J. Physiol.* **228**, 1145–1148.

Pelligrino, D. A., and J. A. Dempsey (1976). Dependence of CSF on plasma bicarbonate during hypocapnia and hypoxemic hypocapnia. *Respir. Physiol.* **26**, 11–26.

Pierce, N. F., D. S. Fedson, K. L. Brigham, S. Permutt, and A. Mondal (1971). Relation of ventilation during base deficit to acid–base values in blood and spinal fluid. *J. Appl. Physiol.* **30**, 677–683.

Plum, F., and J. B. Posner (1967). Blood and cerebrospinal fluid lactate during hyperventilation. *Am. J. Physiol.* **212**, 864–870.

Plum, F., and J. B. Posner (1968). Inhomogeneity of cisternal and lumbar CSF acid–base balance during acute metabolite alterations. *Scand. J. Clin. Lab. Invest., Suppl.* **102**, I-B.

Plum, F., and R. W. Price (1973). Acid–base balance of cisternal and lumbar cerebrospinal fluid in hospital patients. *N. Engl. J. Med.* **289**, 1346–1351.

Plum, F., J. B. Posner, and W. W. Smith (1968). Effect of hyperbaric–hyperoxic hyperventilation on blood, brain and CSF. *Am. J. Physiol.* **209**, 1240–1244.

Pontén, U. (1966). Consecutive acid–base changes in blood, brain tissue and cerebrospinal fluid during respiratory acidosis and baseosis. *Acta Neurol. Scand.* **42**, 455–471.

Pontén, U. (1977). Carbon dioxide tension relations in the brain in various acid–base-conditions. *In* "Acid–Base Homeostasis of the Brain Extracellular Fluid and the Respiratory Control System (H. H. Loeschcke, ed.), pp. 8–15. Publishing Sciences Group, Inc. Littleton, Massachusetts.

Pontén, U., and B. K. Siesjö (1966). Gradients of CO_2 tension in the brain. *Acta Physiol. Scand.* **67**, 129–140.

Pontén, U., and B. K. Siesjö (1967). Acid–base relations in arterial blood and cerebrospinal fluid of the unanesthetized rat. *Acta Physiol. Scand.* **71**, 89–95.

Posner, J. B., and F. Plum (1967). Spinal-fluid pH and neurologic symptoms in systemic acidosis. *N. Engl. J. Med.* **277**, 605–613.

Posner, J. B., A. G. Swanson, and F. Plum (1965). Acid–base balance in cerebrospinal fluid. *Arch. Neurol. (Chicago)* **12**, 479–496.

Razavi, A. K., B. Burns, A. M. Sciuto, G. H. Gurtner, and D. G. Davies (1977). The Wien effect in compensated metabolic acidosis. *Respir. Physiol.* **29**, 25–33.

Reivich, M. (1964). Arterial P_{CO_2} and cerebral hemodynamics. *Am. J. Physiol.* **206**, 25–35.

Robin, E. D., R. D. Whaley, C. H. Crump, A. G. Bickelman, and D. M. Travis (1958). Acid–base relations between spinal fluid and arterial blood with special reference to control of ventilation. *J. Appl. Physiol.* **13**, 385–392.

Schwab, M. (1962). Das Säure-Basen-Gleichgewicht im arteriellen Blut und Liquor cerebrospinalis bei chronischer Niereninsuffizienz. *Klin. Wochenschr.* **40**, 765–772.

Schwab, M., and H. Dammaschke (1962). Atmung, Säure–Basen-Gleichgewicht und Ammoniak/Ammonium im Blut und Liquor cerebrospinalis bei Lebercirrhose. *Klin. Wochenschr.* **40**, 184–199.

Semple, S. J. G. (1965). Respiration and the cerebrospinal fluid. *Br. J. Anaesth.* **37**, 262–267.

Severinghaus, J. W. (1965). Electrochemical gradients for hydrogen and bicarbonate ions across the blood–CSF barrier in response to acid–base balance changes. *In* "Cerebrospinal Fluid and the Regulation of Ventilation" (C. McC. Brooks, F. F. Kao, and B. B. Lloyd, eds.), pp. 247–258. Blackwell, Oxford.

Severinghaus, J. W., and A. Carceleń B. (1964). Cerebrospinal fluid in man native to high altitude. *J. Appl. Physiol.* **19**, 319–321.

Severinghaus, J. W., and N. A. Lassen (1967). Step hypocapnia to separate arterial from tissue P_{CO_2} in the regulation of cerebral blood flow. *Circ. Res.* **20**, 272–278.

Severinghaus, J. W., R. A. Mitchell, B. W. Richardson, and M. M. Singer (1963). Respiratory control at high altitude suggesting active transport regulation of CSF pH. *J. Appl. Physiol.* **18**, 1115–1166.

Severinghaus, J. W., H. Chiodi, E. J. Eger, B. B. Branstater, and T. F. Hornbein (1966). Cerebral blood flow at high altitude. *Circ. Res.* **19**, 274–282.

196   Donald G. Davies

Shannon, D. C., H. Kazemi, N. Croteau, and E. F. Parsons (1970). Cerebral acid–base changes during reduced cranial blood flow. *Respir. Physiol.* **8**, 385–396.

Siesjö, B. K. (1972). The regulation of cerebrospinal fluid pH. *Kidney Int.* **1**, 360–374.

Siesjö, B. K., and Å. Kjällquist (1969). A new theory for the regulation of the extracellular pH in the brain. *Scand. J. Clin. Lab. Invest.* **24**, 1–9.

Siesjö, B. K., and S. C. Sørensen, eds. (1971). "Ion Homeostasis of the Brain." Munksgaard, Copenhagen.

Siesjö, B. K., and N. N. Zwetnow (1970). The effect of hypovolemic hypotension on extra- and intracellular acid–base parameters and energy metabolites in the rat brain. *Acta Physiol. Scand.* **79**, 114–124.

Skinhøj, E. (1966). Regulation of cerebral blood flow as a single function of the interstitial fluid pH in the brain. *Acta Neurol. Scand.* **42**, 604–607.

Sørensen, S. C. (1971). The chemical control of ventilation. *Acta Physiol. Scand., Suppl.* **361**.

Sørensen, S. C., and J. S. Milledge (1971). Cerebrospinal fluid acid–base composition at high altitude. *J. Appl. Physiol.* **31**, 28–30.

Sørensen, S. C., and A. H. Mines (1970). Ventilatory responses to acute and chronic hypoxia in goats after sinus nerve section. *J. Appl. Physiol.* **28**, 832–835.

Sørensen, S. C., and J. W. Severinghaus (1970). Effect of cerebral acidosis on the CSF–blood potential difference. *Am. J. Physiol.* **219**, 68–71.

Swanson, A. G., and H. Rosengren (1962). Cerebrospinal fluid buffering during acute experimental respiratory acidosis. *J. Appl. Physiol.* **17**, 812–814.

Tschirgi, R. D., and J. L. Taylor (1958). Slowly changing bioelectric potentials associated with the blood–brain barrier. *Am. J. Physiol.* **195**, 7–22.

van Heijst, A. N. P., A. H. J. Maas, and B. F. Visser (1966). Comparison of the acid–base balance in cisternal and lumbar cerebrospinal fluid. *Pfluegers Arch.* **287**, 242–246.

Van Vaerenbergh, P. J. J., E. Lacroix, G. Demeester, and I. Leusen (1965). Lactate in cerebrospinal fluid during muscular exercise. *Arch. Int. Physiol. Biochim.* **73**, 729–737.

Vogh, B. P., and T. H. Maren (1975). Sodium chloride and bicarbonate movement from plasma to cerebrospinal fluid in cats. *Am. J. Physiol.* **228**, 673–683.

Wahl, M., P. Deetjen, K. Thurau, D. H. Ingvar, and N. A. Lassen (1970). Micropuncture evaluation of the importance of perivascular pH for the arteriolar diameter on the brain surface. *Pfluegers Arch.* **316**, 152–163.

Weyne, J., and I. Leusen (1971). Bicarbonate, chloride, and lactate in brain during acid–base alterations. *In* "Ion Homeostasis of the Brain" (B. K. Siesjö and S. C. Sørensen, eds.), pp. 352–374. Academic Press, New York.

Weyne, J., G. Demeester, and I. Leusen (1970). Effects of carbon dioxide, bicarbonate and pH on lactate and pyruvate in the brain of rats. *Pfluegers Arch.* **314**, 292–311.

Wichser, J., and H. Kazemi (1975). CSF bicarbonate regulation in respiratory acidosis and alkalosis. *J. Appl. Physiol.* **38**, 504–511.

Woodbury, J. W. (1971). A hypothetical model for CSF formation and blood–brain barrier function. *In* "Ion Homeostasis of the Brain" (B. K. Siesjö and S. C. Sørensen, eds.), pp. 465–471. Academic Press, New York.

CHAPTER 7

Specific Mechanisms for O_2 and CO Transport in the Lung and Placenta

G. H. GURTNER, B. BURNS, H. H. PEAVY, C. J. MENDOZA, R. J. TRAYSTMAN, W. SUMMER, AND A. M. SCIUTO

I. INTRODUCTION

In the past few years we have been involved in a series of experiments which have led us to believe that there is a specific carrier for O_2 and CO in the lung and placenta. The carrier may be cytochrome P-450 as originally proposed by Longmuir (Longmuir and Sun, 1970). Carrier-mediated transport systems share a number of properties which are used as criteria for their presence. In this chapter we will summarize our work by applying these criteria to our experimental results in both lung and placenta. The criteria which are listed below, are taken from Stein's book "The Movement of Molecules Across Cell Membranes" (1967).

Regulation of Ventilation and Gas Exchange
Copyright © 1978 by Academic Press, Inc.
All rights of reproduction in any form reserved.
ISBN 0-12-204650-1

II. CRITERIA FOR CARRIER-MEDIATED TRANSPORT

A. The Rate of Permeation of the Carried Molecule Is Greater than Could Be Reasonably Expected from Physical Principles

The original observation which initiated this series of experiments was that O_2 appeared to cross the placenta at a far greater rate than did inert gases. This study was concerned with the relative rates of transfer of inert gases across the placenta during artificial perfusion of the fetal side of the sheep placenta (Bissonnette and Gurtner, 1972). We could control the partial pressure of gases in the perfusion medium as well as the perfusion rate. Gas tensions were measured in umbilical artery and vein and in a maternal artery and uterine vein using a mass spectrometer. With this technique we could simultaneously measure placental diffusing capacity for several inert gases as well as for O_2. In addition, uteroplacental blood flow was calculated using the Fick principle.

Different perfusion media were used: a dextran solution, blood, and a fluorocarbon emulsion. The latter solution was used because the physical solubility of inert gases and O_2 is very high in these liquids. By using the fluorocarbons, we could change the amount of inert gas or O_2 which reaches the placental capillary bed without changing placental perfusion rate, and compare relative rates of transport under these conditions. We consistently observed that transplacental O_2 flux was greater than inert gas flux when the fluxes were normalized by dividing by the diffusion gradient (Fig. 1).

In Fig. 1 we have plotted the flux of O_2 (J_{O_2}) in ml/minute divided by the P_{O_2} difference between the maternal and fetal veins ΔP_{O_2} (MV–FV) against $J_{Ar}/\Delta P_{Ar}$ (FV–MV). This index of diffusing capacity differs from the conventional definition because the venous P_{O_2} difference is used rather than the mean capillary difference. It is possible to calculate the mean capillary difference for Ar and O_2; however, one would be required to assume a deterministic model for the arrangement of maternal and fetal blood vessels in the placenta. Because it is not known whether the vascular flow arrangement is cocurrent, crosscurrent, pool, or a combination of these, we chose to present the data in the above manner. The absolute value of diffusing capacity would differ with each model; however, the relationship between Ar- and O_2-diffusing capacity remains the same.

The results in Fig. 1 show that the P_{O_2} was sometimes the same in fetal and maternal veins. This is indicated by the value of infinity for $J_{O_2}/\Delta P_{O_2}$ (MV–FV). In the other experiments, $J_{O_2}/\Delta P_{O_2}$ (MV-FV) was much

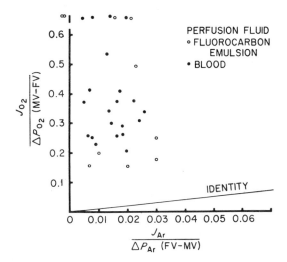

Figure 1.   An index of O_2-diffusing capacity, the transplacental flux of O_2 divided by the difference in P_{O_2} between maternal veins, $J_{O_2}/\Delta P_{O_2}$ (MV–FV), is plotted against a similar index of Ar-diffusing capacity, $J_{Ar}/\Delta P_{Ar}$ (FV–MV). The value of infinity for $J_{O_2}/\Delta P_{O_2}$ (MV–FV) indicates that ΔP_{O_2} (MV–FV) was 0 in these experiments. Data for blood (●) and fluorocarbon (○) perfusion experiments are shown. In all cases O_2 transfer is far larger than Ar transfer.

greater than $J_{Ar}/\Delta P_{Ar}$ (FV–MV). Furthermore, $J_{Ar}/\Delta P_{Ar}$ (FV–MV) was not systematically different during blood and fluorocarbon perfusions.

We interpret these results to mean that O_2 reaches equilibrium between fetal and maternal capillaries in one pass through the placenta. Venous equilibrium can occur only if there is a negligible amount of shunt or variation of $\dot{Q}_M/\dot{Q}_F$ ratios throughout the placenta. This appeared to occur fairly frequently.* In past experiments, the other factors could cause ΔP_{O_2} (MV–FV) to be different from 0. However, $J_{O_2}/\Delta P_{O_2}$ (MV–FV) was always far larger than $J_{Ar}/\Delta P_{Ar}$ (FV–MV). Because $J_{Ar}/\Delta P_{Ar}$ (FV–MV) was similar during blood and fluorocarbon perfusion, we conclude that Ar transfer is diffusion limited. Gurtner and Burns (1975) offer a more detailed discussion of the above experiments.

It is not experimentally feasible to demonstrate this criterion for pul-

---

* In these experiments 10 mg of phenoxybenzamine (dibenzylene) was administered to the fetal–placental unit before the fetus was removed and the perfusion begun. We found that administration of this drug caused vasodilation on the fetal side of the placenta and allowed us to perfuse at nearly normal flows and pressures. It seems possible that the observation of venous equilibrium for O_2 was related to the vasodilation caused by the drug.

monary O_2 and CO transfer because of uncertainties about the magnitude of the membrane-diffusing capacity from morphometric studies. However, we have developed a new approach in which we compare the transfer of O_2 with the simultaneously measured transfer of inert gases to separate any portion of the Alveolar-Arterial *(A-a)* O_2 gradient caused by diffusion limitation from that caused by the distribution of ventilation and perfusion in the lung. This topic is discussed in Section IV.

B.   The Rate of Permeation Is Markedly Reduced by Structurally Analogous Molecules

1.   *Effect on Placental O_2 Transfer of Compounds Which Interfere with Cytochrome P-450*

We have demonstrated that compounds which interact with cytochrome *P*-450 markedly decrease placental O_2 transfer. CO also markedly interferes with O_2 transfer. The effect of diphenhydramine (Benadryl), one of the drugs which interact with cytochrome *P*-450, is shown in Fig. 2. Initially, ΔP_{O_2} (MV–FV) was 0. After two doses of the drug there was a large decrease in $J_{O_2}/\Delta P_{O_2}$ (MV–FV), but no change was observed in the $J_{Ar}/\Delta P_{Ar}$ (FV–MV). Further doses of the drug did affect Ar transfer

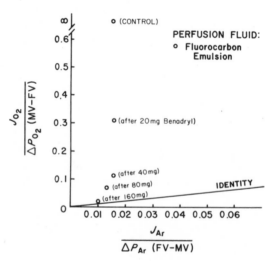

Figure 2. The effect of the drug diphenhydramine (Benadryl), which interacts with cytochrome *P*-450, on the indices of O_2- and Ar-diffusing capacity. Note that the first two doses of the drug decreased $J_{O_2}/\Delta P_{O_2}$ (MV–FV) without affecting $J_{Ar}/\Delta P_{Ar}$ (FV–MV). Each successive dose brings O_2-diffusing capacity closer to Ar-diffusing capacity. Perfusion fluid: fluorocarbon emulsion ($\bigcirc$).

slightly, but decreased O_2 flux even more. After 160 mg of the drug, the O_2- and Ar-diffusing capacities were nearly equal. We believe that this experiment, which is representative of others, demonstrates a dose–response relationship of the specific effect on O_2 transfer of compounds which interact with cytochrome P-450. Because Ar transfer appears to be diffusion limited, nonspecific effects of the drug on membrane permeability would have affected Ar transfer as well. Changes in $\dot{Q}_M/\dot{Q}_F$ ratios would also affect Ar and O_2 transfer in a similar manner.

Other drugs which interact with cytochrome P-450 also decrease placental diffusing capacity. The experimental drug, SKF 525-A, is the most frequently used blocking agent in metabolic studies, and, as discussed below, appears to decrease pulmonary O_2-diffusing capacity.

2. Effect of CO on O_2 Transfer

In some experiments, for reasons which will be explained in the next section, we perfused the fetal side of the placenta with blood containing levels of carboxyhemoglobin (COHb) from 5 to 50%. We found that even low levels of CO reduced $J_{O_2}/\Delta P_{O_2}$ (MV–FV), which we will henceforth redefine as D_{O_2}. D_{O_2} was decreased to 50% of the control level at a fetal COHb of only 8% (Gurtner and Burns, 1976).

D_{O_2} was measured by the steady-state method described above and by a recirculation method in which the rate of O_2 appearance or disappearance was measured from a closed reservoir from which blood was perfused through the fetal side of the placenta and into which the umbilical venous blood was drained. The results of the two methods were similar.

Because of individual variability of placental permeability, D_{O_2} was normalized by dividing by the simultaneously measured diffusing capacity for argon (D_{Ar}). A 50% reduction in D_{O_2}/D_{Ar} was observed at a COHb level of only 8%. The decrease in D_{O_2} cannot be explained by a change in the overall permeability of the placenta, as the normalized permeability to ^3H_2O and to ^{14}C-labeled urea did not change as COHb was increased (Gurtner and Burns, 1976).

The decrease in D_{O_2} cannot be explained by the small reduction in the total O_2 of hemoglobin, because the CO-induced leftward shift in the O_2 caused the O_2 content to increase rather than decrease at the low P_{O_2} levels encountered in the fetal side of the placenta. Similar results were observed when the fluorocarbon emulsions were used in place of blood. We believe that the effect of CO may be of practical importance because similar COHb levels are seen in heavy smokers.

In the recirculation experiments, each perfusion was continued until a steady state occurred for fetal and maternal P_{O_2}. Under these conditions, fetal arterial and venous O_2 content and P_{O_2} values were the same; therefore, no net O_2 exchange occurred across the placenta. The steady-state relationships between fetal and maternal venous P_{O_2} values and COHb content provides evidence that the CO is interfering with a membrane carrier (Fig. 3). In the control condition we found that fetal venous P_{O_2} was higher than maternal venous P_{O_2}. This is compatible with the presence of a crosscurrent or countercurrent gas exchange as proposed by Rankin (1972). As the COHb level was increased, the P_{O_2} difference decreased and reversed sign. At the highest levels studied, maternal venous P_{O_2} was about 20 mm Hg higher than fetal P_{O_2}.

Because the permeability to ^3H_2O and ^{14}C-labeled urea did not change at the different CO levels, it seems reasonable to assume that $\dot{Q}_M/\dot{Q}_F$ distribution also remained constant. Uteroplacental O_2 consumption also remained constant at all CO levels. Under these conditions, the only possible mechanism causing the P_{O_2} differences is a decrease in membrane-diffusing capacity of the placenta.

The possibility that tissue O_2 consumption in the gas-exchange region might affect fetal P_{O_2} has been considered for a number of years. Dawes (1972) described some experiments which were similar to ours, i.e., no transplacental O_2 exchange was present. He measured the relationship between fetal P_{O_2} and maternal P_{O_2} at different maternal P_{O_2} levels, and found that a significant portion of the normal maternal arterial–fetal venous P_{O_2} difference was contributed by placental O_2 consumption alone. Because no measurements of maternal venous P_{O_2} were made, he could

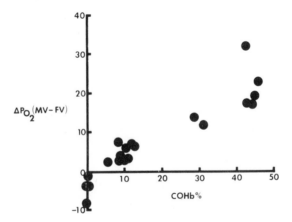

Figure 3. Steady-state P_{O_2} differences between uterine and umbilical venous blood under conditions of no gas exchange. The magnitude of the P_{O_2} differences is related to COHb in the fetal blood. This relationship can be explained if the diffusing capacity of the exchange membrane is decreased by CO while the O_2 consumption of the exchange membrane remains constant.

not conclude that O_2 consumption in the gas-exchange membrane contributed to the P_{O_2} differences; however, he speculated that, since the placenta was an active metabolic organ, such gradients might exist. P_{O_2} gradients could occur within the membrane itself if O_2 consumption of the membrane were large relative to membrane-diffusing capacity. The magnitude of the gradient can be predicted from a modification of Warburg's equation which describes the relationship between membrane P_{O_2} and membrane thickness (Eq. 1).

$$\Delta P_{O_2}(M_{cap}-F_{cap}) = \frac{M}{\alpha D}(\Delta X)^2 \tag{1}$$

where M is the tissue O_2 consumption in ml/minute/gm, αD is the Krogh coefficient, and ΔX is the distance between maternal and fetal capillary.

Equation (1) was derived by integrating the diffusion equation for the steady-state condition in which

$$\frac{d^2 P}{dX^2} = -\frac{M}{\alpha D}$$

In the first integration step

$$\frac{dP}{dX} = -\frac{M}{\alpha D}\Delta X + K_1$$

where K_1, the constant of integration, equals dP/dX at $\Delta X = 0$. This by Fick's first law equals $-V_{O_2}/\alpha DA$. V_{O_2} is the placental O_2 consumption which we assume takes place in the exchange membrane, and equals $MA \, \Delta X$, where A is the area of the exchange membrane and X is its thickness. Using these assumptions,

$$\frac{dP}{dX} = -2\frac{MX}{\alpha D}$$

In the second integration step

$$P_{(X)} = -(M/\alpha D)\Delta X^2 + P_{O_2}(0)$$

where $P_{O_2}(0)$ is the P_{O_2} in the maternal capillary.

In the solution of Eq. 1, α was assumed to be

$$\left(\frac{0.023 \text{ ml } O_2(0° \text{ 760})\text{torr/ml}}{\text{ATM}}\right)\left(\frac{\text{ATM}}{760 \text{ torr}}\right) = 3.026 \times 10^{-5} \text{ ml/ml/torr}$$

ΔX was varied from 0 to 30 μm.

Figure 4 shows the two solutions of Eq. (1) for ratios of $M/\alpha D$ which are tenfold different. The tenfold difference was used because placental D_{O_2} fell to about one-tenth of the control value at the highest COHb level studied (40% COHb).

The value of D in the upper curve of Fig. 4 is 9×10^4 cm^2 minute, which is similar to the diffusion coefficient for O_2 in water. The value of D in the lower curve in Fig. 4 is 10 times larger. We found that no significant membrane gradients occurred unless the value of M was large. In this example, the value of M was taken to be 0.2 ml/minute/gm tissue. This is far larger than the overall M of 0.008 measured by Dawes *et al*. This 25-fold discrepancy between measured O_2 consumption for the entire placenta and the hypothetical value for the exchange membrane would seem to falsify the hypothesis; however, because the gas-exchange membrane makes up only a small portion of the whole placenta and is rich in mitochondria (Björkman, 1965), it seems possible that the local O_2 consumption might be substantially higher than overall O_2 consumption.

3. Mechanisms of Drug and CO Effects on the Carrier

There are two different mechanisms by which drugs and CO can affect the carrier: (a) by competition with O_2 for the heme iron as in the case of CO inhibition, or (b) the drug may bind to the protein portion of the molecule. This allosteric binding in turn affects the rate of reaction at the

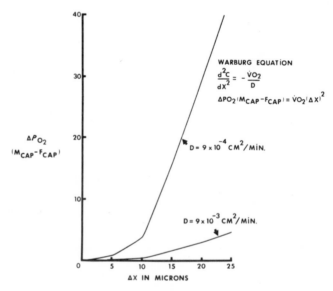

Figure 4. The theoretical relationship predicted by the Warburg equation between maternal–fetal P_{O_2} differences and membrane thickness at two different diffusion coefficients. For a 15-μm membrane, similar to the thickness of the placental exchange membrane, a tenfold decrease in D can cause ΔP_{O_2} to increase from 2 to 20 mm Hg (see text).

heme site (Lipscomb and Gunsalus, 1973), perhaps because the bound drug molecule shields the heme site from the microenvironment. This second mechanism could explain the effects of drugs on O$_2$ transfer.

4. Effect of Drugs on Pulmonary CO Transfer

We have found that the compounds which decrease the O$_2$-diffusing capacity of the placenta also decrease the CO-diffusing capacity of the lung in experimental animals (Burns and Gurtner, 1973).

In 16 normal subjects, we found that diphenhydramine (Benadryl) in a dosage of 50–100 mg caused a 10% reduction in single-breath DL_{CO}, measured using 0.4% CO in the inspired gas ($p < 0.001$) (Table I). The decrease in DL_{CO}, although small, was extremely reproducible because the measurements were made in the supine position at a single lung volume. The variability of DL_{CO} measured under these circumstances has been found to be much smaller than the variability in DL_{CO} measured in the upright position (Gurtner and Fowler, 1971).

However, we could not unequivocally ascribe the decreases to effects

Table I. Changes in Diffusing Capacity and Specific Diffusing Capacity (DL_{CO}/VA) Observed 1 Hour after a Single Oral Dose of Diphenhydramine[a]

Patient	DL_{CO} baseline	% Change	DL_{CO}/ VA baseline	% Change
1	14.1	−8.5	2.6	−12
2	13.9	−10	3.7	−5
3	15.2	−8.5	4.3	−2
4	24.8	−22.0	4.2	−17
5	20.0	−10	3.4	−6
6	19.0	−10.5	3.4	−12
7	22.7	−14	4.5	−16
8	15.0	−8.6	4.2	−12
9	23.5	−15	3.4	−6
10	20.9	−6	3.8	−21
11	19.9	+2	4.1	0
12	28.3	−11.7	4.0	−5
13	16.9	−9	4.1	−10
14	19.3	−8	3.6	−8
15	12.5	−6.4	2.7	0
16	24.1	−11.6	4.6	−5
	Mean	−9.8	Mean	−8.5
	$p < 0.001$		$p < 0.001$	

[a] All measurements were made in the supine position; every effort was made to keep end inspiratory lung volume the same in the two measurements. Both DL and DL/VA decreased significantly.

on a carrier molecule, because the drugs might have caused other changes which could act to decrease diffusing capacity in the absence of a carrier. Because of this uncertainty, we have sought additional evidence for carrier mediation of pulmonary carbon monoxide transport which did not involve the use of drugs. These experiments are described below.

C. The Rate of Permeation Is Not Directly Proportional to Partial Pressure, but Approaches a Saturation Value

1. Saturation Kinetics

A schematic example of this phenomenon is shown in Fig. 5. In Fig. 5, both simple diffusion and facilitated diffusion are assumed to occur. The relationship between flux and partial pressure gradient for simple diffusion predicted by Fick's first law is linear and passes through the origin. The relationship for facilitated diffusion depends on the dissociation curve of the carrier and the kinetics for binding and releasing the carried molecule. In Fig. 5A, a simple hyperbolic relationship is assumed; in Fig. 5B, a sigmoid shape is assumed. We have assumed that the reaction time of O_2 and CO with the carrier is not rate limiting, so that the flux partial pressure relationship resembles the dissociation curve of the carrier.

Diffusing capacity is by definition flux divided by gradient; therefore, it is the slope of the straight line drawn from any point on the total flux curve through the origin. In the bottom panel of Figs. 5A and 5B, diffusing capacity plotted against partial pressure gradient is shown. In Fig. 5A diffusing capacity decreases monotonically as the gradient increases; in Fig. 5B diffusing capacity initially increases, reaches a maximum, and then decreases as partial pressure continues to increase.

At the present time we have data only on saturation kinetics for pulmonary and placental CO transfer. The experimental demonstration of saturation kinetics for placental CO was measured in the same manner and in the same experiments as D_{O_2} during recirculation of fetal perfusion fluid in a closed system (Gurtner *et al.*, 1975a).

The D_{CO} is normalized by dividing each measured D_{CO} by the simultaneously measured diffusing capacity for argon (D_{Ar}). The relationship between normalized D_{CO} and COHb resembles the schematic representation given in Fig. 5A. As mentioned above, the results cannot be explained by a generalized change in placental permeability. In these experiments, the transfer of ^{14}C-labeled urea or [3]H_2O was also measured simultaneously. The permeability of the placenta to these molecules did not change as COHb was increased.

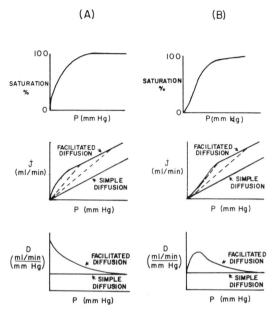

Figure 5. A: A schematic representation of the phenomenon of saturation kinetics in which both simple diffusion and facilitated transport are present. In this example, the dissociation curve for the carrier is assumed to be hyperbolic similar to myoglobin. Flux (J) due to simple diffusion increases directly in proportion to partial pressure. The flux due to the facilitated component approaches a saturation value as partial pressure is increased. The diffusing capacity (D) is the flux divided by the driving pressure and is the slope of the line passing through the origin to any point on the total flux curve. Note that D decreases monotonically as P_{CO} increases. B: This representation is the same as A, except the dissociation curve of the carrier is assumed to be sigmoid in shape, similar to hemoglobin. D first increases, reaches a maximum, and then decreases, similar to the experimentally determined relationship observed between DL_{CO} and end-tidal CO concentration in Fig. 2.

2. Saturation Kinetics for Pulmonary CO Transfer

We have a good deal of data on the phenomenon of saturation kinetics for pulmonary CO transfer. The initial experiments were done on anesthetized, paralyzed dogs using a single-breath technique in which the gas mixture, containing CO and helium, was introduced into the animals' lungs with a large syringe, the airway occluded, and the expired gas collected in a Haldane–Priestly tube after a 10-second breath hold. The results are shown in Fig. 6; they resemble the theoretical relationship in Fig. 5A.

We later measured the alveolar disappearance for CO at the different concentrations and found that part of the change in DL_{CO} which we found

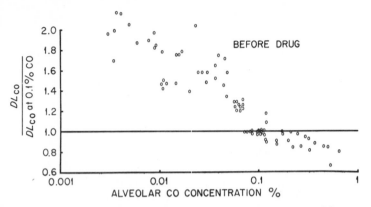

Figure 6. The ratio of single-breath DL_{CO} measured at various alveolar CO concentrations divided by the DL_{CO} measured at 0.1% is plotted against initial alveolar CO concentration. Note the increase in the ratio as CO concentration is decreased. This is the relationship which would pertain if there were a specific pulmonary CO carrier.

in the first series of experiments was due to a saturable absorption of CO to some molecule in the lung tissue. This phenomenon is seen in Fig. 7, which depicts results from an experiment in which alveolar disappearance curves were measured at two CO levels. The rate constants for CO disappearance are similar, but the intercept disappearance curve measured at the lower CO concentration extrapolates back to an intercept at $t = 0$, which is smaller than predicted helium dilution. The alveolar disappearance curve, measured at the lower CO concentration, could be explained by facilitated transport, but also by CO uptake by noncarrier cytochromes.

In an attempt to choose between these alternative hypotheses, we measured steady-state DL_{CO} by the Bates method, at several different inspired CO levels, in anesthetized paralyzed dogs ventilated at constant tidal volume and frequency. Steady-state DL_{CO} measures only gas-to-blood transfer and is unaffected by tissue binding of CO. In each DL_{CO} measurement, inspired, mixed expired, end-tidal, and CO back pressures were measured directly.

The experimental results for 13 dogs are shown in Fig. 8. It should be noted that DL_{CO} initially increases, reaches a maximum, and then decreases as CO level is increased. These results correspond to the theoretical curve of Fig. 5B, in which the dissociation curve of the carrier molecule is sigmoid in shape. Because the directly measured dissociation curve of cytochrome P-450 is sigmoid (Burns *et al.*, 1976), the results are further evidence that cytochrome P-450 is the carrier. If the manifestation of saturation kinetics for transpulmonary CO flux is seen in Fig. 5, the

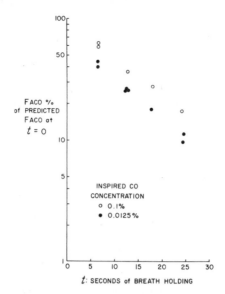

Figure 7. Alveolar disappearance curves for CO were measured at two CO concentrations. Both curves appear to be monoexponential, but the curve measured at 0.0125% CO appears to have a depressed $t=0$ intercept. This is due to absorption of CO by the lung tissue. The amount absorbed is far in excess of the physical solubility of the gas and represents binding to a CO-binding molecule, possibly cytochrome P-450. Inspired CO concentration: $\bigcirc$, 0.14%; $\bullet$, 0.023%.

discrepancy between the results of the single-breath and steady-state DL_{CO} measurements might be explained by CO binding by noncarrier cytochromes. This would affect the single-breath measurements but not the steady-state DL_{CO}.

There appear to be species differences in the manifestation of saturation kinetics. Burns *et al.* (1976) found in rebreathing experiments on sheep that the rate constant for CO disappearance from the lung changed in an inverse relationship with inspired CO level (Table I). These results also support the hypothesis that pulmonary CO transport is partially carrier mediated.

Other criteria given by Stein (1967) are applicable only to mobile carriers or to unidirectional pores reserved specifically for entrance or exit. These are the phenomena of counter-transport and competitive exchange diffusion. These phenomena are due to the presence of a saturating molecule on one side of the membrane which allows transient manifestation of unidirectional flux of another molecule which is also carried. In the experiment mentioned above, CO transfer was from the fetal to the maternal circulation; O_2 transfer was from maternal to fetal circulation.

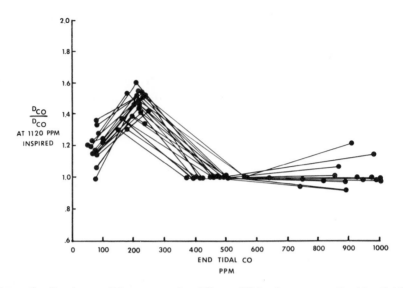

Figure 8. Steady-state DL_{CO} measured at different CO levels was normalized by dividing by the DL_{CO} measured at the inspired CO concentration of 1100 ppm. The normalized DL_{CO} is plotted against end-tidal CO concentration. The decrease in DL_{CO} as end-tidal CO concentration is increased from 200 to 500 ppm is nearly identical with rebreathing single-breath measurements reported in Gurtner *et al*. (1975b), indicating that at these levels of CO the change in DL_{CO} with changes in CO concentration measured by all the methods is caused by facilitated transfer of CO. The increase in steady-state DL_{CO} as CO concentration is increased does not agree with the rebreathing and single-breath measurements. A possible explanation for the discrepancy may involve absorption of CO by noncarrier cytochromes. This would influence only the rebreathing and single-breath measurements.

Under these circumstances, we should have observed counter-transport for O_2, which would have been manifested by an increase in D_{O_2} as COHb increased. The failure to demonstrate this criterion can be interpreted as evidence that cytochrome P-450 acts as a fixed site carrier. This seems reasonable, for the cytochrome is structurally part of the endoplasmic reticulum and cannot be extracted without denaturation.

III. IDENTITY OF THE CARRIER

A. Evidence in Favor of Cytochrome P-450 as the Carrier

The evidence in favor of cytochrome P-450 as the carrier include the following: the effects on gas exchange of compounds which bind to the cytochrome; the reaction kinetics of the cytochrome; and the correlation between the K_m for facilitated transport and the $P50$ of the carrier.

The compounds which bind to the cytochrome markedly decrease transplacental O_2 transfer while not affecting inert gas transfer (Gurtner and Burns, 1972, 1975; Gurtner et al., 1975b; Mendoza et al., 1976). Cytochrome P-450 is present in the liver, lungs, placenta, kidney, and adrenals. This cytochrome reversibly binds both O_2 and CO (Peterson et al., 1972; Peterson and Griffin, 1972); the reaction rate with CO has been measured and is considerably faster than the reaction rate of CO with hemoglobin (Lipscomb and Gunsalus, 1973; Peterson et al., 1972). The O_2 association rate with P-450 for mammalian liver P-450 has been reported to be 20 times faster than the CO association rate (Rösen and Stier, 1973). Compounds which bind to cytochrome P-450 act to slow the association and dissociation with CO, presumably by shielding the CO binding site (Lipscomb and Gunsalus, 1973). This may be the mechanism by which placental O_2 transport is reduced by such compounds.

When the data from Fig. 4 was plotted on a Lineweaver–Burke plot, a K_m (CO concentration at 50% of maximum facilitated flux) value for facilitated flux of CO of 210 ppm or 0.15 mm Hg was calculated. This K_m value agrees fairly well experimentally with our measurements of the $P50$ for cytochrome P-450 in liver (0.15 mm Hg) and in lung (0.26 mm Hg) (Burns et al., 1976).

In addition, saturation kinetics for CO transfer, as well as the reduction in DL_{CO} caused by drugs which bind to cytochrome P-450, can be correlated with the presence of the cytochrome in the lung. This is demonstrated by comparing the measurements made in the newborn lamb, which has less than one-tenth the adult concentration of pulmonary cytochrome P-450, with the same measurements in the adult sheep. These results are shown in Tables II and III.

B. Evidence Against Cytochrome P-450 as the Carrier

There are certain experimental results in the literature which seem to be inconsistent with our working hypothesis that cytochrome P-450 is the carrier.

One argument is that the O_2 affinity of cytochrome P-450 is too large for this molecule to act as an O_2 carrier in the placenta and lung. Although no O_2-binding spectrum has been demonstrated for mammalian cytochrome P-450, there is some indirect evidence which involves drug metabolism that the K_m (related to the P-50 of the cytochrome) is on the order of 1 mm Hg. It is argued that cytochrome could not act as a placental or pulmonary

Table II. Saturation Kinetics for Pulmonary CO Transfer

	$t_\frac{1}{2}$ (sec)		$DL_{CO}{}^a$ (ml/min/mm/Hg)	
	FACO 65 ppm	FACO 650 ppm	FACO 65 ppm	FACO 650 ppm
Adult sheep ($N = 9$)	4.6	5.1	32.2	24.9
		$p < 0.025$		$p < 0.001$
Newborn lambs ($N = 3$)	20	19.66	1.16	1.18
		N.S.		N.S.

^{a} DL_{CO} measured by the rebreathing technique in adult sheep and newborn lambs. Note that DL_{CO} at an initial FACO of 65 ppm was significantly larger than at 650 ppm. This was partly due to an increased rate of CO disappearance at the lower CO concentration, but was also related to an increased volume of distribution of CO in the lung due to the rapid uptake of CO by the carrier (see Gurtner *et al.*, 1975b, for details). No such effects were seen in the newborn lambs who lack cytochrome *P*-450. This is evidence that cytochrome *P*-450 is responsible for the changes in DL_{CO} observed in the adult sheep and that facilitated CO transport can be correlated with the presence of cytochrome *P*-450.

O_2 carrier because it would always be 100% saturated at physiological P_{O_2} values. This argument may not be valid on theoretical grounds, because even if a carrier system is nearly 100% saturated, it is capable of some degree of facilitated transport. Several years ago, a model for anion transport across the red cell membrane was introduced which proposed that there were positively charged pores in the membrane which would preferentially attract anions and exclude cations, causing anion transport to be several orders of magnitude greater than cation transport. Because of

Table III. Drug Effects on DL_{CO} in sheep

	$DL_{CO}{}^a$ (NORMOXIA)	
	Control	SKF 525A
Adult sheep	30.7 ($N = 6$)	20.4 ($N = 6$)
	$P < 0.0025$	
Newborn lambs	1.46($N = 9$)	1.36($N = 6$)
	N.S.	

^{a} DL_{CO} was measured by a rebreathing technique at an initial FACO of 400 ppm before and after administration of SKF 525A buffered to pH 7.4. The adult dose of the drug was 1000 mg, the lamb dose was 100 mg. On the basis of milligrams per kilogram body weight, or milligrams per M^2 body surface area, the lambs actually received a larger dose. Note that DL_{CO} decreases significantly in the adult sheep, but does not change in the lambs who lack cytochrome *P*-450.

the magnitude of the electrical forces, each positive charge in the membrane pores would have to be associated with a negative anion; therefore, no "unsaturated" site would exist. The system could work because a difference in electrochemical potential across the membrane would make the probability of an anion entering or leaving different at the two sides of the membrane. The electrochemical force could be transmitted along the pore like a mechanical force can be transmitted along a line of contiguous croquet balls: When the ball at the head of the line is struck, the greatest movement is observed in that ball at the opposite end. This model could be the direct analog of an O_2 transport system if the positive charges represented the carrier and the anions represented O_2 of CO.

The model described above could explain all the experimental criteria of carrier-mediated transport except the phenomenon of saturation kinetics. It could also explain the latter phenomenon if the rate-limiting factors for transfer included the rate of binding with and dissociation from the carrier as well as the electrochemical potential difference for the carried molecule.

There is some evidence that the O_2 affinity of the cytochrome may not be as large as previously thought. Cytochrome P-450 appears to be comprised of several heme proteins with different properties. If this is the case, it seems possible that the different cytochromes could have different O_2 affinities. This might explain the experimental results of Kampffmeyer and Keise (1964). These investigators measured the relationship between the rate of microsomal drug metabolism and P_{O_2} for several different compounds. All the metabolism was presumably mediated by cytochrome P-450. They were careful to exclude diffusion as the rate-limiting factor in their experiments. They found that the rate of metabolism of certain drugs was 50% maximal at about 1 mm Hg, whereas for others, metabolism was 50% maximal at P_{O_2} levels as high as 28 mm Hg. If the results are due to differences in O_2 affinity, the cytochrome with a K_m of 28 mm Hg would be an almost optimally efficient placental and pulmonary O_2 carrier.

Another argument is that the relative affinity for O_2 and CO of cytochrome $P = 450$ is different from the relative affinity of the carrier. We found that placental O_2 transfer was markedly decreased by low levels of CO in the experiments described above. This sort of inhibition of O_2 transport could only be possible if the carrier had a much higher affinity for CO than O_2. Although the K_m ($P50$) of our pulmonary CO carrier corresponds well to the measured $P50$ of pulmonary cytochrome P-450, the relative O_2 affinities are unknown.

The only information available is on the effects of various O_2–CO mixtures on drug metabolism or steroid synthesis, using liver or adrenal microsomal preparations (Estabrook et al., 1970; Cooper et al., 1973). In most of these experiments, after a control period in which the microsomes were exposed to a low O_2 concentration (usually 4% O_2), CO was added, keeping the O_2 fraction constant. It was found that the metabolism was inhibited by 50% with CO:O_2 ratios which were between O_2 and 1.0. These ratios are far smaller than one would expect from our experimental results. It seems possible that this discrepancy might be explained by the heterogeneity of the heme compounds which make up cytochrome P-450. Because drug metabolism studies were usually performed at low P_{O_2} levels, those varieties of the cytochrome with relatively low O_2 affinity described above could have been overlooked. It also seems possible that those varieties of the cytochrome which mediate drug metabolism might be different from those varieties which mediate O_2 transport.

If cytochrome P-450 were not the carrier, other oxygenases might play a role. Staudinger *et al.* (1965) have described a second type of oxidase which might act as a carrier. They found that the rate of NADPH oxidation and drug metabolism increased by rat and dog liver microsomes in direct proportion to the P_{O_2} of the preparation up to P_{O_2} levels greater than 200 mm Hg. This oxidase was inhibited by SKF 525-A, but was not as sensitive to CO as cytochrome P-450. They speculated that this oxidase was a copper-containing enzyme. Thus, this oxidase, acting as a carrier, could explain some, but not all, of our experimental results.

IV. PHYSIOLOGICAL IMPORTANCE OF CARRIER-MEDIATED TRANSPORT

All of our placental research has been performed on the sheep placenta which, because of the large distances between maternal and fetal vessels and small surface area, poses a formidable barrier with low diffusing capacity for exchange of materials by simple diffusion. We estimate that up to 80% of placental O_2 transfer may be mediated by the carrier (Gurtner *et al.*, 1975b). Bissonnette *et al.* (1975) have demonstrated carrier-mediated transport of CO in the guinea pig placenta which, because of the lack of fetal tissue layers, offers a smaller barrier to simple diffusion. In this placenta, the estimate of percentage of carrier-mediated CO transport is approximately 20% (Stein, 1967).

The role of a carrier in pulmonary oxygen transfer is more difficult to assess. Because of the large surface area for gas exchange, the short distance between gas and blood, and the large P_{O_2} gradient between alveolar gas and mixed venous blood, sufficient O_2 exchange can occur by simple diffusion to satisfy metabolic needs. There is no clear evidence that, under normal physiological conditions, diffusion could become a rate-limiting process in pulmonary oxygen exchange. We have developed a new method which we believe is capable of separating the component of the $(A-a)$ O_2 gradient due to diffusion limitation, if present, from the component due to $\dot{V}/\dot{Q}$ mismatch (Gurtner et al., 1977). In some preliminary experiments we have found that there is no diffusion limitation for O_2 transfer in anesthetized dogs while the animals breathe air; however, diffusion limitation occurs under conditions of alveolar hypoxia, especially when O_2 consumption is increased. Under these circumstances, administration of drugs which bind to cytochrome P-450 increases the portion of the A-a gradient due to diffusion.

REFERENCES

Bissonnette, J. M. and G. H. Gurtner (1972). Transfer of inert gases and tritiated water across the sheep placenta. *J. Appl. Physiol.* **32,** 64–69.

Bissonnette, J. M., W. K. Wickham, and W. H. Drummond (1975). Placental diffusing capacities at varied carbon monoxide tensions. *Physiologist* **18,** 142 (abstr.).

Björkman, N. (1965). Fine structure of the ovine placentome. *J. Anat.* **99,** 283–297.

Burns, B., and G. H. Gurtner (1973). A specific carrier for oxygen and carbon monoxide in the lung and placenta. *Drug Metab. Dispos.* **1,** 374–379.

Burns, B., Y.-N. Cha, and J. M. Purcell (1976). A specific carrier for O_2 and CO in the lung: Effects of volatile anesthetics on gas transfer and drug metabolism. *Chest* **69,** Suppl., 316–321.

Cooper, D. Y., H. Schleyer, S. S. Levin, and O. Rosenthal (1973). Studies on the partially purified heme protein P-450 from the adrenal cortex. *Ann. N.Y. Acad. Sci.* **212,** 227–242.

Dawes, G. S. (1972). Oxygen consumption and carbon dioxide production in the placenta. *In* "Respiratory Gas Exchange and Blood Flow in the Placenta" (L. D. Longo and H. Bartels, eds.), DHEW Publ. No. (NIH)73-361, pp. 267–277. US Dept. of Health, Education and Welfare, Washington, D.C.

Estabrook, R. W., M. R. Franklin, and A. G. Hildebrandt (1970). Factors influencing the inhibitory effect of carbon monoxide on cytochrome P-450-catalyzed mixed function oxidation reactions. *Ann. N.Y. Acad. Sci.* **174,** 218–232.

Gurtner, G. H., and B. Burns (1972). Possible facilitated transport of oxygen across the placenta. *Nature (London)* **240,** 473–475.

Gurtner, G. H., and B. Burns (1975). Physiological evidence consistent with the presence of a specific O_2 carrier in the placenta. *J. Appl. Physiol.* **39,** 728–734.

Gurtner, G. H., and B. Burns (1976). Competition between CO and O_2 for a placental carrier. *Fed. Proc., Fed. Am. Soc. Exp. Biol.* **35,** 830 (abstr.).

Gurtner, G. H., and W. Fowler (1971). Interrelationships of factors affecting pulmonary diffusing capacity. *J. Appl. Physiol.* **30,** 619–624.

Gurtner, G. H., J. Bissonnette, and B. Burns (1975a). Saturation kinetics for placental CO transfer. *Physiologist* **18,** 235. (abstr.).

Gurtner, G. H., H. Peavy, W. Summer, and B. Burns (1975b). Physiological evidence of a specific O_2–CO carrier in the lung and placenta. *Prog. Respir. Res.* **8,** 166–176.

Gurtner, G. H., C. Mendoza, A. M. Sciuto, R. Ayash, R. Lodato, and B. Burns (1977). A simple method for assessment of diffusion limitation of pulmonary O_2 transfer. Fed. Proc., *Fed. Am. Soc. Exp. Biol.* **36**, 591.

Kampffmeyer, H., and M. Kiese (1964). The hydroxylation of analine and *N*-ethylaniline by microsomal enzymes at low oxygen pressures. *Biochem. Z.* **339**, 454–459.

Lipscomb, J. D., and I. C. Gunsalus (1973). Structural aspects of the active site of cytochrome P-450$_{cam}$. *Drug Metab. Dispos.* **1**, 1–5.

Longmuir, I. S., and S. Sun (1970). A hypothetical tissue oxygen carrier. *Microvasc. Res.* **2**, 287–293.

Mendoza, C., H. Peavy, B. Burns, and G. H. Gurtner (1976). Saturation kinetics for pulmonary CO transfer. *Am. Rev. Respir. Dis.* **113**, Suppl., 196.

Peterson, J. A., and B. W. Griffin (1972). Carbon monoxide binding by pseudomonas putida cytochrome P-450. *Arch. Biochem. Biophys.* **151**, 427–433.

Peterson, J. A., Y. Ishimura, and B. W. Griffin (1972). Pseudomonas putida cytochrome P-450: Characterization of an oxygenated form of the hemoprotein. *Arch. Biochem. Biophys.* **149**, 197–208.

Rankin, J. H. G. (1972). The effects of shunted and unevenly distributed blood flows on crosscurrent exchange in the sheep placenta. *In* "Respiratory Gas Exchange and Blood Flow in the Placenta" (L. D. Longo and H. Bartels, eds.), DHEW Publ. No. (NIH) 73-361, pp. 207–226. US Dept. of Health, Education and Welfare, Washington, D.C.

Rösen, P., and A. Stier (1973). Kinetics of CO and O_2 complexes of rabbit liver microsomal cytochrome P_{450}. *Biochem. Biophys. Res. Commun.* **51**, 603–611.

Staudinger, H. J., B. Kerekjarto, V. Ullrich, and Z. Zubrzycki (1965). A study on the mechanism of microsomal hydroxylation. *Oxidases Relat. Redox Syst., Proc. Symp., 1964* pp. 815–837.

Stein, W. D. (1967). "The Movement of Molecules Across Cell Membranes." Academic Press, New York.

CHAPTER 8

Measurement of the Distribution of Ventilation–Perfusion Ratios

PETER D. WAGNER

I. INTRODUCTION

The idea that maldistribution of either inspired gas or pulmonary arterial blood within the lungs can interfere with gas exchange is not new. Early in this century, Krogh and Lindhard (1917) discussed the conse-

217

Regulation of Ventilation and Gas Exchange
Copyright © 1978 by Academic Press, Inc.
All rights of reproduction in any form reserved.
ISBN 0-12-204650-1

quences of ventilatory inequality on gas exchange, but quantitative approaches were not attempted. A few years later, Haldane and Priestley (1935) made similar comments and distinguished between the effects of ventilation–perfusion inequality on oxygen on the one hand and carbon dioxide on the other. They reasoned, falsely, that CO_2 was invulnerable to the effects of maldistribution because of its essentially linear dissociation curve (while hypoxemia was expected because of the distinctly nonlinear dissociation curve of O_2). Without quantitative approaches, however, there could be little progress in the study of ventilation–perfusion relationships; it was not until about 1950 that advances were made.

Working separately (but at about the same time) Fenn et al. (1946) on the one hand and Riley and Cournand (1949, 1951) and Riley, Cournand, and Donald (1951) on the other, developed similar quantitative relationships dealing with alveolar gas exchange. Although the principles were straightforward, embodying only the concept of conservation of mass, the necessary numerical computations were formidable. This led both groups to present their work graphically as the oxygen–carbon dioxide diagram and the four-quadrant diagram, respectively. These efforts are appreciated by current workers as milestones in the study of pulmonary gas exchange, and form the basis upon which most subsequent work has been based.*

Because of the difficulty of the numerical computations, much further progress had to wait until the digital computer became available (in the latter half of the 1960's) to the pulmonary physiologist. The key to computer analysis of gas exchange was recognized by both Kelman (1966, 1967) and Olszowka and Farhi (1968) as the ability to describe the O_2 and CO_2 dissociation curves with digital computer algorithms. Once this had been accomplished, these workers (Kelman, 1968; Olszowka and Farhi, 1969) and West (1969) were able to quantitate the effects of ventilation–perfusion inequality on gas exchange with relatively little effort. It was shown numerically (West, 1969) and later theoretically (Evans et al., 1974) that under essentially all conditions ventilation–perfusion inequality interferes with the exchange of all known gases, irrespective of the shape of their dissociation curve (O_2, CO_2, CO) or their solubility (foreign inert gases). Many questions of clinical importance were answered. Important examples include: (a) the gas exchange behavior of theoretical (but reasonable) distributions of ventilation–

---

* Symbols used in this chapter: P_{O_2}, Partial pressure of oxygen; P_{CO_2}, partial pressure of carbon dioxide; P_A, alveolar partial pressure; $P_{c'}$, end capillary partial pressure; $P_{\bar{v}}$, mixed venous partial pressure; λ, blood:gas partition coefficient; $\dot{V}_A/\dot{Q}$, ventilation–perfusion ratio; $\dot{Q}$, perfusion; Pa, systemic arterial partial pressure; R, retention; $\dot{V}_A$, alveolar ventilation; E, excretion; $\dot{Q}_T$, total pulmonary blood flow; $\dot{V}_E$, minute ventilation; $\dot{V}_{O_2}$, oxygen consumption.

perfusion ratios (West, 1969); (b) the effect of replacing N_2 by a more soluble gas such as N_2O (Farhi and Olszowka, 1968); (c) the effect of theoretically changing the shape, position, or slope of the dissociation curve of the gas in question (West, 1969–1970); (d) the effects of inequality on exchange of inert gases of various solubilities (Colburn et al., 1974); and (e) the effects of breathing elevated concentrations of O_2 on gas exchange in poorly ventilated lung units (Dantzker et al., 1975).

Research of this kind has clearly been very useful in answering questions about the effects on gas exchange of assumed distributions of ventilation–perfusion ratios, but the reverse problem—namely, that of learning as much as possible about the distribution of ventilation–perfusion ratios in an individual from measurements of gas exchange—is of greater importance from both the physiological and clinical standpoint.

The work of Fenn, Rahn, and Otis, and of Riley and co-workers quoted previously led to simple and now well-known ways of describing the distribution (of ventilation–perfusion ratios) in individuals. Using measured arterial and mixed expired O_2 and CO_2 partial pressures, these workers showed how it was possible to quantitatively describe the lung as if it consisted of just three types of gas-exchange units: normal ("ideal"); unventilated (physiological shunt); and unperfused (physiological dead-space). Simple expressions allowed the determination of the precise distribution of bloodflow between normal and unventilated "compartments" and of ventilation between normal and unperfused compartments that would exactly explain the measured arterial and expired P_{O_2} and P_{CO_2} values.

Numerous attempts have been made to improve upon this approach to the description of the distribution of ventilation–perfusion ratios. Notable among them is the method of Lenfant and Okubo (1968) based upon the rise in arterial P_{O_2} during nitrogen washout. Here, mathematical techniques were used to determine a continuous distribution of ventilation–perfusion ratios compatible with the observed data. Peslin et al. (1971) demonstrated some theoretical limitations to this method, but there are also some physiological limits to this approach. In particular, all the hypoxemia is treated as if caused by ventilation–perfusion inequality or shunt, so that any contribution from incomplete diffusion equilibration cannot be identified. In addition, areas of low ventilation–perfusion ratio may collapse during O_2 breathing, thereby changing the distribution as it is being measured. Finally, because of the shape of the oxyhemoglobin dissociation curve, resolution is poor for lung units with ventilation–perfusion ratios above about 1.0.

An alternate approach was suggested by Farhi (1967), Farhi and Yokoyama (1967), and Yokoyama and Farhi (1967) about ten years ago.

They proposed to measure the elimination of three inert gases by the lung under quasi-steady-state conditions. They developed a theoretical basis exactly analogous to that of the O_2–CO_2 diagram of Rahn and Fenn (1955) based on conservation of mass and used it to construct two-compartment models which would explain the elimination data. The gases used by these authors were methane, ethane, and nitrous oxide, gases of medium to low solubility.

Some years ago we realized that the use of more inert gases whose solubilities covered a wider range would permit a still better definition of quantitative ventilation–perfusion relationships, and the multiple inert gas elimination approach was developed. As with most techniques requiring several years for development, the proper order for description of the various aspects of the method is not the same as the actual sequence of their development. This chapter deals in some depth with the current theoretical and experimental aspects of the multiple inert gas approach.

II. THEORETICAL BASIS

A. General Principles

The lung is considered to consist of a population of gas-exchange units (arranged in parallel) each with its own ventilation and blood flow. As an inert gas previously dissolved in dextrose or saline which is being infused intravenously at a constant rate reaches the lungs through the pulmonary artery, it will be partially eliminated by respiration and partially retained in the effluent pulmonary venous blood. Using the steady-state principle of conservation of mass and assuming [reasonably (Forster, 1957; Wagner, 1977b)] that there is diffusion equilibration for inert gases between alveolar gas and end-capillary blood, Farhi (1967) showed that a simple relationship described quantitative gas exchange in any one homogeneous lung unit:

$$\frac{P_A}{P_{\bar{v}}} = \frac{P_{c'}}{P_{\bar{v}}} = \frac{\lambda}{\lambda + \dot{V}_A/\dot{Q}} \tag{1}$$

This expression also presupposes that the inert gas in question is absent from inspired gas.

Invoking simple mixing theory, the mixed arterial blood entering the systemic circulation has an inert gas partial pressure (in relation to the mixed venous value) given by

$$\frac{Pa}{P_{\bar{v}}} = \sum_{j=1}^{j=N} \left(\frac{\dot{Q}_j \lambda}{\lambda + \dot{V}_A/\dot{Q}_j} \right) \tag{2}$$

where $\dot{Q}_j$ are (fractional) perfusion values for each of the N gas exchange units of ventilation–perfusion ratio $\dot{V}_A/\dot{Q}_j$ comprising the entire lung. If several, say M, inert gases are simultaneously infused, then the retention R_i ($\equiv Pa/P_{\bar{v}}$) of the ith gas is given by

$$R_i = \sum_{j=1}^{j=N} \left(\frac{\dot{Q}_j \lambda_i}{\lambda_i + \dot{V}_A/\dot{Q}_j} \right) \qquad i = 1,M \tag{3}$$

Mixed expired gas is treated similarly. Defining E_i as excretion of the ith gas,

$$E_i = \sum_{j=1}^{j=N} \left(\frac{\dot{V}_{A_j} \lambda_i}{\lambda_i + \dot{V}_A/\dot{Q}_j} \right) \qquad i = 1,M \tag{4}$$

Here, $\dot{V}_{A_j}$ are the fractional ventilations of the N lung units.

Irrespective of the values of M and N, Eq. (3) demonstrates a fundamental relationship between two functions. One of the two functions is the curve relating retention R_i to blood gas partition coefficient λ_i, called the retention–solubility curve. The other is the curve relating blood flow $\dot{Q}_j$ to its associated lung unit with ventilation–perfusion ratio $\dot{V}_A/\dot{Q}_j$, called the distribution of perfusion. Equation (4) demonstrates a corresponding relationship between the excretion–solubility curve and the distribution of ventilation. Note that R_i and E_i are related through the principle of mass conservation by:

$$\dot{V}_E E_i = \lambda_i \dot{Q}_T (1 - R_i) \tag{5}$$

and that fractional ventilation $\dot{V}_{A_j}$ is related to fractional perfusion $\dot{Q}_j$ by the relationship

$$\dot{V}_{A_j} = \dot{Q}_j (\dot{V}_A/\dot{Q}_j) \frac{\dot{Q}_T}{\dot{V}_E} \tag{6}$$

Equations (5) and (6) state that: (a) the retention and excretion curves are necessarily related, and (b) the distributions of ventilation and perfusion are necessarily related. In other words, if it were not for factors such as random experimental errors, retention and excretion could be calculated from the distribution either of ventilation or of blood flow. Conversely, either retention or excretion can be used to infer information about both distributions. In practice, because of experimental errors, it transpires that retention data are more reliable than excretion data for insoluble gases. The reverse is true for the soluble gases, and it therefore makes good sense to combine retention and excretion data in obtaining information about both distributions (Evans and Wagner, 1977).

B. Recovery of Information about Ventilation–Perfusion Inequality from Inert Gas Elimination Data

The relationships developed in Eqs. (1)–(6) may be used as the basis for obtaining information about the distributions of ventilation and bloodflow with respect to the ventilation–perfusion ratio from inert gas elimination data. The question of how much information is available has recently received considerable attention (Wagner *et al.*, 1974c; Jaliwala *et al.*, 1975; Olszowka, 1975; Dawson *et al.*, 1976; Wagner, 1977a; Evans and Wagner, 1977; Howard and Bradner, 1977). The related question of how best to recover this information is also an important issue. There is general agreement about the following aspects: (a) The multiple inert gas elimination approach gives more information than previously obtainable. (b) It cannot give the unique distribution present in the lung for two reasons—namely, the number of gases used is finite and their measurement cannot be made without incurring experimental error. (c) Methods exist for placing limits on distributions compatible with a given set of data to allow interpretation of such data. (d) A uniform statement about the amount of information available from inert gas measurement cannot be made—individual data sets will vary in this regard.

In general, two kinds of approaches can be described for obtaining information from a set of inert gas data (Wagner, 1977a; Evans and Wagner, 1977). One can be labeled "bounds analysis," and the other is the determination of a "representative distribution" of ventilation–perfusion ratios. Conceptually, the former can be compared to the notion of variance about a mean, while the latter is equivalent to the mean. Determining a representative distribution is rapid and inexpensive and gives those features of the distribution that are reliable and generally stable mathematically in the presence of error. It is interpreted in the light of the information obtained from bounds analysis which is statistically oriented, and tedious and expensive to use. Both approaches are considered useful, and within each category more than one way exists for treating the problem. Recently developed approaches (Wagner, 1977a; Evans and Wagner, 1977) used in our laboratory will be described.

C. Bounds Analysis

A fuller description of the concepts and methods of this analysis is given elsewhere (Wagner, 1977a; Evans and Wagner, 1977). The concepts are best discussed in a graphical manner both because such an approach is the easiest for the reader and because it relates the current problem to well-established principles of gas exchange for O_2 and CO_2.

While the analysis given here focuses on the respiratory gases O_2 and CO_2 rather than inert gases (for reasons of greater familiarity to most readers), it is directly applicable to two inert gases being eliminated. In fact, the concepts and techniques are directly suited to any number of (inert) gases being eliminated simultaneously.

Consider the O_2–CO_2 diagram of Rahn and Fenn (1955) (Fig. 1). These authors showed how a unique curved line could be slung between known venous and inspired points and that any point on this line was associated with a single value of the ventilation–perfusion ratio. This "$\dot{V}_A/\dot{Q}$ line" is of course the graphical solution to the steady-state mass balance equations in the lung (that is, the Fick principle). The line can be "calibrated" in terms of $\dot{V}_A/\dot{Q}$ ratio, as shown.

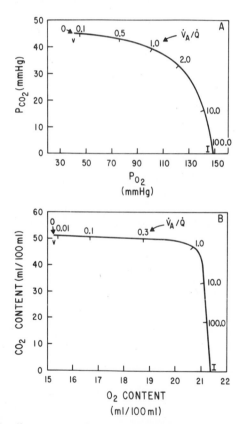

Figure 1. O_2–CO_2 diagrams. A. Standard diagram for P_{O_2} and PCO_2 showing the ventilation–perfusion ratio line calibrated with ventilation–perfusion ratios ($\dot{V}_A/\dot{Q}$). B. Corresponding $\dot{V}_A/\dot{Q}$ line on the O_2–CO_2 content diagram. Note the greater angularity of the latter. Both $\dot{V}_A/\dot{Q}$ lines are concave.

An exact corresponding line exists in another coordinate system, namely that of the corresponding blood contents for O_2 and CO_2 (Fig. 1B). Similar calibration with $\dot{V}_A/\dot{Q}$ values can be performed. This line has a special property—it is *concave*, i.e., its slope decreases (becomes more negative) as $\dot{V}_A/\dot{Q}$ rises. The importance of this concavity is that, because it is hypothesized that all lungs can be thought of as collections of homogeneous compartments situated along the concave line, all combinations of such compartments must give rise to a mixed arterial O_2 and CO_2 content point lying below the line (provided the weight given to each such compartment, i.e., the compartmental perfusions, are all positive). Note that because of the nonlinearity of the O_2 and CO_2 dissociation curves, the O_2–CO_2 content diagram must be used rather than the O_2–CO_2 partial pressure diagram when combining compartments to form the arterial blood.

There is a limit to the area on the O_2–CO_2 content diagram that such combinations of compartments can occupy; it is given by the straight line joining the venous and inspired points. Thus, in Fig. 2 is defined what one might call the region of possible outputs of lung models exchanging O_2 and CO_2. Now consider an arterial "point," that is, a point within the region of possible outputs corresponding to a pair of O_2 and CO_2 contents (the solid circle, Fig. 3). By drawing straight lines (three are shown) through the arterial point, the ventilation–perfusion ratios corresponding to the intersection of each straight line with the $\dot{V}_A/\dot{Q}$ line can be determined. From simple geometrical principles, the fractional perfusions necessarily associated with each of these $\dot{V}_A/\dot{Q}$ compartments can be determined from the lengths of the associated segments in Fig. 3.

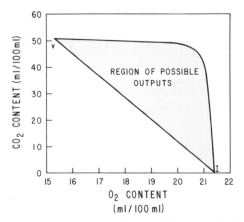

Figure 2. Region of possible outputs. Stippled area defines possible locations of arterial O_2 and CO_2 content pairs formed by positive combinations of compartments along the $\dot{V}_A/\dot{Q}$ line.

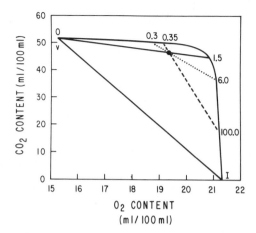

Figure 3. Three possible two-compartment models precisely compatible with the arterial point given by the solid dot. The interval analysis (see text) gives the fractional perfusions of the individual compartments (which are indicated by the intersection of each interval with the $\dot{V}_A/\dot{Q}$ line). Numbers are the $\dot{V}_A/\dot{Q}$ values of these compartments. Rotation of the interval about the arterial point by moving the endpoints along the $\dot{V}_A/\dot{Q}$ line from v to I gives an infinite set of precisely compatible two-compartment models.

Thus, in the examples of Fig. 3, the arterial point could be the result of (a) a shunt of 27% with the remaining 73% of the bloodflow in a compartment of $\dot{V}_A/\dot{Q}$ 1.5; (b) 72% of the bloodflow at a $\dot{V}_A/\dot{Q}$ of 0.3 and 28% at a $\dot{V}_A/\dot{Q}$ of 6.0; or (c) 89% of the bloodflow at a $\dot{V}_A/\dot{Q}$ of 0.35 and 11% at a $\dot{V}_A/\dot{Q}$ of 100.0. Of course, an infinite number of such compartmental pairs can equally well explain the given arterial point (determined by drawing all other straight lines through the arterial point).

Several additional important points arise from this two-compartment approach: First, it can be shown that for each $\dot{V}_A/\dot{Q}$ compartment the perfusions calculated in this manner are the greatest possible perfusions consistent with the given arterial point. Thus, this simple construction permits calculation of the absolute upper bound on compartmental bloodflow for all compartments (one at a time) for any desired arterial point. In more complicated cases than the above two-dimensional one (i.e., when six inert gases are used) the same maximum perfusion calculations can be performed using standard linear programing methods (Dantzig, 1963). The algorithm we used is listed in the appendix (subroutine LPQMAX). Such calculations for three sets of arterial points are given in Fig. 4 [both when the arterial point consists only of O_2 and CO_2 content (open circles), and when it consists of six inert gas retentions (closed circles)]. Second, while an infinite number of two-compartment models can be found to fit the data, there are also many two-compartment

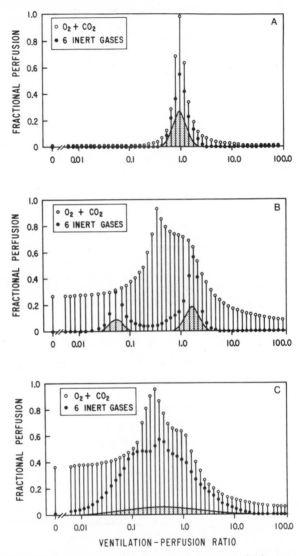

Figure 4. Maximum possible fractional perfusion at several $\dot{V}_A/\dot{Q}$ values for each of 3 arterial points derived from narrow (A), bimodal (B), and broad (C) distributions. Results are given for the two-gas system (O_2 and CO_2 content, ○) and the 6 inert gas system (●). In each case, six forcing functions provide tighter restrictions than two, but in A the differences are of little physiological importance. A large improvement in resolution is afforded by 6 gases for the bimodal case (B), while in C the improvement in extending the data from two to six points is seen mainly at the upper and lower extremes of $\dot{V}_A/\dot{Q}$. All three examples clearly demonstrate the lack of resolution within a narrow range of $\dot{V}_A/\dot{Q}$.

models that will not. Thus, in Fig. 3, the given arterial point cannot be the result of a shunt plus a compartment of $\dot{V}_A/\dot{Q}$ 6.0 (in any combination), because the straight line joining the associated coordinates does not pass through the given arterial point. In other words, definite restrictions can be placed on compartmental combinations compatible with any given arterial point. Third, determination of an infinite number of three- (or more-) compartment distributions that fit the given arterial point is also feasible (Wagner, 1977a). The only requirement is that the selected compartments form a triangle (polygon) which encloses the given arterial point. Fourth, of greatest importance is the concept that the geometrical location of the given data point within the region of possible outputs determines how tight the restrictions are in a given case (Fig. 5). If the arterial point lies precisely on the boundary of the region of possible outputs (point A in Fig. 5), the restrictions are complete; the point (in this two-gas example) represents a homogeneous lung of the associated $\dot{V}_A/\dot{Q}$ and is incompatible with any other compartmental arrangement. Point B in Fig. 5 is close to the boundary in the region of its maximal curvature. While in the strict mathematical sense uniqueness has been lost, fairly severe restrictions can still be placed on the values of compartmental ventilation–perfusion ratio and bloodflow that will explain the point. By performing the rotational analysis of Fig. 3 it can be seen that most of the bloodflow must be in compartments of $\dot{V}_A/\dot{Q}$ close to 1, although small amounts of perfusion cannot be excluded from any region of the spectrum

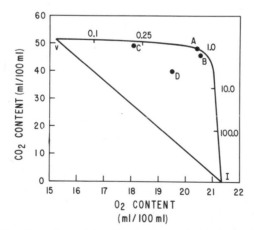

Figure 5.   Four hypothetical arterial points (A–D) are shown; in the text, the severity of restrictions on perfusion at any $\dot{V}_A/\dot{Q}$ is indicated for each point. In general, the closer the arterial point is to the boundary of the region of possible outputs, the tighter the restrictions that can be placed.

of $\dot{V}_A/\dot{Q}$. By contrast, examine point C in Fig. 5, which is equally as close to the boundary as point B, but in a region of very little curvature of the boundary. While essentially all the perfusion could be in the $\dot{V}_A/\dot{Q}$ region close to 0.25, the point C could equally well arise as the result of a two-compartment lung with approximately equal perfusions at $\dot{V}_A/\dot{Q}$ ratios of 0 and about 1. Thus the restrictions on point C in Fig. 5 are not nearly as tight as those on point B. Finally, considering point D in Fig. 5, it is clear that for points deep in the interior of the possible region very little restriction can be placed on the compartmental distribution of perfusion.

This concept is the basis for much of the recent discussion quoted previously concerning the inert gas method. It is clear that with just six data points (six gases) all distributions recovered from sets of inert gas data are defined by no more than six parameters. Consequently, if more complicated cases are treated, as for example that of Olszowka (1975), some desirable features of the distribution are beyond definition. Olszowka's example is similar in kind to that shown in the bottom panel of Fig. 4 and in general corresponds to interior points such as D in Fig. 5. On the other hand, if retention sets lying closer to the boundary of the region of possible outputs are analyzed, most of the important features of the distribution can be identified (using bounds analysis). Even then, however, resolution within any one decade of $\dot{V}_A/\dot{Q}$ is limited.

The linear programing algorithm LPQMAX for finding maximum perfusion of a compartment is easily modified for testing unimodality of a distribution in a given case (Evans and Wagner, 1977). Unimodality of perfusion and of ventilation are separate questions, and the appropriate algorithms LPUNIQ and LPUNIV are listed in the appendix. The specific question asked by these programs is whether a given set of retentions can be explained by a unimodal distribution (or, conversely, whether at least two populations of units of basically different $\dot{V}_A/\dot{Q}$ must be present). The answer is either yes or no. These programs are very useful in interpreting data which suggest that at least two $\dot{V}_A/\dot{Q}$ populations are present, and their use is illustrated later.

The preceding discussion has utilized linear programing as a means of explaining the extent to which important features of distributions can be defined satisfactorily using error-free data of six inert gases. Experimental errors are always present, however, and the following approach is used to allow for the effects of such errors within the above framework.

Figures 6A and 6B show how errors in the inert gas measurements can be handled. Suppose P is a known arterial point (that is, P gives the real O_2 and CO_2 contents of arterial blood). Because of random errors in measurement, it is highly unlikely that an attempt to measure these O_2 and

CO_2 contents would precisely result in the values indicated by P. Statistically, the concentrations actually measured are represented by the cloud of points centered on P. This cloud is generated using appropriate random error values for each gas repeatedly added to P (that is, by what is known as a Monte Carlo simulation). In Fig. 6, the variances for each gas are taken to be equal in terms of distance on each axis, thus resulting in a circular cloud. Unequal variances would result in an elliptical cloud. The

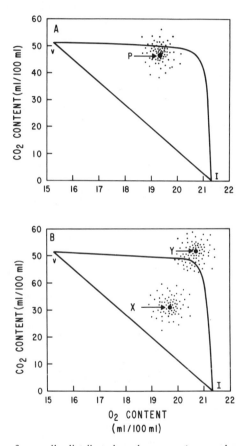

Figure 6. Effects of normally distributed random error (assumed equal for O_2 and CO_2). A. Random error is added to a hypothetical known arterial point P. Note that some error-containing values so formed lie inside and some outside the region of possible outputs. B. Random error is subtracted from measured (error-containing) arterial data points X and Y. X lies deep within the permissible space; Y is an exterior point. The portions of the cloud of values lying within the permissible space in each case indicate in a probabilistic sense the region in which the real arterial point lies.

relative density of this cloud in any region reflects the chance that if a measured, error-containing data set lay in that particular region it really came from the point P. Notice that this cloud has points that lie both inside and outside of the region of possible outputs. The significance of the exterior points in Fig. 6A is that while no lung model could give rise to such points in the absence of errors, introduction of error may well result in a measured set of contents that lie outside the region of possible outputs.

Now consider (Fig. 6B) two different arterial points X and Y that have been measured experimentally. These points will each contain some degree of error, and the problem is to estimate in each case the probable location of the real arterial point that gave rise to X and Y.

For the interior data point X, random error has been subtracted many times from X to form a density cloud which gives the probabilistic description of where the arterial point of the real lung could lie given error of a certain magnitude. Because in this example virtually all such points are found to lie within the permissible region, it is a straightforward matter to consult the χ^2 table for two degrees of freedom (as the data consist of two observations) and to establish the probability that the real arterial point lies within a certain distance of the measured point X. Thus, one could select an appropriate probability, say 90%, and draw a circle of the corresponding radius (obtained from the χ^2 table) around X. Statistically, this area will enclose 90% of the arterial points that through addition of error could have given rise to X.

Each point within that circle may now be explored (graphically in the two-gas case or by the various linear programs referred to earlier) to build up a statistical description of the restrictions on the distributions compatible with the point X.

Unfortunately (from the mathematical standpoint), such a simple scheme for analyzing effects of error is not applicable to the exterior point Y. The reason is evident on inspection of the density cloud of points centered on Y. Many of those points lie outside the permissible region, and it is accordingly not possible to find models that fit these points. Only those points lying within the permissible region require attention as candidates for the real arterial point responsible for Y. Consulting the χ^2 table in this case ignores the restrictions imposed by the geometry, and it is therefore not the appropriate test to use. If the measured data point in practice often lies outside the permissible space, then an alternative scheme must be developed that will locate only those points in the density cloud that lie within the space. While such considerations may not often be necessary for O_2 and CO_2 as illustrated, they become increasingly important as more forcing functions are used. This is because for these more complex methods the relative volume of the permissible space is greatly reduced compared to the simpler case under discussion. Using the method employing six inert gases, measured data points are mostly found to be outside the permissible space.

Given such a data point Y (Fig. 6B), it is not difficult to locate a large number (say, 50) of points lying within the permissible space, by repeatedly subtracting error from Y randomly and retaining only those points that fall within the space. Interior points are distinguished from exterior points by the inability of the latter to be fitted by any compartmental model (using standard quadratic programing methods) (Lawson and Hanson, 1974). This set of 50 interior points has statistically sampled the area from which the real lung giving rise to Y originated. Now we can explore as before the compatible distributions of each of these 50 data points to look for restrictions on the amount of perfusion that could be located in different regions of $\dot{V}_A/\dot{Q}$ spectrum. Such analyses yield both qualitative information on the possible form of the distribution and quantitative probabilistic information on the variability of patterns of distribution.

Figure 7 gives a summary of the above approach as it is applied to

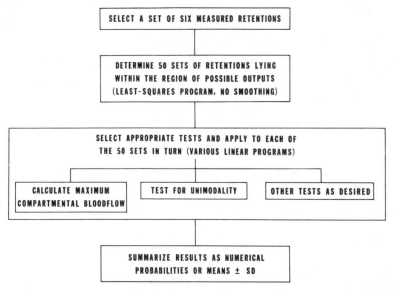

Figure 7. Flow diagram of the integrated scheme for placing of limits on $\dot{V}_A/\dot{Q}$ distributions associated with actual measured retentions. This scheme accounts for both experimental error and nonuniqueness.

actual sets or retentions, and Fig. 8 gives an example of the approach applied to one set of data from a patient with chronic obstructive pulmonary disease. The retentions that are analyzed are what may be called minimum variance retentions—a weighted average of the measured retentions and the retentions calculated from excretions [Eq. (5)]. The weighting differs for each gas and is explained more fully elsewhere (Evans and Wagner, 1977).

Figure 8 gives mean maximum compartmental perfusions plus 1 standard deviation for each of the 50 $\dot{V}_A/\dot{Q}$ compartments. These statistics are taken over the 50 retention sets. For values of $\dot{V}_A/\dot{Q}$ less than 0.01 and greater than 10, mean maximum compartmental perfusion is physiologically negligible and in particular, mean maximum shunt is close to 0, suggesting strongly that there is essentially no shunt present in this patient. In two regions of the $\dot{V}_A/\dot{Q}$ spectrum, mean maximum compartmental perfusion reaches high levels, and in these areas the standard deviations are also high. These findings demonstrate that in those two regions little resolution exists, so that the precise height and width of "modes" of perfusion in these regions cannot be defined. An important finding is that in the intervening region, mean maximum perfusion falls to only 5% of the cardiac output. This shows that there can be very little perfusion in the intervening interval, and the result suggests that testing for unimodality in each of the 50 cases is appropriate. When this was done with the appropriate linear program (LPUNIQ), not one of the 50 sets of the retentions was compatible with a unimodal distribution.

The overall interpretation of the data after executing the scheme in Fig.

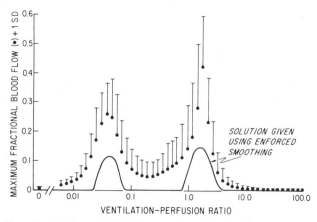

Figure 8. Example of scheme of Fig. 5 for a patient with chronic obstructive lung disease. Mean maximum compartmental bloodflow (+ 1 S.D.) and the distribution recovered using enforced smoothing (described later) are shown. For interpretation see text.

8 is that there is a very high probability that the patient has a bimodal $\dot{V}_A/\dot{Q}$ distribution with considerable amounts of perfusion in low $\dot{V}_A/\dot{Q}$ regions. In each of these two modes, the fine structure is beyond definition, and in fact each may be made up of "sub-modes." There can be virtually no shunt, only a small amount of bloodflow in the region between the two modes, and areas of high $\dot{V}_A/\dot{Q}$ are notably absent.

It is clear that while "bounds analysis" represents thorough evaluation of individual sets of inert gas data, it is not a practical means of analysis of all data. Furthermore, no single or representative distribution is obtained. Our compromise is to analyze all data using a rapid algorithm which gives a representative $\dot{V}_A/\dot{Q}$ distribution, and to interpret such data as necessary using bounds analysis as described above. In this way, a single properly interpretable distribution is obtained in a practical manner.

D. Representative Distributions

There are several ways of obtaining a useful representative distribution from given sets of retentions. Tham (1975) has suggested the use of two logarithmically normal modes as the basic model. There, up to six parameters (means, standard deviations, and height of each mode) are determined so as to best fit the inert gas data in a least-squares sense.

Another approach is to use standard quadratic programing in a multicompartmental model, constraining compartmental perfusions to be nonnegative. Geometrically, this approach will find as the best fit to the given data set Y (Fig. 9) the point K which lies on the boundary of the region of possible outputs. For a system using six inert gases, such an approach gives distributions consisting of three (or fewer) ventilated and

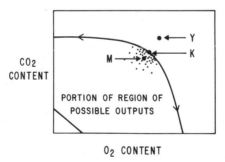

Figure 9. Choice of one representative arterial point for the common case of the measured arterial point (Y) lying outside the region of possible outputs. Standard quadratic programing (least-squares approach) will locate the boundary point (K) closest to Y. The enforced smoothing technique locates a point close to M (the center of mass of the region that in a probabilistic sense is the region of origin of the arterial point of the real lung) and is suggested as an appropriate choice.

perfused compartments (or two such compartments plus shunt and deadspace). A good reason for not using this approach is evident from inspection of Fig. 9. The resulting point (K) lies on the boundary of the region defined previously (Fig. 6B) as the probable region of origin of the real arterial point (which is defined by the Monte Carlo method as the collection of small closed circles in Fig. 9).

Our choice has been to develop an approach for obtaining a representative solution which is representative in that the associated best-fit retentions closely approximate the center of mass (M) of the collection of points in Fig. 9. This is done by incorporating an appropriate amount of smoothing explicitly into the constrained quadratic programing approach referred to above (Evans and Wagner, 1977). The number of $\dot{V}_A/\dot{Q}$ compartments used (50) is sufficient to numerically approximate a continuum. The amount of smoothing introduced to approximate the center of mass as described above is sufficient to stabilize the distributions in the presence of random error. Verification that the center of mass is approximated comes from the bounds analysis approach where the center of mass is determined directly using the Monte Carlo approach (Evans and Wagner, 1977). The smoothing algorithm we use (SMOOTH) is listed in the appendix. In Fig. 8, the curve given by the solid line is the distribution obtained from this algorithm with the smoothing weight (Z) set at its standard value, 40. It is evident that the important features of the bounds analysis approach are reflected by this result. The absence of shunt and of areas of high $\dot{V}_A/\dot{Q}$, and the bimodality and position of the modes all agree well. In interpreting the smooth distribution, it must be recognized that precise height–width characteristics of the modes are beyond resolution, and that small amounts of perfusion might be present in the $\dot{V}_A/\dot{Q}$ region between the two modes.

E.   Additional Theoretical Considerations

The foregoing sections have dealt at some length with the problems of obtaining information about ventilation–perfusion inequality and methods for their solution. Now, some of the more peripheral aspects of the approach will be considered.

F.   Calculations of O_2 and CO_2 Exchange from Recovered Distributions

Both the inert gas method above and computer programs such as those of West (1969) and West and Wagner (1977) are based on the assumption that there is complete partial pressure diffusion equilibration between alveolar gas and end-capillary blood in all lung units. It is generally accepted that inert gases equilibrate extremely rapidly in the lung (Forster, 1957; Wagner, 1977b), and that both O_2 and CO_2 require about an order of magnitude longer for the same degree of diffusion equilibration. Typically, 99% equilibration requires about 0.02 seconds for inert gases and 0.2 seconds or more for O_2 and CO_2. Assuming complete diffusion equilibration for all gases, a distribution calculated from inert gas data can be used to calculate expected values for arterial P_{O_2} and P_{CO_2} if the venous and inspired P_{O_2} and P_{CO_2} are known. This is done by combining the subroutine SMOOTH described previously with West's program (West, 1969; West and Wagner, 1977) or its equivalent.

Should the arterial P_{O_2} calculated in this manner exceed the measured value in a given case (by more than say two standard deviations of the variability known to arise from experimental error), it can be reasonably concluded that mechanisms of hypoxemia are operating in addition to those of ventilation–perfusion inequality, shunt, and hypoventilation (each of which is reflected by inert gases). While in theory bronchial and thebesian shunts could account for such a discrepancy, such a shunt would generally have to be of the order of several percent of the cardiac output. This is considered to be unlikely under most conditions. On the other hand, failure of diffusion equilibration for O_2 could also account for such a discrepancy; thus the inert gas approach can indirectly suggest the presence and importance of diffusion impairment as a factor in the development of hypoxemia. One would expect that if the inspired O_2 level were raised toward 100%, any such discrepancy would worsen if the cause were large bronchial or thebesian shunts, but be reduced if the mechanism were failure of diffusion equilibration.

It is of interest that such a discrepancy has been noted in a few dogs with severe hypoxemia caused by pulmonary edema (Wagner *et al.*, 1975b). In these dogs the discrepancy was abolished by breathing 100% O_2, suggesting that diffusion impairment was a factor. However, even in this extreme situation, the majority of the hypoxemia was due to a combination of shunt and ventilation–blood flow inequality. While such a discrepancy has not been noted in patients with severe chronic obstructive pulmonary disease either at rest or during exercise (Wagner *et al.*, 1977), it has been observed in patients with advanced interstitial fibrosis but only during exercise (Wagner, 1977c). As with the dogs, this presumptive evidence for diffusion impairment suggests only a minor quantitative role for this mechanism in the genesis of hypoxemia, the majority being due to shunt plus ventilation–bloodflow inequality.

G. Relative Contributions of Intrapulmonary and Extrapulmonary Factors in Hypoxemia

Because of the ability to calculate expected values for arterial P_{O_2} and P_{CO_2}, it is possible to analyze in a given case the relative roles of intrapulmonary factors (shunt, ventilation–perfusion inequality) and extrapulmonary factors (O_2 uptake/CO_2 production, hemoglobin, inspired P_{O_2}, cardiac output) in contributing to hypoxemia.

For example, assume a patient with a severe myocardial infarct and low cardiac output state has an arterial P_{O_2} of 50 mm Hg breathing room air (cardiac output 2 liters/minute). Then, with the $\dot{V}_A/\dot{Q}$ distribution determined from inert gas data, it is not difficult to calculate the beneficial theoretical effect on arterial P_{O_2} of restoring cardiac output to, say, 6 liters/minute (keeping the $\dot{V}_A/\dot{Q}$ distribution unchanged). The beneficial effect of increased cardiac output comes from the associated necessary increase in mixed-venous P_{O_2}, which must in turn increase the arterial P_{O_2} if the $\dot{V}_A/\dot{Q}$ distribution is unaltered. Similar calculations can be made to assess the benefit to be expected for increasing $P_{I_{O_2}}$ or the hemoglobin level. Such analyses have been extremely helpful in the assessment of patients with complicated cardiopulmonary diseases, particularly those in the intensive care setting and those in whom arterial hypoxemia is striking in the absence of more than mild abnormalities in measurable lung function.

H. Effects of Molecular Weight on Steady-State Gas Exchange

A continuing issue in studies of gas exchange is that of the influence of molecular weight. It has been known for many years that when inhaled, insoluble gases differ in their quantitative behavior depending on their molecular weights (Farhi, 1969). The relevance of such observations to steady-state gas exchange is very difficult to determine, and the inert gas approach can be used to obtain information in this area so long as either the retentions or the excretions in the particular case to be evaluated are reasonably close to those of a homogeneous lung, which is often the case. The following analysis is used. Consider Eq. (1) again:

$$R = \frac{\lambda}{\lambda + \dot{V}_A/\dot{Q}}$$

A simple linear transformation of the retention–solubility relationship is accomplished by inverting both sides:

$$\frac{1}{R} = \frac{\lambda + \dot{V}_A/\dot{Q}}{\lambda} = 1 + \frac{\dot{V}_A/\dot{Q}}{\lambda} \tag{7}$$

Thus, $1/R$ is a linear function of $1/\lambda$ for a homogeneous lung. This linear transformation can be used to test whether all inert gas retentions obey Eq. (1) (that is, "see" the same effective $\dot{V}_A/\dot{Q}$ value). A heavy gas will have a higher retention than a light gas of the same solubility if molecular weight is important. Because the six gases used (sulfur hexafluoride, mol. wt. 146; ethane, mol. wt. 30; cyclopropane, mol. wt. 42; halothane, mol. wt. 197.5; ether, mol. wt. 74; and acetone, mol. wt. 58) vary by as much as sixfold in molecular weight, the heavy gases should not lie on the same straight line ($1/R$ vs. $1/\lambda$) as the light gases if molecular weight is important. This approach can be applied even when the data came from a lung with some inequality, for the alinearity of the inverse relationship is minor until the inequality is marked. Evaluation of raw data by this approach has never revealed molecular weight-dependent behavior of heavy gases even in chronic obstructive lung disease (Wagner et al., 1977). Thus, while molecular weight can certainly be shown to be of importance in single inspiration/expiration maneuvers, the importance of this behavior in steady-state gas exchange is probably slight, even in disease states.

I. Series Ventilatory Inequality

The inert gas approach is formulated on the assumption that all individual gas-exchange units are arranged in parallel with one another. However, it is probable that not only in normal lungs but especially in some diseased lungs, steady-state P_{O_2} and P_{CO_2} differences exist amongst lung units arranged in series with each other. If such series inequality of ventilation was based on incomplete diffusive gas mixing, it should be demonstrable using the above analysis linearizing the retention–solubility curve. If, on the other hand, such concentration differences existed on the same basis as in the parallel model, a question arises as to whether the pattern of inert gas elimination is intrinsically different from that seen in parallel forms of ventilation–perfusion inequality. If the pattern were different, an analysis based on a parallel model would produce inconsistencies, but the presence of series inequality would be detectable.

It is possible to compare inert gas elimination in series and parallel models of the lung (Wagner and Evans, 1977). When this is done, it is evident that under the conditions appropriate to actual use of the inert gas approach, there exists a parallel model whose quantitative inert gas-exchange pattern cannot be distinguished from a given series model.

It is therefore concluded that the inert gas method can be analyzed on the basis of a parallel model even if series inequality is present, but that series inequality is not identifiable by this approach.

III. EXPERIMENTAL APPLICATIONS

A. Methodology

Details of the methods required for measuring inert gas levels appear extensively elsewhere (Wagner *et al.*, 1974b,d) and do not warrant repetition here. It is worth noting, however, that the fundamental tool for measuring the gases has been the gas chromatograph (GC). While the GC is inexpensive compared to other multigas analyzers [in particular, the mass spectrometer (MS)] and is remarkably reliable and sensitive, the procedure is necessarily time-consuming and limited to discrete sampling (the GC requires entry of individual samples followed by a waiting period for their elution and detection). The use of the MS instead of the GC was considered several years ago, but because of cost, insufficient sensitivity, and unreliability, the matter was never pursued. Recently, however, Mastenbrook and colleagues (1977) have been able to measure the appropriate gases by MS with the necessary sensitivity. Should the MS prove feasible, random errors could be reduced considerably if only by the ability to sample continuously and average the data. More importantly, this would open the door to more demanding nonsteady-state inert gas measurements (which are currently impractical using gas chromatography). Such nonsteady-state studies would provide information on not only ventilation and bloodflow, but on lung gas and tissue volumes (in terms of distribution).

B. Results Obtained Using Steady-State Inert Gas Approach

The inert gas approach has now been applied in many clinical situations, several of which have been reported either in print or at various meetings in abstract. The following account is a brief summary of the principal findings in the most interesting applications. It is designed to give the reader a feel for the diversity of the results and for their implications both physiologically and clinically, rather than a full account in any one case. As with most new techniques, the results obtained to date have raised more questions than they have answered. Recall that representative distributions should be interpreted in the light of the foregoing "bounds" analysis.

C. Normal Subjects

The extent of the $\dot{V}_A/\dot{Q}$ inequality detected by the inert gas method exceeds that obtained from radioactive gas measurements (Fig. 10)

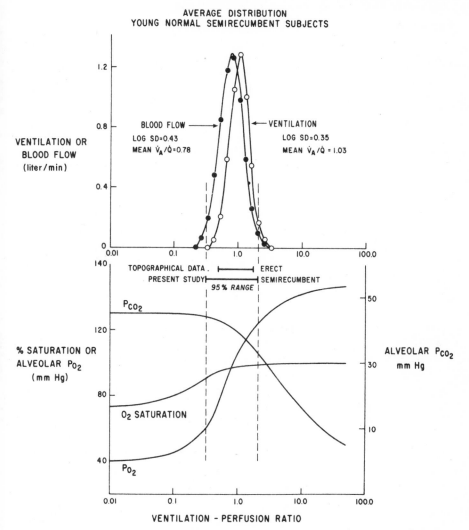

Figure 10. A log normal distribution with mean and standard deviation equal to the average values for young normal subjects. Note that the range of $\dot{V}_A/\dot{Q}$ values detected by inert gas elimination exceeds that determined by radioactive gas methods. Alveolar P_{O_2} is calculated to vary between about 60 and 120 mm Hg over the range of $\dot{V}_A/\dot{Q}$ present.

(Wagner *et al.*, 1974b). This is not surprising in view of the known limitations of the latter approach (averaging counts from small areas and not receiving counts from all areas). This comparison suggests that a measurable $\dot{V}_A/\dot{Q}$ inequality exists within small areas of lung even in normal young volunteers. Figure 10 should, however, be placed in perspective, because even the amount of inequality shown here is associated with an alveolar–arterial P_{O_2} difference of less than 10 mm Hg, far less than that seen in most lung diseases.

Recent measurements in young normal subjects by Gledhill and co-workers (1977) suggest that during moderately heavy exercise the $\dot{V}_A/\dot{Q}$ distribution worsens (the narrow unimodal distribution seen at rest becoming slightly broader). This is consistent with the simultaneously observed and well-known increase in the alveolar–arterial P_{O_2} difference that occurs with heavy exercise. The broadening of the distribution is interesting in that it occurs in the face of reduction in the gravitational component of $\dot{V}_A/\dot{Q}$ inequality (Bake *et al.*, 1968) and thus probably represents an increase in the amount of inequality within small regions of the lung. While the increase in dispersion of the distribution theoretically increases physiological deadspace, the associated large increase in tidal volume (and consequent reduction in the ratio of anatomical deadspace to tidal volume) is more marked, producing the well-known net fall in total measured deadspace.

The mechanism of the increase in the $\dot{V}_A/\dot{Q}$ inequality with exercise is as yet unknown.

Another effect noted in normal volunteers (those having areas of low $\dot{V}_A/\dot{Q}$ breathing air) is the disappearance of low $\dot{V}_A/\dot{Q}$ areas during O_2 breathing and the simultaneous development of shunts involving about the same amounts of bloodflow (Wagner *et al.*, 1974b). O_2-induced atelectasis (Briscoe *et al.*, 1960; Dantzker *et al.*, 1975) is presumed to be the mechanism responsible for these observations. Similar effects have been noted frequently in patients with acute respiratory failure (Wagner *et al.*, 1974a), but rarely if ever in patients with low $\dot{V}_A/\dot{Q}$ regions on the basis of chronic lung diseases (obstructive lung disease, asthma, interstitial diseases). It is possible that in these chronic disease states the phenomenon of collateral ventilation protects otherwise vulnerable lung regions from collapse.

D. Chronic Obstructive Pulmonary Disease

Patients appear to have different patterns of inert gas exchange depending on their clinical features and associated probable pathological findings (Fig. 11A). Those of clinical type A (Burrows *et al.*, 1966), having essen-

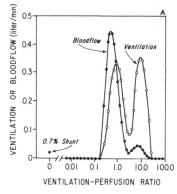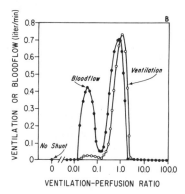

Figure 11. Examples of the distribution of ventilation–perfusion ratios in patients with chronic obstructive pulmonary disease, type A (Fig. 11A) and type B (Fig. 11B). Type A patients tend to have areas of very high $\dot{V}_A/\dot{Q}$, while type B often have areas of very low $\dot{V}_A/\dot{Q}$. Shunt ($\dot{V}_A/\dot{Q}$ = 0) is rarely seen in either type.

tially no sputum production and increased lung compliance, almost always have areas of very high ventilation–perfusion ratio (Wagner *et al.*, 1977). By contrast, areas of very low $\dot{V}_A/\dot{Q}$ are not found and shunt is rarely present. while the total alveolar ventilation may be normal, only a part is associated with well-perfused regions, so that the overall $\dot{V}_A/\dot{Q}$ of these well-perfused regions is lower than normal (about 0.6 instead of about 1.0), explaining the hypoxemia.

The high $\dot{V}_A/\dot{Q}$ areas are probably due to the capillary destruction noted in emphysema, so that areas that are still ventilated may receive extremely little perfusion. The absence of shunt and of low $\dot{V}_A/\dot{Q}$ areas in the face of severe airways obstruction probably reflects both the lack of sputum production and the effectiveness of collateral ventilation in providing gas flow to obstructed areas.

Patients with a chronic productive cough and evidence of cor pulmonale of clinical type B are generally seen to have large amounts of perfusion to areas of very low $\dot{V}_A/\dot{Q}$ (≤ 0.1), but rarely is any appreciable shunt observed (Fig. 11B). High $\dot{V}_A/\dot{Q}$ areas may or may not be present. While it is likely that high $\dot{V}_A/\dot{Q}$ areas in this group also reflect the alveolar destructive process of emphysema, the predominance of the bronchitic component in their clinical presentation makes accurate classification essentially impossible.

An important clinical point is that when given 100% O_2, both groups of chronic obstructive pulmonary disease (COPD) patients failed to elevate their arterial P_{O_2} as expected (of normal subjects) in spite of the very low values of shunt that were observed (Wagner *et al.*, 1977). This apparent paradox is in all probability due mainly to the extremely slow rate of N_2 washout noted in these patients. Such a slow washout greatly delays the eventual rise in P_{O_2} in low $\dot{V}_A/\dot{Q}$ areas, so that after breathing 100% O_2 for even 30 minutes the arterial P_{O_2} does not acurately distinguish between shunting and ventilation–perfusion inequality, and greatly overestimates the shunt.

In both groups of patients both at rest and during sustained exercise (V_{O_2} $\approx$ 500–1200 ml/minute), the arterial P_{O_2} calculated from the measured inert gas data agreed very well with that measured directly, strongly suggesting that diffusion equilibration is adequate to prevent the occurrence of alveolar–end capillary P_{O_2} differences.

A final point pertains to the relationship between the degree of hypoxemia and the pattern of $\dot{V}_A/\dot{Q}$ inequality. It is not possible to predict the pattern of the $\dot{V}_A/\dot{Q}$ distribution from the degree of hypoxemia or hypercapnia. This is due to the complicated interaction between the shape of the $\dot{V}_A/\dot{Q}$ distribution and factors such as total ventilation and cardiac output in determining arterial P_{O_2} and P_{CO_2}.

E. Chronic Interstitial Lung Disease

Nine patients with severe, stable restrictive lung disease of various etiologies have been studied at rest and during exercise (Fig. 12). The

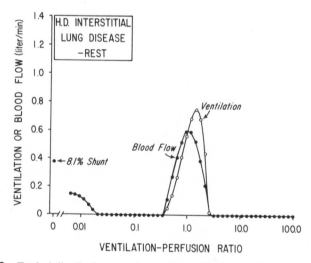

Figure 12. Typical distribution seen in a patient with advanced interstitial lung disease. Note that moderate amount of perfusion are present in extremely poorly ventilated ($\dot{V}_A/\dot{Q}$ < 0.01) or unventilated lung. The pattern is quite different from that seen in obstructive lung disease (Fig. 11). $\dot{V}_E$ = 12.9 liters/min; $\dot{Q}_T$ = 4.6 liters/min.

$\dot{V}_A/\dot{Q}$ pattern was strikingly different from that seen in either normal lungs or in COPD. Units had either normal ventilation–perfusion ratios or were essentially unventilated ($\dot{V}_A/\dot{Q} \leq 0.01$) with no areas of intermediate $\dot{V}_A/\dot{Q}$. Areas of high $\dot{V}_A/\dot{Q}$ were usually not seen. As a result of slightly below-normal values for cardiac output, hypoxemia was sometimes more marked than otherwise expected of patients in whom the effective shunt was generally $\leq 20\%$ of the total bloodflow. This interaction between cardiac output and the amount of $\dot{V}_A/\dot{Q}$ inequality was particularly striking during exercise, where arterial P_{O_2} was 51 mm Hg mean, mixed-venous P_{O_2} was 26 mm Hg, and cardiac output 8 liter/minute ($\dot{V}_{O_2}$ 660 ml/minute mean).

At rest, the observed amount of inequality plus shunt completely accounted for the degree of hypoxemia, but this was not true during exercise, when only about 81% (Wagner *et al.*, 1976a) of the hypoxemia could be thus explained. This may well be an example of the effect of alveolar–end capillary P_{O_2} differences caused by diffusion impairment.

It thus appears that in these patients with advanced generalized interstitial lung disease there are essentially two populations of lung units—those able to maintain normal ventilation–perfusion ratios in spite of obvious mechanical derangement because of the interstitial disease process, and those units, essentially destroyed, associated with zero or near-zero ventilation but some continuing perfusion. The striking absence of units of intermediate to low $\dot{V}_A/\dot{Q}$ is confirmed by the bounds analysis referred to earlier, but is still unexplained. It would undoubtedly require the study of many more patients at various stages of severity to throw light on this intriguing issue.

F. Hypoxemia Following Myocardial Infarction

A number of patients with varying degrees of hypoxemia following acute myocardial infarction have been studied (Wagner *et al.*, 1976b). All showed the same basic $\dot{V}_A/\dot{Q}$ pattern consisting of essentially normal ($\dot{V}_A/\dot{Q}$ about 1) or essentially unventilated ($\dot{V}_A/\dot{Q} \leq 0.05$) units. The pattern is thus similar to the patients with interstitial disease. Here, because the presumed pathological basis of the low $\dot{V}_A/\dot{Q}$ area is edema, it is not surprising to find units either ventilating normally (in relation to bloodflow) or essentially unventilated.

What was surprising was the finding that the magnitude of the effective shunt did not greatly increase with increasing severity of heart failure and was always modest ($\leq 20\%$ of cardiac output and usually $< 15\%$). In spite of this, the inert gas data were compatible with the observed increase in hypoxemia with increasing severity of heart failure. Here again, the important role of a low cardiac output is evident: Our patients with severe heart failure were more hypoxemic than their more fit counterparts because their cardiac output was low rather than because of more severe pulmonary edema.

G. Asthma

An interesting contrast to the above patients is provided by a group of relatively young asthmatic subjects, asymptomatic at the time of study (Wagner *et al.*, 1975a). We were surprised to find moderately severe $\dot{V}_A/\dot{Q}$ inequality in these patients, in spite of essentially no wheezing, reasonable if not normal airways function, and minimal hypoxemia ($P_{O_2} \geqslant 80$ in almost all instances). This constellation of observations shows that significant abnormalities not evident by blood gas measurements, chest X-ray, or measurement of airflow at the mouth can exist in asymptomatic individuals, a conclusion of major importance. We suggest that the pathological basis of this is small airway mucus plugging.

The $\dot{V}_A/\dot{Q}$ distribution pattern in these patients was striking. Almost all showed reproducibly bimodal patterns (normal $\dot{V}_A/\dot{Q}$ and very low $\dot{V}_A/\dot{Q}$, ~ 0.07) with no shunt.

This apparent bimodality has been thoroughly studied by the bounds analysis approach. The results show that the probability of these curves not being bimodal is very small (about 5% or less for each set of data, even if their reproducibility is not taken into account). The bimodal pattern plus the absence of shunt points strongly to the role of collateral ventilation in providing some gas to alveoli beyond obstructed airways.

IV. SUMMARY AND CONCLUSIONS

Numerical analysis of the arterial and expired concentrations of infused inert gases is a powerful tool in investigating gas exchange and mechanisms of hypoxemia. Information not previously available can be obtained. However, it is important to appreciate the necessary limitations of the approach. Because of the limited number of data and errors in their measurements, the distributions obtained are of limited resolution and must be appropriately interpreted. Two kinds of mathematical approaches are described here. They are complementary, each serving a different purpose and each considered to be essential. Interpretation of clinical data using the inert gas method is based on both of these approaches, so that the chances of being misled by the results are small. In spite of these limitations, different groups of patients are found to have different patterns of ventilation–perfusion inequality, so that mechanisms of hypoxemia vary. The measurements to date have resulted in many observations of both physiological and clinical importance and have led to an increased understanding of mechanisms of altered gas exchange in cardiopulmonary disease.

REFERENCES

Bake, B., J. Bjure, and J. Widimsky (1968). The effect of sitting and graded exercise on the distribution of pulmonary blood flow in healthy subjects studied with the ^{133}Xenon technique. *Scand. J. Clin. Lab. Invest.* **22,** 99–106.

Briscoe, W. A., E. M. Cree, J. Filler, H. E. J. Houssay, and A. Cournand (1960). Lung volume, alveolar ventilation and perfusion interrelationships in chronic pulmonary emphysema. *J. Appl. Physiol.* **15,** 785–795.

Burrows, B., C. M. Fletcher, B. E. Heard, N. L. Jones, and J. S. Wootliff (1966). The emphysematous and bronchial types of chronic airways obstruction. A clinicopathological study of patients in London and Chicago. *Lancet* **1,** 830–835.

Colburn, W. E., Jr., J. W. Evans, and J. B. West (1974). Analysis of effect of the solubility on gas exchange in nonhomogeneous lungs. *J. Appl. Physiol.* **37,** 547–551.

Dantzig, G. B. (1963). "Linear Programming and Extensions," pp. 94–108. Princeton, New Jersey.

Dantzker, D. R., P. D. Wagner, and J. B. West (1975). Instability of lung units with low $\dot{V}_A/\dot{Q}$ ratios during O_2 breathing. *J. Appl. Physiol.* **38,** 886–895.

Dawson, S. B., H. Ozkaynak, J. A. Reeds, and J. P. Butler (1976). Evaluation of estimates of the distribution of ventilation–perfusion ratios from inert gas data. *Fed. Proc., Fed. Am. Soc. Exp. Biol.* **35,** 453 (abstr.).

Evans, J. W., and P. D. Wagner (1977). Limits on $\dot{V}_A/\dot{Q}$ distribution from analysis of experimental inert gas elimination. *J. Appl. Physiol.* **42,** 889–898.

Evans, J. W., P. D. Wagner, and J. B. West (1974). Conditions for reduction of pulmonary gas transfer by ventilation–perfusion inequality. *J. Appl. Physiol.* **36,** 533–537.

Farhi, L. E. (1967). Elimination of inert gas by the lung. *Respir. Physiol.* **3,** 1–11.

Farhi, L. E. (1969). Diffusive and convective movement of gas in the lung. *In* "Circulatory and Respiratory Mass Transport" (G. E. W. Wolstenholme and J. Knight, eds.). pp. 277–297. Churchill, London.

Farhi, L. E., and A. J. Olszowka (1968). Analysis of alveolar gas exchange in the presence of soluble inert gases. *Respir. Physiol.* **5,** 53–67.

Farhi, L. E., and T. Yokoyama (1967). Effects of ventilation–perfusion inequality on elimination of inert gases. *Respir. Physiol.* **3,** 12–20.

Fenn, W. O., H. Rahn, and A. B. Otis (1946). A theoretical study of the composition of alveolar air at altitude. *Am. J. Physiol.* **146,** 637–653.

Forster, R. E. (1957). Exchange of gases between alveolar air and pulmonary capillary blood: Pulmonary diffusing capacity. *Physiol. Rev.* **37,** 391–452.

Gledhill, N., A. B. Froese, and J. A. Dempsey (1977). Ventilation to perfusion distribution during exercise in health. *In* "Muscular Exercise and the Lung" (J. A. Dempsey and C. E. Reed, eds.), pp. 325–343. Univ. of Wisconsin Press, Madison.

Haldane, J. S., and J. G. Priestley (1935). "Respiration." Yale Univ. Press, New Haven, Connecticut.

Howard, R. S., and H. Bradner (1977). The $\dot{V}A/\dot{Q}$ resolution of inert gas data. *Bull. Math. Biol.* **39,** 87–98.

Jaliwala, S. A., R. E. Mates, and F. J. Klocke (1975). An efficient optimization technique for recovering ventilation–perfusion distributions from inert gas data. Effects of random experimental error. *J. Clin. Invest.* **55,** 188–192.

Kelman, G. R. (1966). Digital computer subroutine for the conversion of oxygen tension into saturation. *J. Appl. Physiol.* **21,** 1375–1376.

Kelman, G. R. (1967). Digital computer procedure for the conversion of P_{CO_2} into blood CO_2 content. *Respir. Physiol.* **3**, 111–115.

Kelman, G. R. (1968). Computer program for the production of O_2–CO_2 diagrams. *Respir. Physiol.* **4**, 260–269.

Krogh, A., and J. Lindhard (1917). The volume of the dead space in breathing and the mixing of gases in the lungs of man. *J. Physiol. (London)* **51**, 59–90.

Lawson, C. L., and R. J. Hanson (1974). "Solving Least Squares Problems," pp. 169–174 and 190. Prentice-Hall, Englewood Cliffs, New Jersey.

Lenfant, C., and T. Okubo (1968). Distribution function of pulmonary blood flow and ventilation–perfusion ratio in man. *J. Appl. Physiol.* **24**, 668–677.

Mastenbrook, S. M., Jr., T. A. Massaro, and J. A. Dempsey (1977). Feasibility of mass spectrometry for multiple inert gas elimination measurements. *Fed. Proc., Fed. Am. Soc. Exp. Biol.* **36**, 609.

Olszowka, A. J. (1975). Can $\dot{V}_A/\dot{Q}$ distributions in the lung be recovered from inert gas retention data? *Respir. Physiol.* **25**, 191–198.

Olszowka, A. J., and L. E. Farhi (1968). A system of digital computer subroutines for blood gas calculations. *Respir. Physiol.* **4**, 270–280.

Olszowka, A. J., and L. E. Farhi (1969). A digital computer program for constructing ventilation–perfusion lines. *J. Appl. Physiol.* **26**, 141–146.

Peslin, R., S. Dawson, and J. Mead (1971). Analysis of multicomponent exponential curves by the Post–Widder's equation. *J. Appl. Physiol.* **30**, 462–472.

Rahn, H., and W. O. Fenn (1955). "A Graphical Analysis of the Respiration Gas Exchange." Am. Physiol. Soc., Washington, D.C.

Riley, R. L., and A. Cournand (1949). 'Ideal' alveolar air and the analysis of ventilation-perfusion relationships in the lungs. *J. Appl. Physiol.* **1**, 825–847.

Riley, R. L., and A. Cournand (1951). Analysis of factors affecting partial pressures of oxygen and carbon dioxide in gas and blood of lungs: theory. *J. Appl. Physiol.* **4**, 77–101.

Riley, R. L., A. Cournand, and K. W. Donald (1951). Analysis of factors affecting partial pressures of oxygen and carbon dioxide in gas and blood of lungs: Methods. *J. Appl. Physiol.* **4**, 102–120.

Tham, M. K. (1975). Letter to Editor. *J. Appl. Physiol.* **38**, 950.

Wagner, P. D. (1977a). A general approach to the evaluation of ventilation–perfusion ratios in normal and abnormal lungs. *Physiologist* **20**, 18–25.

Wagner, P. D. (1977b). Diffusion and chemical reaction in pulmonary gas exchange. *Physiol. Rev.* **57**, 257–312.

Wagner, P. D. (1977c). Ventilation–perfusion inequality and gas exchange during exercise in lung disease. *In* "Muscular Exercise and the Lung" (J. A. Dempsey and C. E. Reed, eds.), pp. 345–356. Univ. of Wisconsin Press, Madison.

Wagner, P. D., and J. W. Evans (1977). Conditions for equivalence of gas exchange in series and parallel models of the lung. *Respir. Physiol.* **31**, 117–138.

Wagner, P. D., D. R. Dantzker, R. Dueck, R. R. Uhl, R. Virgilio, and J. B. West (1974a). Continuous distributions of ventilation–perfusion ratios in acute and chronic lung disease. *Clin. Res.* **22**, 134A (abstr.).

Wagner, P. D., R. B. Laravuso, R. R. Uhl, and J. B. West (1974b). Continuous distributions of ventilation–perfusion ratios in normal subjects breathing air and 100% O_2. *J. Clin. Invest.* **54**, 54–68.

Wagner, P. D., H. A. Saltzman, and J. B. West (1974c). Measurement of continuous distributions of ventilation–perfusion ratios: Theory. *J. Appl. Physiol.* **36**, 588–599.

Wagner, P. D., P. F. Naumann, and R. B. Laravuso (1974d). Simultaneous measurement of eight foreign gases in blood by gas chromatography. *J. Appl. Physiol.* **36**, 600–605.

Wagner, P. D., D. R. Dantzker, V. E. Iacovoni, R. F. Schillaci, and J. B. West (1975a). Distributions of ventilation–perfusion ratios in asthma. *Am. Rev. Respir. Dis.* **111,** 940 (abstr.).

Wagner, P. D., R. B. Laravuso, E. Goldzimmer, P. F. Naumann, and J. B. West (1975b). Distributions of ventilation–perfusion ratios in dogs with normal and abnormal lungs. *J. Appl. Physiol.* **38,** 1099–1109.

Wagner, P. D., D. R. Dantzker, R. Dueck, J. L. dePolo, K. Wasserman, and J. B. West (1976a). Distribution of ventilation–perfusion ratios in patients with interstitial lung disease. *Chest* **69,** 256 (abstr.).

Wagner, P. D., D. R. Dantzker, V. W. Tornabene, M. M. LeWinter, and J. B. West (1976b). Effects of ventilation–perfusion inequality on arterial P_{O_2} following acute myocardial infarction. *Clin. Res.* **24,** 160A (abstr.).

Wagner, P. D., D. R. Dantzker, R. Dueck, J. L. Clausen, and J. B. West (1977). Ventilation–perfusion inequality in chronic obstructive pulmonary disease. *J. Clin. Invest.* **59,** 203–216.

West, J. B. (1969). Ventilation–perfusion inequality and overall gas exchange in computer models of the lung. *Respir. Physiol.* **7,** 88–110.

West, J. B. (1969–1970). Effect of slope and shape of dissociation curve on pulmonary gas exchange. *Respir. Physiol.* **8,** 66–85.

West, J. B., and P. D. Wagner (1977). Pulmonary gas exchange. *In* "Bioengineering Aspects of the Lung" (J. B. West, ed.), pp. 361–457. Dekker, New York.

Yokoyama, T., and L. E. Farhi (1967). Study of ventilation–perfusion ratio distribution in the anesthetized dog by multiple inert gas washout. *Respir. Physiol.* **3,** 166–176.

APPENDIX: FORTRAN LISTINGS OF QUADRATIC AND LINEAR SUBROUTINES

Subroutine SMOOTH. This is the least-squares (quadratic) program that finds the best fit to a set of retentions. Smoothing is incorporated into the variable WT that is passed in from the calling program (Evans and Wagner, 1977). NCALL is an integer variable recognizing the sequence of calling of subroutine SMOOTH and is used only as a flag for suppression of print statements. NGASES is the number of inert gases (up to 9 allowed by present dimensioning). NVAQS is the number of virtual $\dot{V}_A/\dot{Q}$ compartments (50 is allowed by present dimensioning). FACT is the conversion factor between units of solubility (ml/100 ml/mm Hg) and the blood:gas partition coefficient. It is given by $(P_B - P_{H_2O}/100$, where P_B is barometric pressure and P_{H_2O} saturated water vapor pressure in mm Hg. PC is the array of blood:gas partition coefficients. BSAVE is the array of retentions weighted for each gas according to variance (Evans and Wagner, 1977). A is the $\lambda_i(\lambda_i + \dot{V}_A/\dot{Q}_j)$ matrix [Eq. (1)], $i = 1$, NGASES and $j = 1$, NVAQS, weighted both by smoothing (WT) and according to the variance of each gas. F is the array of flags all set to 1.0 initially that label a $\dot{V}_A/\dot{Q}$ compartment as having (1.0) or not having (0.0) perfusion. H is a corresponding array of variables, all set to 0.0 initially, used in determining which compartments are to be used in the analysis. $\dot{Q}$ is the set of compartmental perfusions recovered from the least-squares analysis. E is the residual sum of squares, AD the array of best-fit retentions, and RD the array of residuals. Thus, RD = BSAVE − AD for each gas. The input variables to SMOOTH are thus NCALL, NGASES, NVAQS, FACT, PC, BSAVE, A, F, H, and WT. Values for the remaining variables are produced by the subroutine.

The routine should be used in conjunction with the compartmental weights incorporating smoothing (U) and the inert gas weight reflecting variance in the data (W) (Evans and Wagner, 1977).

Subroutine LPQMAX. This subroutine is the linear program that finds maximum compartmental perfusion in each of the compartments in turn. The input variables given in the CALL list are NGASES (the number of inert gases used); NVAQS (the number of compartments used); FACT (the same conversion factor as used in subroutine SMOOTH); VT (total ventilation); QT (total cardiac output); ITEST (a flag that is created internally); S and PC (respectively, solubilities and partition coefficients of the inert gases); R (the retentions to be analyzed, which must be exact values obtained according to the scheme of Fig. 7); VQ (the ventilation–perfusion ratios of the compartments); and QMAX (the determined array of maximum bloodflow in each of the compartments).

Subroutine LPFEAS is a subroutine which is used by LPQMAX and which is the basis of the linear program.

Subroutine LPUNIQ determines whether the perfusion distribution can be fitted by a unimodal curve. The variables required for operation of this subroutine are much the same as those for LPQMAX. VA is the same as VT; VAQ is the same as VQ; and Q is the array of compartmental bloodflows of the compatible unimodal distribution if it exists. NIN is not currently used but could contain the sequence number of the set of retentions undergoing analysis.

Subroutine LPUNIV is the corresponding subroutine determining whether a unimodal distribution of ventilation is compatible with the data. The variables in the CALL list are the same as for LPUNIQ, except for the variable E which is the set of excretions rather than retentions.

```
      SUBROUTINE SMOOTH(NCALL,NGASES,NVAQS,FACT,PC,BSAVE,A,F,H,Q,
    1 WT,E,AD,RD)
      DIMENSION S(10),PC(10),RD(10),AD(10),B(10),F(50),WT(50)
      DIMENSION Q(50),VAQ(50),C(10,10),A(50,10),RBAR(10),H(50)
      DIMENSION BSAVE(10)
      DO 4848 I=1,10
      B(I)=0.0
      RBAR(I)=0.0
      DO 4848 J=1,10
      C(I,J)=0.0
4848  CONTINUE
      SSQPRE = 1000000.0
      SSQPRE = SSQPRE**4
      NGLS1 = NGASES - 1
      NV = NVAQS -1
      ITER = 0
      REP = 2.0
50    CONTINUE
      DO 702 I=1,NGASES
      B(I) = BSAVE(I)
702   CONTINUE
      DO 100 I=1,NGASES
      DO 110 J=1,I
      C(J,I) = 0.0
      DO 120 K=1,NVAQS
      IF(F(K).EQ.0.0) GO TO 120
      C(J,I) = C(J,I) + A(K,I)*A(K,J)
120   CONTINUE
110   CONTINUE
100   CONTINUE
      DO 200 I=1,NGASES
      C(I,I) = 1.0 + C(I,I)
200   CONTINUE
      DO 220 I=1,NGASES
      C(I,NGASES+1) = B(I)
220   CONTINUE
      DO 300 I=1,NGLS1
      I1 = I + 1
      DO 310 J=I1,NGASES
      N1 = NGASES + 1
      DO 320 K=J,N1
      C(J,K) = C(J,K) - C(I,J)*C(I,K)/C(I,I)
320   CONTINUE
      M = NGASES
310   CONTINUE
300   CONTINUE
      RD(NGASES) = C(NGASES,NGASES+1)/C(NGASES,NGASES)
      M = NGASES
      DO 330 I=1,NGLS1
      RD(NGASES-I) = C(NGASES-I,NGASES+1)
      M=NGASES
      RD(NGASES-I) = C(NGASES-I,NGASES +1)
      M=NGASES
      NN1 = NGASES - I + 1
      DO 340 K=NN1,NGASES
      RD(NGASES-I) = RD(NGASES-I) - C(NGASES-I,K)*RD(K)
      M = NGASES
340   CONTINUE
      RD(NGASES-I) = RD(NGASES-I)/C(NGASES-I,NGASES-I)
      M = NGASES
330   CONTINUE
```

```
            DO 420 J=1,NVAQS
            Q(J) = 0.0
            DO 430 I=1,NGASES
            Q(J) = Q(J) + RD(I)*A(J,I)
430         CONTINUE
420         CONTINUE
            IF(REP.LT.3.0) GO TO 4564
            SUMWB = 0.0
            SUMB = 0.0
            DO 4561 J=1,NV
            IF(Q(J).LT.0.0) GO TO 4561
            IF(F(J).GT.0.0) GO TO 4561
            SUMB = SUMB + Q(J)*Q(J)
            IF(J.EQ.1) SUMWB = -Q(1)*Q(1)
4561        CONTINUE
            SUMWB = SUMWB + SUMB
            SUMCC = 0.0
            DO 4562 I=1,NGASES
            SUMC = 0.0
            DO 4563 K=1,NV
            IF(F(K).GT.0.0) GO TO 4563
            IF(Q(K).LE.0.0) GO TO 4563
            SUMC = SUMC + A(K,I)*Q(K)
4563,       CONTINUE
            SUMCC = SUMCC + SUMC*SUMC
4562        CONTINUE
            T = SUMB/(SUMCC + SUMWB)
4564        CONTINUE
            REP = 3.0
            XMIN = 1.0
            DO 810 I=1,NVAQS
            IF(F(I).GT.0.0.AND.Q(I).LT.0.0) GO TO 820
            GO TO 810
820         REP = 2.0
            Y = H(I)/(H(I) - Q(I))
            IF(XMIN.GT.Y) XMIN = Y
810         CONTINUE
            IF(REP.EQ.3.0) GO TO 3000
            DO 830 I=1,NVAQS
            IF(F(I).EQ.0.0) GO TO 830
            IF(Q(I).GE.0.0) GO TO 825
            Y = H(I)/(H(I) - Q(I))
            IF(Y.EQ.XMIN) F(I) = 0.0
825         H(I) = (1.0 - XMIN)*H(I) + XMIN*Q(I)
830         CONTINUE
            GO TO 50
3000        CONTINUE
            SUM1 = 0.0
            DO 1099 I=1,NGASES
            SUM1 = SUM1 + RD(I)*RD(I)
1099        CONTINUE
            SUM2 = 0.0
            DO 2099 J=1,NV
            SUM2 = SUM2 + Q(J)*Q(J)*F(J)
2099        CONTINUE
            SSQ = SUM1 + SUM2
            IF(SSQ.GE.SSQPRE) GO TO 4098
            SSQPRE = SSQ
            DO 840 I=1,NVAQS
            IF(F(I).GT.0.0.AND.Q(I).EQ.0.0) F(I) = 0.0
            IF(F(I).GT.0.0) H(I) = Q(I)
            IF(F(I).GT.0.0) F(I) = 1.0
            IF(F(I).EQ.0.0.AND.Q(I).GT.0.0) REP = 2.0
            IF(F(I).EQ.0.0.AND.Q(I).GT.0.0) H(I) = T*Q(I)
            IF(F(I).EQ.0.0.AND.Q(I).GT.0.0) F(I) = 1.0
            IF(F(I).EQ.0.0) H(I) = 0.0
```

```
840       CONTINUE
          ITER = ITER + 1
          IF(ITER.EQ.99) GO TO 550
          IF(REP.EQ.2.0) GO TO 50
4098      CONTINUE
          E = 0.0
          DO 390 I=1,NGASES
          AD(I) = BSAVE(I) - RD(I)
          IF(I.GT.NGLS1) GO TO 390
          E = E + RD(I)*RD(I)
390       CONTINUE
          DO 850 I=1,NVAQS
850       Q(I) = Q(I)/WT(I)
          IF(E.GT.0.02.AND.NCALL.EQ.1) RETURN
550       WRITE (5,600) ITER
600       FORMAT('    ITERATION NUMBER =',I3,/)
          SUMQ = 0.0
          DO 4001 J=1,NVAQS
          IF(F(J).EQ.0.0) Q(J) = 0.0
          SUMQ = SUMQ + Q(J)
4001      CONTINUE
          WRITE (5,5002) SUMQ
5002      FORMAT('   TOTAL BLOOD FLOW =',F10.6,//)
          WRITE (5,650)
650       FORMAT('      SOLUBILITY              RETENTIONS      BEST FIT
     1 ERROR',//)
4004      CONTINUE
          DO 3005 I=1,NGASES
          S(I) = PC(I)/FACT
          WRITE (5,655) S(I),BSAVE(I),AD(I),RD(I)
655       FORMAT(F14.5,F22.7,F15.7,F15.10)
3005      CONTINUE
          WRITE (5,630) E
630       FORMAT(//'   REMAINING SUM OF SQUARES =',E14.8,/)
          RETURN
          END
```

```
      SUBROUTINE LPQMAX(NGASES,NVAQS,FACT,VT,QT,ITEST,S,PC,R,VQ,QMAX)
      DIMENSION QMAX(50),A(8,57),B(10),C(60),S(10),PC(10),R(10),VQ(50)
      DIMENSION V(50),Q(50),INB(60),INBSAV(60),IBV(10),IBVSAV(10)
      DIMENSION VAQ(10),QQ(10),AA(8,57),II(7),KK(7)
      DOUBLE PRECISION A,AA,PC,VQ,R,DMIN,TMIN,TOL,TOL1,TESTR,X,B,C,VT,QT
      DO 830 I=1,8
      DO 830 J=1,57
      A(I,J)=0.0
      AA(I,J)=0.0
  830 CONTINUE
      TOL=-0.00000000001
      TOL1=0.000000001
      NV=NVAQS-1
      N1=NGASES+1
      N2=NGASES+2
      N3=NV+N1
      N4=NVAQS+N1
      R(N1)=1.0
      DO 4 J=1,NV
      A(N1,J)=1.0
      DO 4 I=1,NGASES
      A(I,J)=PC(I)/(PC(I)+VQ(J))
    4 CONTINUE
      DO 5 J=NVAQS,N3
      JJ=J-NV
      DO 5 I=1,N2
      A(I,J)=0.0
      IF(I.NE.JJ) GO TO 5
      A(I,J)=1.0
    5 CONTINUE
      A(N2,N4)=0.0
      DO 6 I=1,N1
      A(I,N4)=R(I)
      A(N2,N4)=A(N2,N4)-R(I)
    6 CONTINUE
      DO 7 J=1,NV
      A(N2,J)=0.0
      DO 7 I=1,N1
      A(N2,J)=A(N2,J)-A(I,J)
    7 CONTINUE
      CALL LPFEAS(NGASES,NVAQS,ITEST,INBSAV,IBVSAV,II,KK,A)
      IF(ITEST.EQ.0) TYPE 4611
 4611 FORMAT(///'   THERE IS NO FEASIBLE SOLUTION IN LPQMAX'//)
      IF(ITEST.EQ.0) RETURN
C        HERE IS COMP MAX ROUTINE
      DO 500 J=1,N3
      IF(A(N2,J).LE.TOL1) GO TO 500
      DO 501 I=1,N1
  501 A(I,J) = 0.0
  500 CONTINUE
      DO 502 J=1,N4
  502 A(N2,J) = 0.0
      DO 600 JMAX=1,NV
      DO 4848 I=1,N1
 4848 IBV(I) = IBVSAV(I)
      DO 4849 J=1,N4
 4849 INB(J) = INBSAV(J)
      DO 503 I=1,N2
      DO 503 J=1,N4
  503 AA(I,J) = A(I,J)
```

```
         AA(N2,JMAX) = -1.0
         NFLAG = 0
         DO 504 I=1,N1
         IF(JMAX.NE.IBV(I)) GO TO 504
         NFLAG = 1
         GO TO 506
504      CONTINUE
506      CONTINUE
         IF(NFLAG.EQ.0) GO TO 507
         DO 505 I=1,N1
         IF(A(I,JMAX).EQ.0.0) GO TO 505
         IFLAG = I
505      CONTINUE
         DO 508 J=1,N4
         AA(N2,J) = AA(N2,J) + AA(IFLAG,J)
508      CONTINUE
507      CONTINUE
510      DMIN = 0.0
         DO 511 J=1,NV
         JJ = INB(J)
         IF(AA(N2,JJ).GE.DMIN) GO TO 511
         DMIN = AA(N2,JJ)
         JPIVOT = JJ
         JMARK = J
511      CONTINUE
         IF(DMIN.LT.TOL) GO TO 6000
400      CONTINUE
         DO 5004 L=1,N1
         II(L)=NVAQS
         DO 5005 I=1,N1
         NCOMP=IBV(I)
         IF(L.EQ.1) GO TO 5006
         IF(NCOMP.LE.II(L-1)) GO TO 5005
5006     IF(NCOMP.GE.II(L)) GO TO 5005
         II(L)=NCOMP
         KK(L)=I
5005     CONTINUE
5004     CONTINUE
         GO TO 7009
         WRITE (5,951) JMAX
951      FORMAT(///' HERE ARE THE RESULTS MAXIMIZING PERFUSION IN COMPARTMEN
     1   T ',I2,//)
7009     CONTINUE
         DO 5007 L=1,N1
         IORD=II(L)
         KORD=KK(L)
         VAQ(L)=VQ(IORD)
         QQ(L)=AA(KORD,N4)
5007     CONTINUE
C5007    WRITE (5,59) IORD,VQ(IORD),AA(KORD,N4)
C  59    FORMAT(I10,F50.10,F53.10)
         MFLAG=0
         DO 3001 J=1,7
         IF(VAQ(J).NE.VQ(JMAX)) GO TO 3001
         MFLAG=1
         QMAX(JMAX)=QQ(J)
         GO TO 3002
3001     CONTINUE
3002     CONTINUE
         IF(MFLAG.EQ.1) GO TO 5008
         QMAX(JMAX)=0.0
5008     CONTINUE
         GO TO 600
6000     CONTINUE
         TMIN = 1000000.0
         TMIN = TMIN*TMIN
```

```
            LFLAG = 0
            DO 513 I=1,N1
            IF(AA(I,JPIVOT).LE.TOL1) GO TO 513
            TESTR = AA(I,N4)/AA(I,JPIVOT)
            IF(TESTR.GE.TMIN) GO TO 513
            TMIN = TESTR
            IPIVOT = I
            LFLAG = 1
513         CONTINUE
            IF(LFLAG.EQ.0) GO TO 400
            X = AA(IPIVOT,JPIVOT)
            DO 514 J=1,N4
            AA(IPIVOT,J) = AA(IPIVOT,J)/X
            C(J) = AA(IPIVOT,J)
514         CONTINUE
            DO 515 I=1,N2
            B(I) = AA(I,JPIVOT)
            IF(I.EQ.IPIVOT) GO TO 516
            DO 517 J=1,N4
            AA(I,J) = AA(I,J) - C(J)*B(I)
517         CONTINUE
516         CONTINUE
515         CONTINUE
            INB(JMARK) = IBV(IPIVOT)
            IBV(IPIVOT) = JPIVOT
            GO TO 510
600         CONTINUE
            RETURN
            END
```

```
          SUBROUTINE LPFEAS(NGASES,NVAQS,ITEST,INBSAV,IBVSAV,II,KK,A)
          DIMENSION II(7),KK(7)
          DIMENSION INB(60),IBV(10),A(8,57),IBVSAV(10),INBSAV(60)
          DIMENSION B(10),C(60)
          DOUBLE PRECISION A,B,C,TESTR,X,TOL1,TOL,DMIN,TMIN,W
          NV=NVAQS-1
          N1=NGASES+1
          N2=NGASES+2
          N3=NV+N1
          N4=NVAQS+N1
          TOL1=0.000000001
          TOL=-TOL1
          JPIVOT = 0
          IPIVOT = 0
          DO 8 J=1,NV
8         INB(J) = J
          DO 9 I=1,N1
9         IBV(I)=NV+I
100       DMIN = 0.0
          DO 10 J=1,NV
          JJ = INB(J)
          IF(A(N2,JJ).GE.DMIN) GO TO 10
          DMIN = A(N2,JJ)
          JPIVOT = JJ
          JMARK = J
10        CONTINUE
          IF(DMIN.LT.TOL) GO TO 99
          W = -A(N2,N4)
          IF(W.GE.TOL1) GO TO 52
          DO 5000 L=1,N1
          II(L)=NVAQS
          DO 5001 I=1,N1
          NCOMP=IBV(I)
          IF(L.EQ.1) GO TO 5002
          IF(NCOMP.LE.II(L-1)) GO TO 5001
5002      IF(NCOMP.GE.II(L)) GO TO 5001
          II(L)=NCOMP
          KK(L)=I
5001      CONTINUE
5000      CONTINUE
          DO 5848 I=1,N1
          IBVSAV(I) = IBV(I)
5848      CONTINUE
          DO 5849 J=1,N4
5849      INBSAV(J) = INB(J)
          GO TO 98
99        CONTINUE
          TMIN = 1000000.0
          DO 11 I=1,N1
          IF(A(I,JPIVOT).LE.0.0) GO TO 11
          TESTR = A(I,N4)/A(I,JPIVOT)
          IF(TESTR.GE.TMIN) GO TO 11
          TMIN = TESTR
          IPIVOT = I
11        CONTINUE
          X = A(IPIVOT,JPIVOT)
          DO 12 J=1,N4
          A(IPIVOT,J) = A(IPIVOT,J)/X
```

```
               C(J) = A(IPIVOT,J)
     12        CONTINUE
               DO 14 I=1,N2
               B(I) = A(I,JPIVOT)
               IF(I.EQ.IPIVOT) GO TO 15
               DO 13 J=1,N4
               A(I,J) = A(I,J) - C(J)*B(I)
     13        CONTINUE
     15        CONTINUE
     14        CONTINUE
               INB(JMARK) = IBV(IPIVOT)
               IBV(IPIVOT) = JPIVOT
               GO TO 100
     98        CONTINUE
               ITEST=1
               RETURN
     52        CONTINUE
               ITEST=0
               RETURN
               END
```

```
      SUBROUTINE LPUNIQ(NGASES,NVAQS,FACT,VA,QT,NIN,S,PC,R,VAQ,Q)
      DIMENSION S(10),PC(10),R(10),Q(50),VAQ(50),A(8,57),B(10),C(60)
      DIMENSION II(7),KK(7)
      DIMENSION RET(10),QQ(50),INB(60),INBSAV(60),IBV(10),IBVSAV(10)
      DOUBLE PRECISION PC,VAQ,A,VA,QT,R
      DO 4536 J=1,NVAQS
 4536 QQ(J)=0.0
      NV=NVAQS-1
      RNV=NV
      NV2=(NVAQS-2)/2
      KQMAX=NV2+1
      KQORIG=KQMAX
      NV3=NVAQS-2
      ITEST=0
      ISIGN=-1
      KOUNT=0
      N1=NGASES+1
      N2=NGASES+2
      N3=NV+N1
      N4=NVAQS+N1
      R(N1)=1.0
      DO 100 KCOMP=1,15
      DO 102 KM=1,2
      K1=KQMAX+1
      DO 107 I=1,NGASES
  107 A(I,1)=PC(I)/(PC(I)+VAQ(1))
      DO 108 J=2,KQMAX
      DO 108 I=1,NGASES
      A(I,J)=0.0
      DO 1020 M=J,KQMAX
 1020 A(I,J)=A(I,J) + PC(I)/(PC(I)+VAQ(M))
  108 CONTINUE
      DO 103 J=K1,NV
      DO 103 I=1,NGASES
      A(I,J)=0.0
      DO 104 M=K1,J
  104 A(I,J)=A(I,J) + PC(I)/(PC(I)+VAQ(M))
  103 CONTINUE
      A(N1,1)=1.0
      DO 105 J=2,KQMAX
  105 A(N1,J)=K1-J
      DO 106 J=K1,NV
  106 A(N1,J)=J+1-K1
      DO 5 J=NVAQS,N3
      JJ=J-NV
      DO 5 I=1,N2
      A(I,J)=0.0
      IF(I.NE.JJ) GO TO 5
      A(I,J)=1.0
    5 CONTINUE
      A(N2,N4)=0.0
      DO 6 I=1,N1
      A(I,N4)=R(I)
      A(N2,N4)=A(N2,N4)-R(I)
    6 CONTINUE
      DO 7 J=1,NV
      A(N2,J)=0.0
      DO 7 I=1,N1
    7 A(N2,J)=A(N2,J)-A(I,J)
      CALL LPFEAS(NGASES,NVAQS,ITEST,INBSAV,IBVSAV,II,KK,A)
```

```
      IF(ITEST.EQ.0) GO TO 49
      DO 303 L=1,7
      IORD=II(L)
      KORD=KK(L)
      QQ(IORD)=A(KORD,N4)
303   CONTINUE
      SUM=0.0
      DO 456 J=1,KQMAX
      SUM=SUM+QQ(J)
      QQ(J)=SUM
456   CONTINUE
      SUM=0.0
      DO 457 J=K1,NV
      JJ=K1+NV-J
      SUM=SUM+QQ(JJ)
      QQ(JJ)=SUM
457   CONTINUE
      DO 459 I=1,NGASES
      RET(I)=0.0
      DO 459 J=1,NV
459   RET(I)=RET(I)+PC(I)*QQ(J)/(PC(I)+VAQ(J))
      TYPE 463,KQMAX
463   FORMAT(' A FEASIBLE UNIMODAL SOLUTION EXISTS FOR KQMAX =',
     1I4,///,'        COMP               VA/Q             GIVEN Q
     1   UNIMODAL Q',/)
      Q(NVAQS)=0.0
      QQ(NVAQS)=0.0
      DO 466 J=1,NVAQS
466   TYPE 461,J,VAQ(J),Q(J),QQ(J)
461   FORMAT(I10,3F20.6)
      TYPE 464
464   FORMAT(////'        GAS        PARTITION COEFF         GIVEN R
     1   UNIMODAL FIT',/)
      DO 462 I=1,NGASES
462   TYPE 461,I,PC(I),R(I),RET(I)
      IF(ITEST.EQ.1) GO TO 101
49    KOUNT=KOUNT+1
      KQMAX=KQORIG + KCOMP*(ISIGN**KOUNT)
102   CONTINUE
100   CONTINUE
      TYPE 5311
5311  FORMAT('  NO FEASIBLE UNIMODAL DISTRIBUTION OF BLOODFLOW FITS THE
     1DATA')
101   CONTINUE
      RETURN
      END
```

```
      SUBROUTINE LPUNIV(NGASES,NVAQS,FACT,VA,QT,NIN,S,PC,E,VAQ,Q)
      DIMENSION S(10),PC(10),VAQ(50),Q(50),V(50),E(10),A(8,57),B(10)
      DIMENSION C(60),INB(60),INBSAV(60),IBV(10),IBVSAV(10),VV(50)
      DIMENSION EXC(10),II(7),KK(7)
      DOUBLE PRECISION VA,QT,VAQ,PC,A,E
      DO 4536 J=1,NVAQS
4536  VV(J)=0.0
      NV=NVAQS-1
      RNV=NV
      VALV=0.0
      DO 66 J=2,NV
      V(J)=Q(J)*VAQ(J)*QT/VA
      VALV=VALV + V(J)
 66   CONTINUE
      V(NVAQS)=1.0-VALV
      NV2=(NVAQS-2)/2
      KVMAX=NV2+8
      KVORIG=KVMAX
      NV3=NVAQS-2
      ITEST=0
      ISIGN=-1
      KOUNT=0
      N1=NGASES+1
      N2=NGASES+2
      N3=NV+N1
      N4=NVAQS+N1
      E(N1)=1.0
      DO 100 KCOMP=1,15
      DO 102 KM=1,2
      K1=KVMAX+1
      DO 107 I=1,NGASES
107   A(I,1)=0.0
      DO 108 J=2,KVMAX
      DO 108 I=1,NGASES
      A(I,J)=0.0
      DO 1020 M=J,KVMAX
1020  A(I,J)=A(I,J) + PC(I)/(PC(I)+VAQ(M))
108   CONTINUE
      DO 103 J=K1,NV
      DO 103 I=1,NGASES
      A(I,J)=0.0
      DO 104 M=K1,J
104   A(I,J)=A(I,J) + PC(I)/(PC(I)+VAQ(M))
103   CONTINUE
      A(N1,1)=1.0
      DO 105 J=2,KVMAX
      A(N1,J)=0.0
      DO 109 M=J,KVMAX
109   A(N1,J)=A(N1,J) + VA/(QT*VAQ(M))
105   CONTINUE
      DO 106 J=K1,NV
      A(N1,J)=0.0
      DO 110 M=K1,J
110   A(N1,J)=A(N1,J) + VA/(QT*VAQ(M))
106   CONTINUE
      DO 5 J=NVAQS,N3
      JJ=J-NV
      DO 5 I=1,N2
```

```
          A(I,J)=0.0
          IF(I.NE.JJ) GO TO 5
          A(I,J)=1.0
    5     CONTINUE
          A(N2,N4)=0.0
          DO 6 I=1,N1
          A(I,N4)=E(I)
          A(N2,N4)=A(N2,N4)-E(I)
    6     CONTINUE
          DO 7 J=1,NV
          A(N2,J)=0.0
          DO 7 I=1,N1
    7     A(N2,J)=A(N2,J)-A(I,J)
          CALL LPFEAS(NGASES,NVAQS,ITEST,INBSAV,IBVSAV,II,KK,A)
          IF(ITEST.EQ.0) GO TO 49
          DO 303 L=1,7
          IORD=II(L)
          KORD=KK(L)
          VV(IORD)=A(KORD,N4)
  303     CONTINUE
          SUM=0.0
          DO 456 J=2,KVMAX
          SUM=SUM+VV(J)
  456     VV(J)=SUM
          SUM=0.0
          DO 457 J=K1,NV
          JJ=K1+NV-J
          SUM=SUM+VV(JJ)
  457     VV(JJ)=SUM
          VV(1)=0.0
          DO 459 I=1,NGASES
          EXC(I)=0.0
          DO 459 J=1,NV
          EXC(I)=EXC(I)+PC(I)*VV(J)/(PC(I)+VAQ(J))
  459     CONTINUE
          TYPE 463,KVMAX
  463     FORMAT('   A FEASIBLE UNIMODAL SOLUTION EXISTS FOR KVMAX =',
         1I4,///,'        COMP              VA/Q            GIVEN V
         1    UNIMODAL V',/)
          SUMV=0.0
          DO 560 J=2,NV
  560     SUMV=SUMV+VV(J)
          VV(NVAQS)=1.0-SUMV
          DO 466 J=1,NVAQS
  466     TYPE 461,J,VAQ(J),V(J),VV(J)
          TYPE 464
  464     FORMAT(////'        GAS        PARTITION COEFF          GIVEN E
         1      UNIMODAL FIT',/)
          DO 462 I=1,NGASES
  462     TYPE 461,I,PC(I),E(I),EXC(I)
  461     FORMAT(I10,3F20.6)
          IF(ITEST.EQ.1) GO TO 101
   49     KOUNT=KOUNT+1
          KVMAX=KVORIG + KCOMP*(ISIGN**KOUNT)
  102     CONTINUE
  100     CONTINUE
          TYPE 5311
 5311     FORMAT(//////' NO FEASIBLE UNIMODAL DISTRIBUTION OF VENTILATION
         1FITS THE DATA')
  101     CONTINUE
          RETURN
          END
```

CHAPTER 9

Lung Surfactant Mechanics: Some Unresolved Problems

J. HILDEBRANDT

I. INTRODUCTION

It has been 50 years since von Neergaard (1929) noted the important role of surface tension in lung mechanics. Although great strides have been made in understanding the chemistry, physics, physiological func-

Regulation of Ventilation and Gas Exchange

tion, and turnover of the alveolar lining, many fundamental aspects of its properties, origin, and pathophysiology remain in a speculative state, and some in serious dispute. I will review briefly the historical development of our concepts of the function and properties of the lining and try to highlight some areas of current thought and research activity. This survey is intended to supplement and extend, but not repeat, a recent monograph on a similar topic (Hoppin and Hildebrandt, 1976).

II. HISTORICAL DEVELOPMENTS

A. Surface Effects in the Lung

Von Neergaard obtained data of the type shown in Fig. 1 in which the pressure–volume relationships of excised lungs filled with air and then

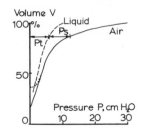

Figure 1. Deflation curves of mammalian lungs. Solid line: air-filled; dashed line: saline-filled; dotted line: gas trapping. Tissue component of recoil pressure is *Pt;* surface component is *Ps.*

with an isosmotic saline solution were compared. The results demonstrated in a simple and direct way that eliminating the air–lung interface (or at least reducing its interfacial tension nearly to zero) greatly reduced lung recoil. He interpreted the curve obtained with liquid as representing the recoil of the lung's tissue elastic elements (*Pt*). The additional component of recoil arising from the surface tension at the interface (*Ps*) acted in parallel with *Pt*, therefore additively. (His picture persists to this day, and although many doubt the total simplicity of this interpretation, no reliable modifications have yet been offered). He went one step further, in that he measured the surface tension (γ) of lung liquid, obtaining a value of about 35 mN/m (equivalent to dynes/cm)* or roughly half that of pure water. This allowed him to conclude that the interface had some detergent-like properties.

---

* mN/m = milli Newton/meter = dynes/cm.

However, it appears von Neergaard did not exploit his findings to nearly the extent that he might almost immediately have done. For example, by reflecting on the shape and position of his two curves (admittedly his data were crude), he might have deduced a most important property of the lining, which was not formally demonstrated until 30 years later. Thus, one notices that the curves converge monotonically. If one were to think of alveoli as a mass of bubbles with *constant* surface tension, these curves would tend to *diverge* as the lung deflated ($Ps = 2\gamma/r$ predicting that Ps increases or r decreases). One is therefore forced to suggest that γ must instead be decreasing; in fact, because Ps approaches zero, γ would also become very small. Allowing alveoli to become nonspherical and interdependent would not lead to a different conclusion. For example, Fig. 2A diagrams alveoli that are hexagonal in cross section. Force due to surface tension is developed parallel to the flat alveolar walls, and brings about a retractive force in the entire network. Should the alveolus somehow collapse like an accordion rather than isotropically (Fig. 2B), it still

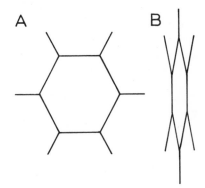

Figure 2. Hexagonal array of interdependent alveoli. A: Uniformly inflated. B: Deflated without change in surface area.

develops a retractive force in the vertical direction. Consequently, when Ps approaches zero in an elastic structure, one may conclude that γ must be very small irrespective of alveolar geometry. Of course, in order to exert recoil at the trachea, alveolar gas must be continuous with the tracheal air. In other words, following airway closure (dotted line, Fig. 1) a vanishing Ps would not reflect absence of recoil in alveoli but rather absence of continuity along the airways. Airway closure and trapping do occur under certain circumstances, and their effects must always be borne in mind.

264   J. Hildebrandt

B. Calculation of Surface Area

1. The Energy Principle

Pressure–volume (P–V) curves such as von Neergaard provided were essentially rediscovered in the early 1950's, and the initial thinking at that time concerning γ paralleled his own remarkably closely. Radford (1954) again began by assuming that γ had a fixed value during lung deflation, but made an important advance through a simple application of thermodynamics. He noted that the external P–V work done by the interface as the lung emptied spontaneously could be directly equated to the change in surface energy. For each small change in volume (dV) the increment in work (dW) (shown in Fig. 3A) would therefore be $Ps\ dV = \gamma\ dA$, where dA is change in alveolar surface area. The total work done would be

$$\int_{V_0}^{V_{max}} Ps\ dV = \int_{A_0}^{A_{max}} \gamma\ dA$$

the first integral being the area between the saline and air deflation curves. Radford then reasoned that if γ were constant (he felt there was no reason to suspect otherwise) one could use this scheme to find alveolar surface area indirectly. This would provide a novel and totally independent estimate of A. The equation then reduced to

$$\int_{V_0}^{V_{max}} Ps\ dV = \gamma\ (A_{max} - A_0)$$

Hence, to find $A_{max} - A_0$ he need only integrate P–V data planimetrically, and divide by γ. He chose $\gamma = 50$ mN/m, because it seemed reasonable that a fluid not unlike plasma should wet the alveolar surface. Upon applying this method to several species, he concluded that prior anatomical estimates of A, based on morphometric techniques, were about *ten times too large*. He was reluctant to accept the possibility that one of his assumptions might be greatly in error.

2. Anisotropy

The preceding calculation required no explicit assumptions about alveolar geometry, or about changes in alveolar shape with lung expansion. Subsequent developments from Radford's argument did rely upon a relationship between alveolar surface area and lung volume. *Isotropic* deflation of alveolar spaces, of any initial shape whatsoever, yields the simplest relation: $A = KV^{2/3}$ (Fig. 3B). A number of morphometric methods applied to alveolar geometry have yielded data which scatter around this curve. Another possibility is "accordion" deflation, wherein

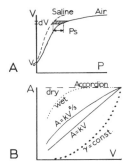

Figure 3. Calculation of alveolar surface area and surface tension. A: Element of work, *dW*, done by the air–liquid interface when the lung volume reduced by *dV* is *Ps dV*, also equal to surface tension γ times change in surface area, *dA*. B: Possible area–volume relationships of the lung. For explanation, see text.

alveolar walls begin forming pleats and fold up *without* significant shortening. In its pure form in a nonsticky lung, the accordion could produce *no* change at all in area during deflation (dashed line, Fig. 3B). On the other hand, if the pleats were moist and began to stick to each other, causing the smaller alveolar spaces to collapse entirely, a rapid reduction in *interfacial* area could result after partial lung deflation (dotted line in Fig. 3B).

The accordion model is still revived occasionally and deserves a few additional comments. First, alveolar walls having folds could not exert retractive forces, as they are actually under compression. Yet, the whole lung *always* exerts some recoil (see Fig. 1), as do individual elements of lung tissue when elongated up to approximately twice their resting lengths (Fukaya *et al.,* 1968; Sugihara *et al.,* 1971). Conversely, tissue which is elastic does not curl or pleat unless its length is less than its resting length, which occurs near the residual volume (RV). It therefore seems unlikely that folding without shortening would occur in the lung. Second, the normal lung is surprisingly stable, i.e., resistant to adhesion of alveolar walls, or to total alveolar collapse (Young *et al.,* 1970; Mead *et al.,* 1970). Atelectasis and instability are observed only in anomalous circumstances, perhaps more so in excised rat lungs than elsewhere (e.g., Gil and Weibel, 1972).

Radford could readily have extended his calculation to allow an estimate of the way in which A varied with V. For example, by a stepwise lowering of the upper limit of integration (V_{max}) in the equation

$$\frac{1}{\gamma} \int_{V_0}^{V_{max}} Ps \; dV = A_{max} - A_0$$

one obtains corresponding successive values of A_{max}. Since *Ps* falls rather sharply near total lung capacity (TLC), calculated area would also drop rapidly, as depicted in Fig. 3B (open circles). The resulting relationship displays a curvature unexpected from the preceding discussion. It might be compatible with atelectasis beginning immediately from TLC, or other gross distortions in alveolar ducts. After contemplating a plot such as this, one might be led to suspect that perhaps Ps becomes rapidly smaller not primarily because of the dwindling surface area, but rather because of a diminishing γ.

C.   Variable Surface Tension

1.   Bubbles and Balances

A concept of alveolar surface tension which differed radically from Radford's view appeared the following year. Pattle (1955) deduced from observations of the shape of bubbles derived from edema foam that the alveolar surface was lined with a lipoproteinaceous material acting much like a poorly soluble monolayer developing a high film pressure (Π) approaching that of the aqueous subphase (γ_0). The net resultant surface tension ($\gamma = \gamma_0 - \Pi$) was therefore near zero.

An explanation which neatly resolved the totally disparate conclusions about alveolar γ (zero in one case, and 35–50 mN/m in the other) came quickly thereafter. Clements (1957) noted that indeed *all* estimates of γ, high and low, could be correct, because when lung lining material was compressed *in vitro* on a surface balance, the initial γ of near 50 could be reduced to 5–10 mN/m (Fig. 4). This was a property already well known in

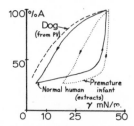

Figure 4.   Relationship between area and surface tension. Solid line: extract of normal lung; dashed line: computed from $P-V$ data; dotted line: extract from surfactant-deficient lung.

surface chemistry for many years, but new to lung mechanics. It immediately provided a basis for a better understanding of both normal lung function, and of abnormalities associated with acute losses of lung compliance (e.g., ARDS and IRDS)* wherein the $\gamma-A$ curve might be shifted

---

* ARDS and IRDS denote, respectively, adult and infant respiratory distress syndromes.

toward higher minimum γ. A second feature apparent from these *in vitro* studies was the clear absence of reversibility, helping to explain some of the large hysteresis regularly found in lung *P–V* curves. The reason for the γ–A hysteresis of surfactant remains somewhat unclear (see below).

2. Computed Surface Tension

Brown (1957), a colleague of Clements, promptly showed that Radford's method could be modified just slightly to derive γ–A relations from *P–V* curves roughly compatible with the new *in vitro* data. He applied the equation $\Delta W_i = Ps_i \Delta V_i = \overline{\gamma}_i \Delta A_i$ to each (*i*th) strip of the *P–V* curve in succession (Fig. 5), ΔW_1 being the surface work done when the lung deflated an amount ΔV_1, etc., and $\overline{\gamma}_1$ the mean surface tension in the first interval. However, A was not measured, so it was necessary to propose a reasonable approximation, for example, to assume isotropic deflation (see Fig. 3B). Thus, taking the derivative dA/dV of $A = KV^{2/3}$, he obtained $\Delta A_1 = 2K \Delta V_1/3$, and $\Delta W_1 = \overline{\gamma}_1 2K \Delta V_1/3 (V_1)^{1/3}$. In order to reduce the number of unknowns by one, he made the further initial assumption that $\overline{\gamma}_1$ (at TLC) was 50. Thereafter, K and all subsequent $\overline{\gamma}_i$ could be computed, as shown in Fig. 5. This method gave results somewhat different

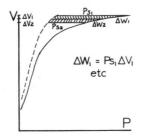

Figure 5. Method for calculating successive values of γ along a deflation curve, as proposed by Brown (1975).

from the *in vitro* data, but sufficiently close to confirm the notion that γ dropped sharply to very low values during lung deflation, close to zero (Brown *et al.*, 1959). One may also note as an aside that Radford's approach was really identical to the above, except that his strip element effectively incorporated the entire vital capacity. Had he chosen a $\overline{\gamma}$ of 5 mN/m, which may be considered a good estimate of the mean γ for the *entire* deflation curve (cf. Fig. 7), his A would have turned out to match the morphometric estimates quite closely; i.e., it would have been a factor of about 10 larger.

III.   FACTORS INVOLVED IN LUNG STABILITY

A.   Alveolar Stability

1.   Independent Alveoli

An important application of the finding that γ was a strong function of surface area, and hence of volume, was quickly perceived by Clements *et al.* (1958, 1961). This relates to the problem of maintaining the patency of millions of alveoli of differing sizes and shapes which are effectively connected in parallel. For example, even *two* soap bubbles cannot be deflated in parallel: One bubble always gains most of the total volume while the other collapses. However, a multiple parallel bubble system may deflate stably, provided the surfaces are lined by an appropriate surfactant film (Hildebrandt, 1974). In this case, as one bubble begins to collapse, its surface tension falls, and so does its recoil pressure, thus braking further collapse. Similarly, the many alveoli of the lung may be considered to be stabilized by this mechanism.

2.   Interdependent Alveoli

Whether other factors may be more important than low surface tension in protecting alveolar stability is not totally clear. Mead *et al.* (1970) pointed out that attachments to adjacent alveoli effectively "stiffen" each unit and guard against its collapse. In other words, each unstable unit is suspended by a network of neighboring interalveolar septa. In this way the specific compliance of the unit may be reduced by a factor of about three. This factor would render the early stability computations made by Clements and co-workers, based on independent bubbles rather than interdependent alveoli, overly stringent, because they relied *only* on film compressibility to achieve stability. In fact, Fung (1975a,b) has argued on theoretical grounds that alveolar septal stability should be totally independent of γ. However, this runs counter to experience with animal lungs, where γ can be altered by interstitial edema (Cook *et al.*, 1959) or by ventilation at room temperature (Faridy *et al.*, 1966; Nagao *et al.*, 1977). Whenever compliance falls appreciably as a result of changes in surface forces, focal subpleural atelectasis is commonly observed. Also, alveolar instability was originally (Avery and Mead, 1959) and still is (Farrell and Avery, 1975) considered a primary functional defect of the lungs of infants afflicted with hyaline membrane disease (IRDS).

3.   Stability in Polyhedral Alveoli

It is likely that the theoretical prediction of Fung, based on an essentially "dry" model of parenchyma, fails to account for observed properties because of the way surface tension effects were incorporated. His model considers γ simply as a force *parallel* to the tissue recoil forces (Fig. 6A). In reality, rounded interfaces must be present at all alveolar edges and corners (Fig. 6B), producing force components *normal* to the walls. Then, whenever the slightest asymmetry appears in the corner geometry, a tendency to collapse occurs. For example, the pair of adjacent walls subtending the smallest angle will be drawn into apposition (Fig. 6C) or "zipped up." The process is spontaneous, as a net reduction in surface area implies a lower surface free energy. The mechanism may be best understood in terms of subphase pressures. Each corner (edge) pool of liquid is under a *negative* hydrostatic pressure equal to $P_{sub} = \gamma/r$. If all γ are equal, but one radius of curvature is smaller than the other two (Fig. 6B: $r_1 = r_2 > r_3$), a more negative corner pressure P_3 results. Flexible alveolar walls would tend to collapse toward P_3, but are normally restrained from doing so by tension in the walls. Pressure differences arising from inequalities in corner angles θ could be accentuated by inequalities in γ (e.g., $\gamma_3 > \gamma_1 = \gamma_2$) or by the presence of unequal amounts of alveolar fluid or infiltrates which enhance uneven r. Normally, the inequalities in P_{sub} are small at low lung volumes, because all γ are near zero. As a consequence, the collapsing tendency is too slight to produce atelectasis. However, when low γ is not achieved, the differences in P_{sub} are proportionately amplified. This model of parenchymal mechanics therefore predicts a strong and direct effect of the magnitude of γ on alveolar instability. Clearly, at higher lung volumes the larger traction in the wall elements will act to "unzip" and reverse atelectasis. A more comprehensive analysis of this model has not yet been developed; indeed, because of

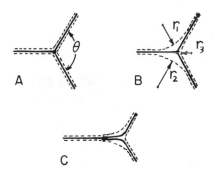

Figure 6. Surface forces at an alveolar intersection. Solid lines: interalveolar septa; dashed lines: surfactant lining separated from septal wall by subphase of varying thickness. A: Minimal subphase, sharp corner. B: Fluid at corners, giving rise to various radii of curvature, r. C: Adhesion of adjacent septa caused by surface forces.

the many possible combinations of γ, θ, r, and tissue tension, it may prove difficult to generalize.

B. Airway Stability

Related in many respects to alveolar collapse is airway collapse. However, although higher γ is observed to be associated with alveolar instability, it is apparently associated with greater airway stability. Thus, stiff lungs may be deflated to lower than normal lung volumes before airway closure limits further deflation. The explanation seems to be that the outward traction on small airways, which is proportional to γ, prevents airway narrowing sufficiently to inhibit meniscus formation (Macklem, 1971). On the other hand, evidence has been obtained from rat lungs to support the concept that foam can be produced in small airways, which then brings about small airway closure by obstruction (Frazer and Weber, 1976). Nevertheless, it seems menisci would also have to form at some point in the terminal airways or alveolar ducts as a necessary step in bubble generation. Excised lungs are more prone to gas trapping at 37°C than at 22°C, yet vital capacity maneuvers can be performed repeatedly *in vivo* without airway obstruction. Details of the mechanism of gas trapping, including the role of temperature, bronchiolar tone, airway fluid volume, and its viscosity or surface tension largely remain to be clarified.

IV. *In Vitro* vs *In Situ* MEASUREMENTS OF SURFACE TENSION

The chemistry and physics of the alveolar lining are more readily examined *in vitro* than in the lung itself. Accordingly, our knowledge of both the composition and many of the physical properties of surfactant has been derived almost entirely from studies either of extracts of whole lung homogenates, or preferably, from alveolar wash material with minimal cell disruption. Nevertheless, because of potential *in vitro* alterations in the chemical nature of the surface layer and subphase, and in physical interrelationships of these with the adjacent epithelial cell layer, it would seem prudent to confirm as many of these properties as possible *in situ*.

A. Estimates from *P–V* Data

Brown's calculation (1957) already described provided the first comparison between *in vitro* and *in situ* estimates of γ. A more detailed analysis was published some time later by Bachofen *et al.* (1970). They introduced a simplification in the calculation which eliminated the necessity for strip planimetry. Thus, as in Fig. 5, the area of any strip is $dW = P\,dV = \gamma\,dA$, and $dA = \frac{2}{3}kV^{-1/3}\,dV$. Therefore, $P\,dV = \frac{2}{3}kV^{-1/3}\,\gamma\,dV$. By dropping dV from both sides of this equation, they obtained $\gamma = 3V^{1/3}\,P/2k$. Because

$$\gamma_{max} = \frac{3}{2k}V_{max}^{1/3}\,P_{max}$$

it follows that

$$\frac{\gamma}{\gamma_{max}} = \left(\frac{P}{P_{max}}\right)\left(\frac{V}{V_{max}}\right)^{1/3}$$

where the subscript max denotes peak inflation, and γ_{max} must be arbitrarily assumed, e.g., 50 mN/m. Figure 7 (dashed line), shows typical data from

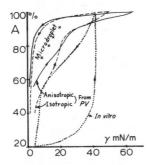

Figure 7. Comparison of γ–A relationships. Dotted line: *in vitro;* dashed line: calculated from P–V curves, assuming $A = KV^{2/3}$ (isotropic); solid line: calculated from same P–V data, assuming $A = KV^{0.44}$ (anisotropic); crosses: direct measurements using spreading of microdroplets (Schürch *et al.*, 1976).

cat lung calculated in this fashion by Bachofen *et al.* (1970). It is evident that although the overall properties of many *in vitro* studies were confirmed, there are some interesting differences. The tension becomes lower faster than suspected from surface balance studies, and the hysteresis is generally less, particularly on the expansion curve from low lung volumes.

1. Critique of Assumptions Relating P–V Data to γ–A Estimates

One may question whether the γ–A curves computed from P–V data offer improved reliability over *in vitro* methods. The computations rest on several important assumptions: All volume changes are isotropic, i.e., no configurational changes occur; $\gamma_{max} = 50$; at a given volume, the alveolar duct configuration is unaffected when air is replaced by saline; and saline reduces all surface forces to zero, but does not affect the tissue recoil. Each of these must be considered briefly.

a. Alveolar Shape.   It is known from morphometric studies such as those of Klingele and Staub (1970) that alveolar shape *does* change significantly with air inflation, especially over the lower half of the vital capacity. Here, the mouths of alveoli undergo relative widening as the ducts expand. The correspondence between air and saline filling in respect to these geometrical alterations is not known. Other approaches relating surface area to volume by stereological techniques have given somewhat variable results, yielding exponents in the equation $A = KV^n$ ranging from 0.41 (Forrest, 1970) through 0.66 (D'Angelo, 1972) to 1.0 (Gil and Weibel, 1972). Tsunoda *et al.* (1974) recomputed the Bachofen data using their own n of 0.44, believing that this would illustrate the effect of one type of fairly gross anisotropy. Although the corrections were not substantial (dotted line, Fig. 7), they tended to bring the *in vitro* and calculated curves into greater *discordance*. Therefore, from these studies it would appear that anisotropy might not be of prime importance in explaining the discrepancy between the two sets of data.

b. Maximum Tension.   The choice of γ_{max} affects only the *scale* and not the basic shape of the $\dot{\gamma}-A$ function. Nevertheless, the quantity is of great interest from the standpoint of understanding the lung's surface characteristics. However, γ_{max} may be difficult to define (let alone measure), just as TLC is arbitrarily defined for animals and excised lungs (e.g., peak transpulmonary pressure of 25 cm H_2O, etc.). Further increments in pressure, or longer equilibration periods at a fixed chosen pressure, or repeated cycles to the same pressure, all result in additional volume increments. Practically, the selected pressure is limited by the ability of the lungs to withstand rupture or tissue microdamage, and this varies with age and species.

Estimates of γ_{max} from lung wash or extract preparations generally fall in the neighborhood of 45 mN/m, but this is dependent on quantity of surfactant added and peak area chosen. The calculation of Tsunoda *et al.* (1974) based on $P-V$ data and thicknesses of alveolar walls suggested γ_{max} could be as high as 65 mN/m. From the oil droplet data of Schürch *et al.* (1976), described more fully below, one may estimate γ_{max} by extrapolating linearly to TLC, giving a value as low as 25 mN/m. A recent study of bubbles (expressed from rat lungs) (Pattle, 1977) suggests γ_{max} may be closer to 35 mN/m. At the moment, therefore, the most direct methods favor lower peak surface tensions, and 35 mN/m might be a reasonable average. Clearly, better methods are needed to establish absolute values of interfacial tension at TLC, and intermediate volumes as well.

The final two assumptions may significantly influence the quantity Ps, particularly above 80% TLC, and involve basic concepts important in and of themselves.

c. Alveolar Duct Configuration. Consider the effect of alveolar duct configuration first on total tissue recoil, taking the saline-filled lung as a point of reference. Each alveolar mouth is ringed by a connective tissue fiber bundle whose function it is to provide support for the free edges of protruding alveolar walls. Without this "chicken-wire" net of fibers, the septa would simply retract or tear, leaving essentially nonalveolated alveolar ducts. The radial traction developed by the septal tissue is low in the fluid-filled lung. However, when surface forces are added, the radial stresses on the rings may double or triple, and more energy must be stored in this elastic tissue. On the other hand, somewhat less energy would be stored in the septa themselves, for they would be shortened by surface tension. Because the septa have low recoil, the latter reduction in stored energy should be small. Consequently, surface forces must bring about some distortion of the tissue recoil curve at higher pressures, signifying a net increase in potential energy. Greater energy storage would occur not only at alveolar mouths, but in other parenchymal boundaries, such as blood vessels and airways. Under these circumstances a tissue recoil curve cannot be found experimentally, and the saline tissue recoil curve represents only a lower bound. (The appendix illustrates a simple two-dimensional analogy of this type of physical system.) Therefore, Ps would be overestimated at the same time that dV/dA is slightly underestimated by assuming isotropy. Surface tension ($\gamma = Ps \, dV/dA$) might therefore be slightly overestimated.

However, near TLC another form of distortion could occur. If the alveolar mouths reached an elastic limit of extension, say at 90% TLC, further inflation would increase septal area disproportionately, such that the isotropic assumption would overestimate dV/dA. Hence, γ could seem too large (cf. Fig. 7). Many possible combinations of distortion exist with varying effects on Ps and dV/dA, a few of which are considered in the appendix. Little is presently known about the details of lung mechanics at the level of the alveolar ducts.

d. Saline Effects. Finally, it is necessary to consider possible effects of saline. It is commonly assumed that interfacial tension is eliminated by the presence of aqueous solutions in the lung. However, Bienkowski and

Skolnick (1974) raised the possibility that two separate interfaces (air/surface and surface/tissue) acted at the alveolar–air boundary, and saline eliminated both. Consequently, the effects of γ(air/surface) might be overestimated, because Ps might also include a component from γ(surface/tissue). They suggested that mineral oil should eliminate only $\gamma(a/s)$ and leave $\gamma(s/t)$ intact. The γ–A curves they computed on this basis more closely resembled *in vitro* curves than those shown by Bachofen *et al.* (1970). Whether this concept represents an advance remains problematic. The method introduces unsupported new assumptions over and above those already discussed. It is, of course, possible that the subphase is a compressed gel kept "dry" by forces similar to those maintaining the negative pulmonary interstitial pressure described by Guyton *et al.* (1976). If so, interesting new properties could be expected at the interfaces and, as well, the gel could require additional forces to bring about its own thinning and stretching. These aspects of surface mechanics have apparently not yet been investigated, perhaps being regarded as "second-order" phenomena.

Another possible effect of saline in lungs has also received scant attention. As intimated above, interstitial space is thought to consist of fluid channels interspersed among a matrix of gel and fibrous elastin and collagen (cf. Fig. 14 below). This fluid is likely under suction (negative pressure) from two sources, the curved corner interfaces (Fig. 6) and the lymphatic pumps, although evidence *against* negative interstitial pressure has recently been summarized by Staub (1977). Deforming the gel requires forces which probably give rise to some "tissue hysteresis." In addition, the negative pressure itself (if present) must generate some retractive elastic force in the tissue. Because lungs immersed in saline rapidly undergo some swelling by absorption through the pleura (Y. Tsuya and J. Hildebrandt, unpublished), one may presume that the saline-filled lung undergoes similar interstitial swelling as well as rapid loss of any negative interstitial pressure. The extreme thinning of alveolar septa near TLC requires high forces: the interstitial material must be deformed from an initial thickness of about 10 μm near minimal volume to less than 4 μm at TLC (Tsunoda *et al.*, 1974). One can think of the two faces of each septum as being "drawn in" by increasingly negative pressures. Consequently, saline filling may, be relieving the "suction effect" of interstitial pressure, eliminate a component of "tissue" recoil, thus causing an underestimate of Pt, and an overestimate of Ps and therefore of γ. The existence of this phenomenon has not yet found experimental support. It would provide a means for explaining the possible development of negative interstitial pressure even in the absence of surface phenomena or lymph pumps.

In the presence of permeable capillaries, small amounts of fluid could shift relatively quickly across the endothelium whenever interstitial pressure fell. To what extent (if any) this effect could contribute to "stress relaxation" is not known.

B. Direct Measurements of Surface Tension

We are left at this point with doubts about the reliability of estimates of γ derived from $P-V$ data as well as from *in vitro* studies. Lacking have been direct measurements of γ *in situ*, as a function of volume and volume history. An important and exciting step toward achieving this end was recently reported by Schürch *et al.* (1976). The technique they employed was an elegant application of well-known principles of surface physics, but in a manner and to a situation not heretofore achieved.

1. Spreading of Microdroplets

The method of Schürch *et al.* (1976) is illustrated in Fig. 8. When an oil droplet is placed on the surface of another liquid, it will not spread unless $\gamma(a/s)$ is greater than the sum of the horizontal components of $\gamma(a/o)$ and $\gamma(o/s)$. By selecting the proper oil, one may therefore estimate $\gamma(a/s)$ at the point where the droplet begins to spread into a film. Schürch *et al.* (1976) calibrated four liquids (three fluorocarbons and one oil) on a surface balance containing lung surfactant, using the hanging plate to measure $\gamma(a/s)$. Spreading for the test liquids was observed at 9, 13, 16, and 20 mN/m, respectively. They then placed 10 μm diameter droplets of these liquids on the surfaces of subpleural alveolar septa by means of micropipets having tip diameters of 1–3 μm. As lung volumes were altered they could observe the point of spreading by microscope. Data were taken at volumes and pressures near the major deflation limb in excised rat and cat lungs kept at 37°C. Their mean values are shown as four crosses in Fig. 7. The results suggest that γ may lie somewhere between the estimates

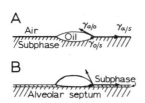

Figure 8. Microdroplet method of measuring surface tension. A: Droplet of immiscible liquid floating on a second liquid whose interfacial tension, $\gamma a/s$, is to be determined. Droplet will spread when $\gamma a/s > \gamma a/o + \gamma o/s$ (horizontal components). B: Droplet on alveolar septum, with thin subphase. Contact angles may differ from A.

obtained from $P-V$ and *in vitro* methods. Over the range which the test liquids were able to cover (up to 87% TLC), there was no evidence of the sharp rise in γ which characterizes the functions derived from $P-V$ data. In fact, as already mentioned, γ_{max} extrapolates (linearly) to as low as 25 mN/m, which happens to lie very close to the "equilibrium surface tension" (γ_{eq}) described in a number of *in vitro* studies (Clements, 1962; Tierney, 1965; King and Clements, 1972). Neither was the lower limit of γ_{min} reached by the droplet. However, extrapolating to 20% TLC would give about 4 mN/m, somewhat above the estimates of 0–1 mN/m obtained for γ_{min} by various bubble and balance techniques. In general, the droplet method appears to give good direct evidence that $\gamma(a/s)$ in the lung *does* fall to very low values, a point which has recently been disputed (Reifenrath and Zimmerman, 1973; Reifenrath, 1975).

2. Possible Errors

A few reservations concerning these data may be borne in mind. First, the lungs were excised, perhaps allowing some alteration of surface activity. Second, most measurements were made on the initial segments of reinflation limbs, following deflation from 25 cm H_2O. This would tend to raise γ slightly. Furthermore, peak inflation pressures higher than 25 cm H_2O might have resulted in a further left shift of the deflation curves, and lower γ. Third, the calibration procedure assumes that $\gamma(o/s)$ is the same in the lung as *in vitro*, which need not be the case if the subphase were a gel. Fourth, the contact angles *in situ* may be significantly altered compared to the calibration setting, as shown in Fig. 8B. The droplet can settle into the subphase of the lung only about 0.1 μm or less, hence must "sit above" the surface, resting on epithelium. This might allow a *lower* $\gamma(a/s)$ to spread the droplet than determined by calibration, hence γ would be overestimated. Most of the foregoing factors would tend to *reduce* the actual γ slightly from the values reported by Schürch *et al.* (1976). Although the magnitude of their overestimate is not predictable, a total error of 5 mN/m is not inconceivable. This would only serve to strengthen their argument that γ_{min} does attain the low levels claimed 20 years ago.

V. STABILITY OF THE SURFACE FILM

A. Temperature

The same oil drop experiment (Schürch *et al.*, 1976) yielded information about another surfactant property, that of lining stability, which is also still in serious dispute. Initial studies of dynamic and static characteristics at body temperature revealed the *in vitro* surface layer to be remarkably

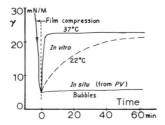

Figure 9. Time course of changes in γ following a rapid film compression. *In vitro* curves at 37°C (solid line) and 22°C (dashed line). Dotted line from *P–V* data, or from bubbles expressed directly from lung; 22° or 37°C.

unstable whenever compressed below γ_{eq} (Tierney, 1965; Tierney and Johnson, 1965). In earlier studies where film stress relaxation was reported at room temperature (Clements *et al.*, 1961), this feature was not particularly disturbing, because the time constant of 30–60 minutes (Fig. 9) was not incompatible with the time course of changes in lung compliance in artificially ventilated animals (Mead and Collier, 1959). However, the data at 37°C, where the time constants were measured in seconds or minutes (Fig. 9) (confirmed by Schoedel *et al.*, 1969; Lempert and Macklem, 1971; Slama *et al.*, 1971), have made it difficult to imagine how low γ could ever be maintained *in vivo*. The problem was approached via *P–V* measurements (Horie and Holdebrandt, 1971; Horie *et al.*, 1974) by recording stress (pressure) relaxation at several fixed volumes on deflation limbs, at temperatures of 22°, 37°, and 47°C. These authors reasoned that if γ rose quickly by amounts such as the 20 dynes reported in the literature, then recoil pressure should recover in the order of 6 cm H_2O in the same time periods. They found instead an almost negligible pressure recovery *in situ* of less than 1 cm H_2O (Fig. 9), and the recovery was furthermore virtually independent of temperature. These data suggested that with respect to film stability, lung wash was *grossly* different from lung lining. This conclusion was confirmed by the droplet studies of Schürch *et al.* (1976), who noted that at a fixed volume (functional residual capacity, FRC), γ remained less than 9 mN/m for 30 minutes, and rose only about 1 mN/m per 20 minutes.

B. Natural Selection

A possible explanation for the discrepancy might, as Bachofen *et al.* (1970) suggested, be a difference in predominant molecular species in the two systems. Goerke and Clements (1973) have shown that pure dipalmitoylphosphatidylcholine (DPPC) could stably withstand compression to less than 5 mN/m at temperatures up to 41°C, above which it appeared to "melt." Perhaps the surface layer *in situ* is somehow able to extrude or exclude other constituents, selectively retaining DPPC, as Schürch *et al.* (1976) suggest.

1. Nonselective Adsorption

"Natural selection" was recently given persuasive support in a stimulating article by Clements (1977). He was led to this conclusion after noting that the lung lining (*P–V* data) in several important respects resembles purified surfactant (*in vitro*) only during *inflation* from the gas-free state, but better resembles DPPC during *deflation*. The main lines of evidence may be summarized as follows. First, King and Clements (1972) had found the time constant for *adsorption* of purified surfactant from subphases *in vitro* to be short, e.g., 10 minutes, whereas this time for DPPC was exceedingly long. Furthermore, the adsorption process was nearly independent of temperature (*T*) from 10° to 45°C. Similarly, the time constant for stress relaxation in rat lungs at 50% TLC after inflation from the degassed state was found to be short (about 2 minutes) and nearly independent of *T*. Clearly, the parallel between adsorption dynamics of surfactant and whole lung relaxation on the inflation limb is suggestive of a common mechanism. Perhaps many species of phospholipids are able to adsorb nonselectively to the air interface and do so in a short period of time. This interpretation may be complicated by the fact that, on the first inflation curve, not all the pressure decay in whole lungs need be due to lining dynamics (adsorption), because gradual alveolar recruitment and airway opening, plus tissue relaxation, are proceeding concurrently.

2. Selective Escape

Clements (1977) goes on to show that the converse process to adsorption—*escape*—bears a different parallel to lung properties. As previously emphasized, it is physiologically important to be able to maintain low γ for long periods of time if alveolar stability is to be preserved. The pressure recovery experiments described above (Horie *et al.*, 1974) demonstrated this to be the case in the lung, whereas purified surfactant failed to hold a low value. On the other hand, DPPC *did* behave properly, having a very long time constant for escape of more than 200 seconds at 37°C. Clements (1977) also pointed out that the admixture of unsaturated lipids or cholesterol to DPPC greatly accelerated the escape process, shortening the time constant to much less than 1 minute at 37°C. A notable temperature dependence was observed, the escape process having a Q_{10} of about

5. Consequently, Clements was tempted to conclude that the lung lining was *converted predominately to DPPC upon deflation from TLC.* Formidable steps remain to be explained, such as how the selection process occurs so readily on the alveolar surface, but poorly *in vitro.* Perhaps the mysterious apoproteins (King, 1977) play a role. On the other hand, *in vitro* experiments may simply serve as a poor model of phospholipid escape *in situ,* where the volume of the subphase is minute, and its physical state and composition may not favor diffusion.

C. The Thermal Transition of DPPC

Clements (1977) has pointed out one other fascinating parallel between the properties of DPPC and "deflation surfactant." When Ps (from rat lungs, after a 2 minute equilibration at an FRC of 40% TLC) was plotted against temperature, an interesting thermal transition appeared around 41°C in the deflation limb (Fig. 10A). Near this temperature, hysteresis (pressure difference between inflation and deflation limbs) became relatively small over the span of just a few degrees by virtue of a right-shift in recoil of the deflation limb. The parallel with a fairly sharp "melting" of DPPC mentioned above was striking, whereas purified surfactant shows a very broad temperature transition (Fig. 10B). Again, DPPC corresponds

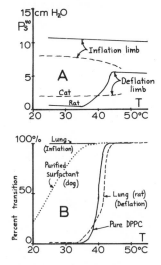

Figure 10. Temperature dependence of surface tension. A: Ps from inflation and deflation limbs of rat lung at 40% TLC, showing thermal transition above 41°C. B: Comparison of thermal transitions of lung, purified surfactant, and pure DPPC.—, Clements (1977); ---, Haire *et al.* (1974).

well to lung lining during deflation. The correspondence shown in Fig. 10 between "inflation lining" and purified dog surfactant is not so satisfying. Furthermore, temperature data from cat lung (Horie *et al.*, 1974) failed to show a transition on the deflation limb, but did suggest a gradual transition above 37°C on the inflation curves (lower recoil at higher temperature), roughly opposite to the findings reported in rats (Fig. 10A). Nevertheless, the suggestion made by Clements (1977) offers some hope of gaining a clearer insight into the complex mechanisms at work at the normal alveolar surfaces:

> When we breathe in, they may liquefy, and surface tension may increase to levels slightly above equilibrium; when we exhale to FRC, the surfaces may turn into almost pure, solid DPPC, decreasing surface tension nearly to zero and defending our lungs against atelectasis. In each cycle, a little surfactant may be used up and be removed and replaced.

VI. DEPLETION OF THE LINING MATERIAL

The final sentence of the above quotation from Clements (1977) serves to introduce another unsettled topic. It seems quite reasonable to claim that somehow "a little surfactant may be used up" by each inflation–deflation cycle. However, the background of this suggestion derives from a fairly controversial and interesting area of surfactantology.

The Stiff Lung

1. Metabolic Factors

In 1965, Schoedel reported a somewhat unusual effect: Deeply ventilating an excised lung led to a rapid fall in compliance. He interpreted the fall to be indicative of mechanical changes in the surfactant. Faridy *et al.* (1966) quite independently investigated the same phenomenon, feeling that the change represented a *depletion* of surfactant, and that recovery of normal high compliance depended on metabolically dependent synthesis or release of new surfactant. Their interpretation was supported by the observation that recovery required warming *and* the presence of O_2 in the lung. Subsequently, it was shown that other metabolic inhibitors such as KCN and iodoacetate also inhibited recovery (Katz *et al.*, 1971). On this basis the metabolic hypothesis gained and held favor. It should be remembered that in the hands of some investigators, neither N_2 nor KCN in lungs inhibited recovery (Gruenwald, 1966; Lingelbach *et al.*, 1968). On these grounds, Lingelbach *et al.* (1968) proposed that aerobic cell metabolism played an unimportant role, that folding or film condensation could take place instead, and that recovery could be readily explained by new spreading of inactivated materials. However, the latter dissident results were generally regarded as anomalies which would hopefully fall into the metabolic schema eventually.

2. *Physical Factors*

The phenomenon has been reexamined recently in several studies, with results consistently supporting Schoedel's original "change of state" hypothesis. (Perhaps the metabolic data may now be viewed as anomalous, which hopefully will be resolved in time!) Horie *et al.* (1978) undertook a comprehensive reinvestigation of factors affecting lung stiffening and recovery in rabbit lungs. They confirmed the basic requirements for stiffening established by others, namely, "room temperature," low end-expiratory pressure (zero is most effective), and large tidal volume (50% TLC works well). With respect to recovery, warming to body temperature was also confirmed to be essential, but the presence of O_2 was *not*. Excised lungs *could* be made stiff at body temperature provided they were edematous, in this case by virtue of saline absorption through the pleura, and these lungs were nonrecovering. Edema evidently led to changes different or considerably more drastic than those brought about by ventilation alone. Nagao *et al.* (1977) examined the temperature dependence of stiffening in greater detail. They discovered a sharp transition region in the vicinity of 26°C, above which stiffening would *not* occur in normal lungs. The transition bore some resemblance to the sharp thermal transition for pure DPPC described by Goerke and Clements (1973), albeit occurring some 15°C lower than the DPPC transition. In another study, Nagao *et al.* (1978) compared the rheological properties of normal and stiff lungs. They were struck by the similarity of the stress relaxation and tidal hysteresis areas (minor loops) seen on the inflation limb of normal lungs and those seen on the inflation *and* on a large part of the deflation limbs after stiffening. In terms of Clements' (1977) "self-purification" hypothesis, the lining behaved like a mixed film over the majority of the $P-V$ cycle, as though deficient in the major stabilizing constituent (DPPC). Perhaps only at low lung volumes was the surface area reduced sufficiently to display the effects of the remaining DPPC.

The picture emerging is that below 26°C the DPPC fraction may aggregate when highly compressed by low end-expiratory volumes and not be replaced rapidly enough by adsorption from the subphase. The DPPC may thus be "depleted" from the interface by a relatively small number of breathing cycles (e.g., 100–500). The rate of depletion is greater the farther the lungs are cooled (Sugiyama *et al.*, 1978), apparently signifying additional diminution of molecular mobility or surface fluidity. If this model is correct, recovery should only take as long as is required to attain temperatures greater than 26°C. Sugiyama *et al.* examined this possibility by recording $P-V$ curves of stiff lungs after successively shorter periods of warming by immersion in saline of various temperatures. In a 37°C bath, deflation curves had returned to near normal within 5–10 minutes. In a 28°C bath, recovery was slower, probably because of the fact that rewarming through the pleura occurred with a smaller temperature gradient. These processes were not affected by the absence of O_2. The "physical" model of surfactant depletion does not rule out slow loss of surface material via airways, consumption by macrophages, etc., whose replacement by metabolically dependent processes certainly must occur. In other words, the physical stiffening mechanism applies to a short time scale; depends almost entirely on ventilatory parameters, temperature, and state of hydration, but operates against the background of gradual surfactant turnover which is dependent on oxidative pathways.

VII. EFFECTS OF SURFACE TENSION ON PULMONARY VASCULAR RESISTANCE AND INTERSTITIAL PRESSURE

Pattle's original paper (1955) stressed the physiological importance of low interfacial tension in the lung in terms of preventing alveolar filling with fluids. He reasoned that should γ become high the suction created at alveolar curvatures would draw fluid from capillaries into alveoli. In addition to affecting capillary transudation, the fluid interstitial pressure might also be expected to help determine the diameters of capillaries and extraalveolar vessels. This is because the total (net) perivascular pressure is the sum of two components: that due to solid elements, and another due to the fluid pressure permeating the solids. Negative or zero fluid interstitial pressures would tend to minimize the interstitial volume, thus permitting maximum vascular distention. On the other hand, positive fluid pressures favor interstitial swelling and would permit vascular narrowing as perivascular cuffs or sleeves develop. Finally, the solid pressure is itself partly dependent on surface tension, for the presence of an interface causes configurational changes both gross (airway and alveolar duct dimensions) and fine (alveolar wall). These additional effects of surface tension in the lung will now be briefly discussed.

A. Pulmonary Vascular Resistance

1. Dependence on Alveolar Pressure

The now familiar concept of vascular "zones" in the lung (West et al., 1964; Hughes et al., 1968) implies a rather simple model of viscous and

Starling resistances in the pulmonary circulation. The site of vascular collapse (the waterfall of Permutt *et al.*, 1961) is presumably at the capillary level. West *et al.* (1964) defined the lung region where alveolar pressure (P_{alv}) exceeded pulmonary arterial pressure (Pa) as Zone I. This region (the apices in upright man) would be virtually unperfused because the capillary transmural pressure there is negative, at least as defined by $Pa - P_{alv}$. In Zone II, P_{alv} is less than Pa, but partial collapse could occur at the outflow ends of the capillaries (Banister and Torrance, 1960). In both Zones I and II the venous pressure (P_V) is less than P_{alv}. Waterfall conditions occur in Zone II, because variations in P_V are not reflected in any changes in flow. In Zone III P_V exceeds P_{alv} such that all capillaries are distended and the Starling flow-limiting mechanism does not operate.

One would therefore anticipate that as the lung is inflated and P_{alv} increases, so Pa would need to be increased proportionally to maintain a given flow. Furthermore, Pa should exceed P_{alv} by an amount equal to the pressure drop along the arterial vessels. This "extraalveolar" resistance reaches a minimum near midlung volume as these vessels expand in width, but before lengthening and narrowing at higher volumes. Indeed, Banister and Torrance (1960) reported an almost equal rise in Pa per increase in tracheal pressure (P_{alv}). However, the problem becomes rapidly more complex (and interesting) when these vascular–lung mechanical interrelationships are examined more closely. Figure 11 shows data replotted from the work of Bruderman *et al.* (1964). Pa is shown as a function of the volume (V) and inflation pressure (P_{alv}) of their isolated lungs. Venous outflow pressure (P_V) was zero (base of lung), and

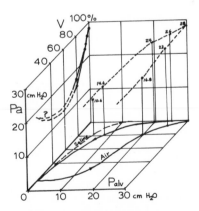

Figure 11. Dependence of pulmonary artery pressure, Pa, on alveolar inflation pressure, P_{alv}, and lung volume, V. The line in space (dashed) lies on a surface describing the relationship at one fixed flow rate (50 ml/minute, dog lungs). Projection of the surface onto the Pa–V plane gives an almost single-valued function. (Data of Bruderman *et al.*, 1964.)

flow rate of perfusate (saline) was constant. The dependence of P_{alv} on V is determined by the lung's mechanical properties, except for a small interaction with Pa (Frank *et al.*, 1959). Thus, Pa becomes the dependent variable. One notices that, on the deflation limb, Pa generally does exceed P_{alv} as required by the idea of an alveolar capillary sluice. On the other hand, Pa is always 2–3 cm H_2O less than P_{alv} on the major inflation limb. Furthermore, Pa was measured from the base of the lungs, such that mean Pa would actually be several cm H_2O less than the values shown, thus serving to further widen the gap between Pa and P_{alv}. Lloyd and Wright (1960) also concluded that flow continued in regions of lung where P_{alv} exceeded Pa by at least 5 cm H_2O.

The data on the inflation limb in Fig. 11 are difficult to explain. Alveolar surface tension seems to be acting in such a way that it *distends* capillaries. The morphology of alveolar septa generally reveals capillaries as bulging *into* the gas space, implying that γ would have the opposite effect. Spherical alveoli would develop the proper curvature to be consistent with the findings. Although the "grape" model has not been supported for many years, it may be that the blood vessels situated at alveolar intersections (corner vessels) which *are* effectively distended by surface tension play an important role in these experiments. This concept would require that their resistance be both significant and in series with the main bed. In other words, even when most capillaries in the septa are squeezed off by the alveolar "pressure clamp," the increased resistance in the total capillary segment would still have to be relatively small and perhaps be offset by a decreased corner resistance.

2. *Dependence on Lung Volume*

Another important feature about the mechanics of the pulmonary vasculature may be noted from Fig. 11. Although Pa clearly depends on lung *volume* (the surface generated by the data points rises along the V axis), there is only a small slope along the P_{alv} axis, signifying lack of dependence between the variables Pa and P_{alv}. In fact, when the surface is projected onto the $Pa–V$ plane, an essentially single-valued function is obtained. This is all the more surprising, because the range of Pa covers the span from well below P_{alv} to well above it. It is in the neighborhood of $Pa = P_{alv}$ that, on the basis of the action of the capillary pressure clamp, one would expect the greatest influence of P_{alv} on blood flow. The implication is that vascular resistance is determined almost entirely by lung *distention*, irrespective of the pressure required to effect lung expansion.

The generality of this conclusion (from Fig. 11) is limited by the fact that only the upper lung volumes were carefully explored by Bruderman *et al.* (1964). However, a partial extension of the idea to lower volumes may be deduced from the results of Thomas *et al.* (1961a,b). Figure 12 shows three views of paths on the mathematical surface relating the independent variable, in their case the pulmonary vascular resistance (R) to V and P_{pl}. In their apparatus lungs were inflated by negative pleural pressure (P_{pl}) rather than positive P_{alv}. Also, instead of maintaining a fixed flow as in Fig. 11, they maintained Pa a fixed level (20 cm H_2O) above P_{alv}. Under these conditions capillary collapse caused by the pressure clamp could not occur. Nevertheless, geometric distortion of both alveolar and extraalveolar vessels would take place, and one might expect that large differences in γ between inflation and deflation (hysteresis) should exert some effect on vascular geometry. Figure 12A shows the $P-V$ hysteresis of one of their excised dog lungs. This may be regarded as a view looking down on the $R-V-P_{pl}$ surface. Next, Fig. 12B looks at the same surface from the "front," in other words, as a projection on the $R-P_{pl}$ plane. The obvious "dependence" of R on P_{pl} in this plane might tempt one to conclude that γ exerted a marked effect on R. However, Thomas *et al.* (1961a,b) also made a "side" view of the surface, with some unexpected results (Fig. 12C). The $R-V$ relation was almost single valued, implying that the surface was *flat* along the P_{pl} axis (cf. Fig. 11). The dependence of R on P_{pl} was therefore illusory. They further showed that $R-V$ data from saline-filled lungs fell within the range obtained from air-filled lungs. At low lung volumes the elevated resistance could be explained by a narrowing of large vessels (interdependence), and perhaps by increased tortuosity including that of alveolar vessels. At high lung volumes all vessels would be lengthened and narrowed, leading to great geometrical distortion and a sharply increasing resistance.

A note of caution concerning comparability of data is in order. The resistance of the pulmonary circuit is known to be highly nonlinear as indicated earlier, being a function of V, Pa, P_V, and perhaps P_{alv}. Thus, a

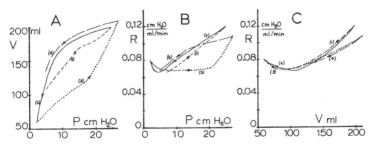

Figure 12. Dependence of pulmonary vascular resistance, R, on pleural pressure and volume of excised dog lungs. Projections of the surface on three planes are shown. (Data of Thomas *et al.*, 1961.)

single R–V function does not exist: Other flow conditions would produce other relationships. A thorough study of all variables has not been reported. The piecemeal approach, although experimentally practical and capable of defining the general features of the system, nevertheless requires lengthy qualitative discussions comparing results whenever new data are presented, or whenever old data are interpreted in a new light.

To summarize, from the fact that lung recoil is increased as γ increases (thus necessitating a higher P_{alv} to inflate the lungs), and from the fact that the fragile capillaries lie within alveolar walls, one would conclude that blood flow should diminish or cease, at a given lung volume V and driving pressure Pa, as γ is varied from 0 up to γ_{max}. These two extremes in γ should be represented by saline-filled lung and inflation curve of air-filled lung, respectively. The evidence reviewed supports only a weak dependence. The negative finding raises a number of very important questions relating to vascular anatomy and transmission of pressures and stresses within the parenchyma. One implication would be that lung "zones" are not sharply definable in terms of relative magnitudes of Pa, P_{alv} and P_V. Perhaps the local *volume* gradients from apex to base in upright humans and the resultant gradient of resistance, coupled with the hydrostatic gradient in Pa, are the primary determinants of local perfusion, rather than Pa in relation to P_{alv}.

B.   Interstitial Pressure

Some aspects of this fascinating question have been raised earlier in connection with saline effects on lung recoil. The magnitude of the pressure in the interstitial spaces remains unsettled, both in peripheral tissue as well as in the lung. Evidence for negative interstitial pressure has been presented (e.g., Guyton *et al.*, 1976), as it has for zero or slightly positive pressure (Wiederhielm, 1972; Staub, 1977). The following discussion will focus on possible ways in which surface tension might influence interstitial pressures.

Based on several arguments, it seems likely that pressures negative with respect to alveolar pressure do exist locally in the lung. Whether these are transmitted to sites of vascular permeability where they might influence transudation is at present unclear.

1.   *Peribronchial and Perivascular Pressure*

The least controversial loci of negative pressure are the peribronchial and perivascular spaces. These have for some time been recognized as the sites of initial fluid accumulation in pulmonary edema (Staub *et al.*, 1967),

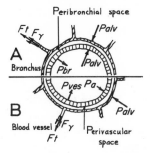

Figure 13. Peribronchial and perivascular forces. A: Peribronchial membrane is under radial traction from tissue attachments, Ft, and surface forces, F_γ. Intrabronchial pressure is balanced by alveolar pressure. B: Blood vessels are subject to similar forces, except intravascular pressure varies independently of P_{alv}.

implying that pressure there is least. Figure 13 depicts diagramatically the forces involved. In the case of the bronchus, P_{alv} is applied to both the intraluminal and extraluminal surfaces, thus having virtually no net effect. The remaining balance of forces equates the recoil of the airway (P_{br}) to the radial pressures ($Pt + P\gamma$) developed by tissue and surface forces, respectively. At low lung volume the size of the airway may exceed the size of the parenchymal "hole" which it effectively replaces, in which case the outward peribronchial pressure would be less than pleural pressure. At high lung volumes the converse may be true. [In the absence of bronchial tone, as in excised dog lungs, the resting bronchial size may exceed this "hole" size even near TLC (T. Takishima, personal communication)]. At any rate, the peribronchial pressure is likely to be generally negative, and more so as γ increases. The peribronchial *fluid* pressure could be much *more negative* than this, because the solid elements in the space might well be quite compressed.

Perivascular pressure is subject to exactly parallel treatment, with the important distinction that transluminal pressures will not as a rule cancel. At the base of the lung Pa may be much greater than P_{alv}, thus distending the vessel; at the apex, $Pa \simeq P_{alv}$. On this basis, perivascular pressure at the lung bases would tend to be less negative than peribronchial pressure. However, the unstressed sizes of the vessels, relative to the size of the "hole," and vascular compliance, could significantly affect the final balance of forces. However, the kerosene experiments of Howell *et al.* (1961), and the latex experiments of Macklin (1946), do suggest that large vessels are distended by inflation, that the perivascular pressure would be almost always negative, and increasingly negative as transpulmonary pressure is increased by lung inflation or by loss of surface activity.

2. Parenchymal Interstitial Pressure

Another site where pressure is virtually certain to be negative is the alveolar corner (see Figs. 6 and 14). Whenever $\gamma > 0$, the corner pressure is negative in the amount γ/r (up to $2\gamma/r$ where two curvatures exist). If $\gamma = 5mN/m$, and $r = 10\,\mu m$, P becomes -5 cm H_2O. With lung expansion γ might increase five- to tenfold, and r decrease because of thinning of the alveolar fluid lining layer. As a result, P could readily fall to -25 cm H_2O, or even less. Fluid pressures such as these would, if directly transmitted to capillary walls, have important (perhaps catastrophic) effects on trans-capillary fluid fluxes. If the anatomical structures between subphase and immediate pericapillary spaces acted as a *rigid* semipermeable membrane, hydrostatic pressures from the subphase would not be transmitted to fluid pockets in the interstitial space (Fig. 14). The relative protein concentrations, reflection coefficients, etc., would determine the steady-state fluid interstitial pressure. However, the interstitial space is capable of swelling; therefore, the membranes are not rigid, and subphase pressure could theoretically be transmitted. In fact, interstitial fluid pressure could be even *more* negative than subphase pressure if the solid interstitial elements (fibers, gel) were under compression. The latter picture is consonant with the view of Guyton *et al.* (1976) of pulmonary interstitial mechanics. The interstitial space would be kept "dry," and the solid elements conceivably under compression, by such forces as the lymphatic pump. It would be capable of forcing fluid "uphill" from a region where hydrostatic pressure might be -10 cm H_2O, to the less negative pleural cavity. Some reabsorption of fluid into the lower pressure venules could also occur.

On the other hand, the negative corner pressure could be dissipated in other ways to entirely prevent its appearance in the interstitial space. For example, if sharp corners became more rounded by tissue distortion when

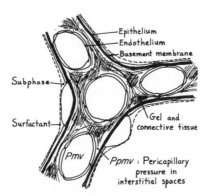

Figure 14.   Schematic representation of parenchymal interstitial space.

γ increased, two effects would result. First, the greater radius of curvature would lessen the negative pressure developed. Second, solid elements at the corners could be placed under tension (negative solid pressure). Consequently, one cannot predict *a priori* what the influence of surface tension on interstitial pressure will be. The implanted capsules developed in Guyton's laboratory (Meyer *et al.*, 1968) could be sensing a true negative interstitial pressure. However, the capsules could also be coupled to the subphases of adjacent alveoli, in which case corner pressure would be sensed. At this point in time it appears reasonable only to say that, because edema fluid (presumably leaked from parenchymal capillaries) accumulates in peribronchial spaces, the parenchymal interstitial pressure should be *less* negative than peribronchial pressure, and the latter is perhaps in the order of pleural pressure (all pressures considered with respect to alveolar pressure).

3. *Transudation*

A number of predictions can be made from the hypothesis that interstitial pressure becomes more negative as γ increases. For example, transcapillary fluid flux should increase after surfactant depletion. Albert *et al.* (1977) have recently tested this prediction using an isogravimetric technique. A lobe of a living dog was suspended by a sling to allow continuous weighing. Lobar artery and vein were connected to a reservoir whose height could be adjusted until lobe weight remained constant. In the control state, at a transpulmonary pressure (TPP) of 30 cm H_2O, isogravimetric Pa (P_{isog}) was equal to P_{alv}. After stiffening the lung by cooling and depleting surfactant, TPP at the same lung volume was increased to 50 cm H_2O, and P_{isog} became 14 cm H_2O less than P_{alv}. This result was interpreted to signify that interstitial pressure had become 14 cm H_2O more negative, and that capillary pressure must be reduced by an equal amount to maintain zero fluid flux. One would certainly agree that peribronchial and perivascular pressures become more negative, although the effect on parenchymal interstitial pressure is less certain (see above). However, a secondary fall in interstitial pressure could result if fluid were drawn out of parenchyma to form cuffs by the more negative pressure in perivascular and peribronchial spaces. This interpretation reaches the same conclusion as did Albert *et al.* (1977), albeit via an indirect mechanism. The sites of leakage in their experiment may actually have been at venules and arterioles (capillaries could have been collapsed by a transmural gradient of 14 cm H_2O), whose perivascular pressures may be more directly affected by increased parenchymal traction. In this case, distant drainage need not be involved.

Nakahara *et al.* (1976) have also reported the results of some iso-gravimetric experiments. Their dog lobes were inflated to 5 cm H_2O, at which volume P_{isog} was found to be 4 cm H_2O higher than P_{alv}. Combining these results with those of Albert *et al.* (1977) gives the plot shown in Fig. 15 (solid line). Although the data are sparse, a clear trend emerges: At low TPP (low γ) a small positive capillary pressure is needed to balance the remaining osmotic and hydrostatic forces, whereas at high γ a definitely negative capillary pressure must be applied. If the oncotic pressures are the same in the three cases shown, the interstitial pressure must become more negative with increasing γ in order to balance the falling capillary pressure. An estimate of interstitial pressure may be made as follows. The net fluid filtration out of vessels is described by

$$\dot{Q}_f = K[(P_{mv} - P_{pmv}) - \sigma(\Pi_{mv} - \Pi_{pmv})]$$

where subscripts *mv* denote microvascular and *pmv* perimicrovascular, Π is osmotic pressure, σ is the reflection coefficient, and K is conductance. Under isogravimetric conditions, $\dot{Q}_f = 0$, $P_{mv} \equiv P_{isog}$, and the equation simplifies to $P_{pmv} = P_{isog} - \sigma(\Pi_{mv} - \Pi_{pmv})$. Taking $\Pi_{mv} \approx 32$ and $\Pi_{pmv} \approx 18$ (Staub, 1977), one obtains $P_{pmv} = P_{isog} - 14\sigma$. This equation is plotted in Fig. 15 for $\sigma = 0.3$, 0.5, and 1.0. If $\sigma = 1.0$, then $P_{pmv} \approx -10$ cm H_2O at FRC, compatible with capsule data (Guyton *et al.*, 1976). On the other hand, Wangensteen *et al.* (1977) have found σ to be between 0.3 and 0.5

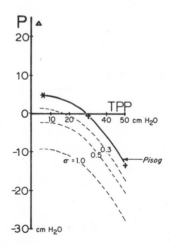

Figure 15. Plot of isogravimetric pressure, P_{isog}, as function of transpulmonary pressure (solid line). Dashed lines are computed perimicrovascular pressures assuming various reflection coefficients, σ. Δ:Guyton and Lindsey (1959); *:Nakahara *et al.* (1976); +:Albert *et al.* (1977);– –: P_{pmv} (relative to P_{alv}).

for adult rabbit lungs. In this case P_{pmv} would be only very slightly negative at mid lung volumes, approach -7 cm H_2O near TLC, and reach -15 to -18 cm H_2O with abnormally high surface tensions. These estimates are subject to uncertainties in Π_{pmv} and σ, and to verification of the preliminary data for P_{isog}. Furthermore, as already mentioned, the P_{isog} measured may be greatly influenced by the most negative pressure locus (peribronchial and perivascular) and only indirectly reflect perimicrovascular pressure.

A final point about isogravimetric experiments may be made. In isolated lungs lymph flow can usually be taken as negligible. As a result, the normal flushing of protein (mainly albumin) from the interstitial space is absent, allowing equilibration of osmotic forces between interstitium and plasma. As a result, P_{isog} may be less than in an intact situation. Lymphatic function in the study of Albert *et al.* (1977) was not assessed. On the other hand, in the presence of good lymphatic flow, a net positive driving force (higher P_{isog}) would be the rule, rather than a zero balance producing no transcapillary fluid flux. These factors complicate the interpretation of isogravimetric data. For example, Fig. 15 shows the critical value of left atrial pressure determined by Guyton and Lindsey (1959), above which pulmonary edema occurs. This could be thought of as the highest P_{isog} compatible with the capacity of the lymphatics to clear transudate. In other words, P_{isog} may range from a low value where steady-state $\dot{Q}_f = 0$, to much higher values where steady-state $\dot{Q}_f$ is equal to maximal lymph flow.

VIII. SUMMARY AND CONCLUSIONS

It may at first seem discouraging to realize that what we really ''know'' concerning the action of surface tension in lungs, and the factors affecting the magnitude of this tension, is small compared to the number of questions and uncertainties remaining to be resolved. On the other hand, one might be encouraged somewhat by the fact that at least it is possible to write at some length upon the subject, and more often than not, to reach into the literature for illuminating data. The field may be described as passing through a stage of ''enlightened ignorance.'' But even this is a tremendous advance, because we may be at the point where most of the reasonable or possible hypotheses concerning each problem area have been thought about. Furthermore, we are now in the position where bounds can usually be placed on most quantities. The broad outline of the role of surface tension in lung and vascular mechanics seems fairly reliable. Narrowing the bounds and completing many of the remaining steps may not be easy, as judged by the painful rate of progress over the past 20 years.

APPENDIX: MODEL OF ANISOTROPIC EXPANSION OF ALVEOLAR DUCT

A simplified model will be considered which illustrates the phenomenon of tissue distortion caused by surface tension effects. Pressure–volume (P–V) relations may be replaced by force–length (F–L) for ease of presentation without influencing the argument. Alveolar septa are represented by a wet elastic sheet, and the fibrous elastic bundles at the alveolar mouth by a spring (Fig. 16). Neglect hysteresis in all elements, and take γ to be constant. Assume that compressive stresses for folding and buckling are negligible, and that below the resting length of the sheet the surface tension cannot exert a retractive force (i.e., area does not decrease during wrinkling).

The analysis can best be carried out graphically. For simplicity, assign linear material properties to the spring and the dry sheet, as shown in Fig. 17 (solid lines). Because the two elements are in series, the total length is the sum of the individual lengths, added horizontally. This sum would represent the "saline" curve. Next, add $F\gamma$ due to surface tension to the sheet (forces add vertically), and then again add lengths of spring and sheet. The resultant F–L curve would represent the "air" curve. Subtracting saline from air gives "F_s," an estimate of surface forces. It is immediately apparent that F_s does not accurately estimate F_γ. However, following the procedure employed in P–V analysis, set $dW_s = F_s dL = \gamma\, dA$, and, assuming isotropy ($A = KL$), then $dA = K\, dL$. Therefore, $\gamma = F_s/K$, showing that γ would be computed to be simply proportional to F_s. We may not know the internal structure of the system; thus it is necessary to guess γ_{max}. Like F_γ, the F_s curve is constant beyond L_1, the inflection point of the air curve, so that a proper choice of γ_{max} could, over this range, give reliable estimates of γ. However, the true F_γ curve rises

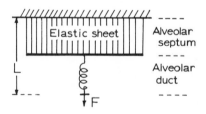

Figure 16.   Two-dimensional model of alveolar duct mechanics.

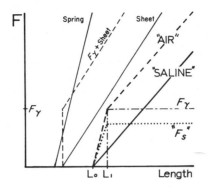

Figure 17. Graphical analysis of force–length relationships of the duct model (see text).

abruptly from zero at L_1, unlike F_s. Increasing the spring compliance further lowers the plateau value of F_s, and widens the sloping ramp segment of F_s as L_1 moves to the right. The region between L_0 (resting length) and L_1, where only spring extension occurs, therefore gives quite misleading information about γ. Indeed, if one takes γ proportional to F_s, one might suspect that γ falls to zero below L_1. It is the sharp deviation from isotropy which underlies the erroneous conclusion in this interval, i.e., dA/dL is not constant during the extension, as might be assumed.

An extension of this model to include nonlinear elastic elements emphasizes the point. Figure 18 shows again the material properties in solid lines, and their sum as the "saline" curve. Sheet and spring are made piecewise linear for simplicity. Next, surface forces are added in parallel with the sheet as before, giving the "air" curve. "F_s" is found by subtracting saline from air curves. Making the assumption of isotropy as above leads to γ proportional to F_s. We would therefore see an *apparent*

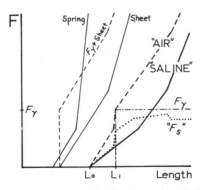

Figure 18. Graphical analysis of the model when force–length characteristics of the elastic elements are nonlinear. Surface tension is assumed constant (see text).

gradual reduction in surface forces toward minimal volume, whereas γ was actually being held fixed throughout. If the sheet becomes much less extensible than the spring (example partially illustrated), F_s shows a *fall* near TLC, similar to the foregoing fall near L_0. Many possibilities concerning duct distortion resulting from various combinations of material properties exist, leading to many possible F_s curves. However, a detailed knowledge of dL/dA would always allow one to calculate γ from F_s, correctly.

ACKNOWLEDGMENTS

I am indebted to Ken Beck, Hiroshi Inoue, Yih-Loong Lai, Steve Scherba, Yasuo Tsuya, and Dean Wilson for critical readings and suggestions.

This work was supported by research grants HL 14854 and HL 20773 from the National Institute of Health.

REFERENCES

Albert, R. K., S. Lakshminarayan, and J. Butler (1977). Increased surface tension favors pulmonary edema. *Clin. Res.* (in press).

Avery, M. E., and J. Mead (1959). Surface properties in relation to atelectasis and hyaline membrane disease. *Am. J. Dis. Child.* **97,** 517–523.

Bachofen, H., J. Hildebrandt, and M. Bachofen (1970). Pressure–volume curves of air- and liquid-filled excised lungs—Surface tension *in situ. J. Appl. Physiol.* **29,** 422–431.

Banister, J., and R. W. Torrance (1960). The effects of the tracheal pressure upon flow: Pressure relations in the vascular bed of isolated lungs. *Q. J. Exp. Physiol.* **45,** 352–367.

Bienkowski, R., and M. Skolnick (1974). On the calculation of surface tension in lungs from pressure–volume data. *J. Colloid. Interface Sci.* **48,** 350–351.

Brown, E. S. (1957). Lung area from surface tension effects. *Proc. Soc. Exp. Biol. Med.* **95,** 168–170.

Brown, E. S., R. P. Johnson, and J. A. Clements (1959). Pulmonary surface tension. *J. Appl. Physiol.* **14,** 717–720.

Bruderman, I., K. Somers, W. K. Hamilton, W. H. Tooley, and J. Butler (1964). Effect of surface tension on circulation in the excised lungs of dogs. *J. Appl. Physiol.* **19,** 707–712.

Clements, J. A. (1957). Surface of lung extracts. *Proc. Soc. Exp. Biol. Med.* **95,** 170–172.

Clements, J. A. (1962). Surface phenomena in relation to pulmonary function. *Physiologist* **5,** 11–28.

Clements, J. A. (1977). Functions of the alveolar lining. *Am. Rev. Respir. Dis.* **115,** 67–71.

Clements, J. A., E. S. Brown, and R. P. Johnson (1958). Pulmonary surface tension and the mucus lining of the lungs: Some theoretical considerations. *J. Appl. Physiol.* **12,** 262–268.

Clements, J. A., R. F. Hustead, R. P. Johnson, and I. Gribetz (1961). Pulmonary surface tension and alveolar stability. *J. Appl. Physiol.* **16,** 444–450.

Cook, C. D., J. Mead, G. L. Schreiner, N. R. Frank, and J. M. Craig (1959). Pulmonary mechanics during induced pulmonary edema in anesthetized dogs. *J. Appl. Physiol.* **14**, 177–186.

D'Angelo, E. (1972). Local alveolar size and transpulmonary pressure *in situ* and in isolated lungs. *Respir. Physiol.* **14**, 251–266.

Faridy, E. E., S. Permutt, and R. L. Riley (1966). Effect of ventilation on surface forces in excised dogs' lungs. *J. Appl. Physiol.* **21**, 1453–1462.

Farrell, P. M., and M. E. Avery (1975). Hyaline membrane disease. *Am. Rev. Respir. Dis.* **111**, 657–688.

Forrest, J. B. (1970). The effect of changes in lung volume on the size and shape of alveoli. *J. Physiol. (London)* **210**, 533–547.

Frank, N. R., E. P. Radford, Jr., and J. L. Whittenberger (1959). Static volume–pressure interrelations of the lungs and pulmonary blood vessels in excised cats' lungs. *J. Appl. Physiol.* **14**, 167–173.

Frazer, D. G., and K. C. Weber (1976). Trapped air in ventilated excised rat lungs. *J. Appl. Physiol.* **40**, 915–922.

Fukaya, H., C. J. Martin, A. C. Young, and S. Katsura (1968). Mechanical properties of alveolar walls. *J. Appl. Physiol.* **25**, 689–695.

Fung, Y. C. (1975a). Stress, deformation, and atelectasis of the lung. *Circ. Res.* **37**, 481–496.

Fung, Y. C. (1975b). Does the surface tension make the lung inherently unstable? *Circ. Res.* **37**, 497–502.

Gil, J., and E. R. Weibel (1972). Morphological study of pressure–volume hysteresis in rat lungs fixed by vascular perfusion. *Respir. Physiol.* **15**, 190–213.

Goerke, J., and J. A. Clements (1973). Relative stability of air/water films of palmitoyl, myristoyl- and dipalmitoyl-phosphatidyl-cholines at 37°C. *Physiologist* **16**, 323.

Gruenwald, P. (1966). Effect of age on surface properties of excised lungs. *Proc. Soc. Exp. Biol. Med.* **122**, 388–392.

Guyton, A. C., and A. W. Lindsey (1959). Effect of elevated left atrial pressure and decreased plasma protein concentration on the development of pulmonary edema. *Circ. Res.* **7**, 649–657.

Guyton, A. C., A. E. Taylor, R. E. Drake, and J. C. Parker (1976). Dynamics of subatmospheric pressure in the pulmonary interstitial fluid. *Lung Liquids, Ciba Found. Symp.* **38**, (New Ser.), 77–96.

Hildebrandt, J. (1974). Anatomy and physics of respiration. *Physiol. Biophys.* **2**, 297–324.

Hoppin, F. G., Jr., and J. Hildebrandt (1976). Mechanical properties of the lung. *In* "Lung Biology in Health and Disease" (C. Lenfant, ed.), Vol. 3, pp. 83–162. Dekker, New York.

Horie, T., and J. Hildebrandt (1971). Dynamic compliance, limit cycles, and static equilibria of excised cat lung. *J. Appl. Physiol.* **31**, 423–430.

Horie, T., R. Ardila, and J. Hildebrandt (1974). Static and dynamic properties of excised cat lung in relation to temperature. *J. Appl. Physiol.* **36**, 317–322.

Horie, T., R. Ardila, K. Nagao, and J. Hildebrandt (1978). Recovery of normal recoil in excised rabbit lungs after repeated inflation. *J. Appl. Physiol.* (in press.)

Howell, J. B. L., S. Permutt, D. F. Proctor, and R. L. Riley (1961). Effect of inflation of the lung on different parts of pulmonary vascular bed. *J. Appl. Physiol.* **16**, 71–76.

Hughes, J. M. B., J. B. Glazier, J. E. Maloney, and J. B. West (1968). Effect of lung volume on the distribution of pulmonary blood flow in man. *Respir. Physiol.* **4**, 58–72.

Katz, P., D. Gail, and D. Massaro (1971). Metabolic factors affecting lung surfactant function. *Clin. Res.* **19**, 54.

King, R. J. (1977). Metabolic fate of the apoproteins of pulmonary surfactant. *Am. Rev. Respir. Dis.* **115**, 73–79.

King, R. J., and J. A. Clements (1972). Surface active materials from dog lung. II. Composition and physiological correlations. *Am. J. Physiol.* **223**, 715–726.

Klingele, T. G., and N. C. Staub (1970). Alveolar shape changes with volume in isolated, air-filled lobes of cat lung. *J. Appl. Physiol.* **28**, 411–414.

Lempert, J., and P. T. Macklem (1971). Effect of temperature on rabbit lung surfactant and pressure–volume hysteresis. *J. Appl. Physiol.* **31**, 380–385.

Lingelbach, E., R. Rüfer, and C. Stolz (1968). Die Abhängigkeit der Oberflächenkräfte isolierter Rattenlungen von Atmung, Temperatur und Stoffwechwel. *Pfluegers Arch.* **304**, 315–321.

Lloyd, T. C., Jr., and G. W. Wright (1960). Pulmonary vascular resistance and vascular transmural gradient. *J. Appl. Physiol.* **15**, 241–245.

Macklem, P. T. (1971). Airway obstruction and collateral ventilation. *Physiol. Rev.* **51**, 368–436.

Macklin, C. C. (1946). Evidences of increase in the capacity of the pulmonary artery and veins of dogs, cats, and rabbits during inflation of the freshly excised lung. *Rev. Can. Biol.* **5**, 199–210.

Mead, J., and C. Collier (1959). Relation of volume history of lungs to respiratory mechanics in anesthetized dogs. *J. Appl. Physiol.* **14**, 669–678.

Mead, J., T. Takishima, and D. Leith (1970). Stress distribution in lungs: A model of pulmonary elasticity. *J. Appl. Physiol.* **28**, 596–608.

Meyer, B. J., A. Meyer, and A. C. Guyton (1968). Interstitial fluid pressure. V. Negative pressure in the lungs. *Circ. Res.* **22**, 263–271.

Nagao, K., R. Ardila, M. Sugiyama, and J. Hildebrandt (1977). Temperature and hydration: Factors affecting increased recoil of excised rabbit lung. *Respir. Physiol.* **29**, 11–24.

Nagao, K., R. Ardila, and J. Hildebrandt (1978). Rheological properties of excised rabbit lungs stiffened by repeated hyperinflation. *J. Appl. Physiol.* (in press.)

Nakahara, K., P. D. Snashall, and N. C. Staub (1976). Isogravimetric microvascular pressure in the isolated perfused dog lung lobe: An estimate of perimicrovascular tissue pressure. *J. Physiol.* (*London*) **265**, 34P–35P.

Pattle, R. E. (1955). Properties, function and origin of the alveolar lining layer. *Nature* (*London*) **175**, 1125–1126.

Pattle, R. (1977). The relation between surface tension and area in the alveolar lining film. *J. Physiol.* (*London*) **269**, 591–604.

Permutt, S., B. Bromberger-Barnea, and H. N. Bane (1961). Alveolar pressure, pulmonary venous pressure and the vascular waterfall. *Med. Thorac.* **19**, 47–68.

Radford, E. P., Jr. (1954). Method for estimating respiratory surface area of mammalian lungs from their physical characteristics. *Proc. Soc. Exp. Biol. Med.* **87**, 58–61.

Reifenrath, R. (1975). The significance of alveolar geometry and surface tension in the respiratory mechanics of the lung. *Respir. Physiol.* **24**, 115–137.

Reifenrath, R., and I. Zimmerman (1973). Surface tension properties of lung alveolar surfactant obtained by alveolar micropuncture. *Respir. Physiol.* **19**, 369–393.

Schoedel, W. (1965). Einflüsse von Beatmung und Zigarettenrauch auf das statische Druck–Volumen-Diagramm isolierter Rattenlungen. *Pfluegers Arch. Gesamte Physiol. Menschen Tiere* **284**, 176–183.

Schoedel, W., H. Slama, and E. Hansen (1969). Zeitabhängige Veränderungen des Filmdruckes alveolarer Oberflächenfilme im Langmuir-Trog. *Pfluegers Arch.* **306**, 20–32.

Schürch, S., J. Goerke, and J. A. Clements (1976). Direct determination of surface tension in the lung. *Proc. Natl. Acad. Sci. U.S.A.* **73**, 4698–4702.

Slama, H., W. Schoedel, and E. Hansen (1971). Bestimmung der Oberflächen-eigenschaften von Stoffen aus den Lungenalveolen mit einer Blasenmethode. *Pfluegers Arch.* **322**, 355–363.

Staub, N. C. (1977). Extravascular forces in lung affecting fluid and protein exchange. *Am. Rev. Respir. Dis.* **115**, 159–163.

Staub, N. C., H. Nagano, and M. L. Pearce (1967). Pulmonary edema in dogs, especially the sequence of fluid accumulation in lungs. *J. Appl. Physiol.* **22**, 227–240.

Sugihara, T., C. J. Martin, and J. Hildebrandt (1971). Length–tension properties of alveolar wall in man. *J. Appl. Physiol.* **30**, 874–878.

Sugiyama, M., S. Nishijima, K. Nagao, and J. Hildebrandt (1978). Effect of temperature on lung volumes, recoil, and in recovery after hyperventilation. (Submitted for publication).

Thomas, L. J., Jr., Z. J. Griffo, and A. Roos (1961a). Effect of negative-pressure inflation of the lung on pulmonary vascular resistance. *J. Appl. Physiol.* **16**, 451–456.

Thomas, L. J., Jr., A. Roos, and Z. J. Griffo (1961b). Relation between alveolar surface tension and pulmonary vascular resistance. *J. Appl. Physiol.* **16**, 457–462.

Tierney, D. F. (1965). Pulmonary surfactant in health and disease. *Dis. Chest* **47**, 247–253.

Tierney, D. F., and R. P. Johnson (1965). Altered surface tension of lung extracts and lung mechanics. *J. Appl. Physiol.* **20**, 1253–1260.

Tsunoda, S., H. Fukaya, T. Sugihara, C. J. Martin, and J. Hildebrandt (1974). Lung volume, thickness of alveolar walls, and microscopic anistropy of expansion. *Respir. Physiol.* **22**, 285–296.

von Neergaard, K. (1929). Neue Auffassungen über einen Grundbefriff der Atemmechanik. Die Retraktionskraft der Lunge, abhängig von der Oberflächenspannung in den Alveolen. *Z. Gesamte Exp. Med.* **66**, 373–394.

Wangensteen, O. D., E. Lysaker, and P. Savaryn (1977). Pulmonary capillary filtration and reflection coefficients in the adult rabbit. *Microvasc. Res.* **14**, 81–97.

West, J. B., C. T. Dollery, and A. Naimark (1964). Distribution of blood flow in isolated lung; relation to vascular and alveolar pressures. *J. Appl. Physiol.* **19**, 713–724.

Wiederhielm, C. A. (1972). The interstitial space. *In* "Biomechanics. Its Foundations and Objectives" (Y. C. Fung, N. Perrone, and M. Anliker, eds.), pp. 273–286. Prentice-Hall, Englewood Cliffs, New Jersey.

Young, S. L., D. F. Tierney, and J. A. Clements (1970). Mechanism of compliance change in excised rat lungs at low transpulmonary pressure. *J. Appl. Physiol.* **29**, 780–785.

SUBJECT INDEX

A

Acetazolamide, potential difference vs. pH and, 180
Acid-base abnormalities, extracellular fluid and, 168
Acid-base balance, oxygen supply and, 93
Acid-base values, for ectotherms, 118
Acidosis, metabolic or lactic, 32
Adenosine triphosphate
  ammonia levels and, 78
  in glutamine formation, 76
Aerobic metabolic rate, 31–32
Air, oxygen replacement in, 100
Air-breathers
  altered ambient gas composition and, 98–100
  humans as, 98–99
Air-breathing ectotherms, respiratory control in, 93–126
  see also Ectotherms
Air-breathing vertebrates, adaptation of to aquatic life, 94–98
Air convection requirement, for ectotherms, 120
Airway stability, 270
  see also Lung
Alligator, arterial P_{CO_2} values for, 102
Alligator mississippiensis, 102, 105, 117
Alveolar CO concentration, 207–208
Alveolar disappearance curves, for carbon monoxide, 209
Alveolar duct
  anisotropic expansion of, 292–294

configuration of, 273
  two-dimensional model of, 292
Alveolar gas, airway continuity and, 263
Alveolar shape, lung surface tension and, 272
Alveolar stability, 268–270
Alveolar surface area, calculation of, 264–266
  see also Lung; Lung surfactant mechanism
Alveolar surface tension
  bubbles and balances in, 266–267
  computed, 267
  hexagonal array of, 263
  interdependent, 268
  polyhedral, 268–270
Ama calva, 99
Ammonia
  asterixis and, 72
  and brain nucleic acids, 76
  in cardiac failure, 72
  in chronic obstructive pulmonary disease, 69–72
  in citrate α-ketoglutarate conversion, 74–75
  gastrointestinal tract as source of, 80–81, 86
  in glucose and pyruvate metabolism, 74
  hypercapnia and, 83
  in Krebs cycle, 73–74
  metabolic changes and, 78–79
  metabolic effects of, 73–80
  neural toxicity of, 70

Bufo marinus, 124
Bulbar poliomyelitis, 131
Bulbopontine pacemaker, 16
Bullfrog
  gas exchange in, 97
  skin CO_2 conductance and loss in, 125

C

Carbon dioxide
  in ammonia infusion in sinoaortic
    chemodenervated animal, 84–85
  ectotherm response to, 107
  as humoral exercise stimulus, 49–50
  interpulmonary, 107
  ventilatory response to, 70
  as ventilatory stimulus in exercise, 54–55
Carbon dioxide changes, in humoral exercise, 48–50
Carbon dioxide concentration, respiration
  rate and, 19
Carbon dioxide pressures, lumbar vs. cisternal, 169
Carbon dioxide responses and receptors, in
  ectotherms, 104–109
Carbon dioxide sensitivity, of sleeping respiratory system, 139–140
Carbon monoxide
  alveolar disappearance curves for, 209
  in placental O_2 transfer, 201–204
Cardiac failure, ammonia level and, 72
Carotid body chemoreceptors, 7
Carrier-mediated transport
  see also Placental O_2 transfer; Pulmonary
    CO transfer
  Fick principle and, 198
  identity of carrier in, 210–214
  of oxygen and carbon monoxide, 198–210
  permeation rate vs. partial pressure in,
    206–210
  physiological importance of, 214–215
Catecholamines, and excess ventilation in
  severe exercise, 58
Caudal medulla, 8–9
  in ventilatory control, 6–10
Caudal pons
  apneustic center and, 10
  transection of, 14
Central circulation, pressure changes in,
  47–48

Central nervous system
  integration of chemoreceptor stimuli by,
    15–23
  ventilation regulation by, 1–25
Cerebral blood flow
  cerebral ECF acidity and, 187–188
  cerebrospinal fluid arterial P_{CO_2} and,
    173–175
Cerebral extracellular fluid
  hydrogen in homeostasis of, 167–189
  regulation of, 168–177
Cerebral extracellular fluid acidity, cerebral
  blood flow regulation and, 187–188
Cerebral hemispheres, ventilation increase
  and, 52
Cerebrospinal acid-base measurement, 170
Cerebrospinal bicarbonate, in respiratory
  acidosis, 185–186
Cerebrospinal fluid
  acid-base measurements in, 168, 170–171
  and active transport of bicarbonate to
    blood, 178
  ammonia level of, 73, 76–77
  cerebral venous P_{CO_2} and, 170–172
  changes in composition of, 107
  "charged membrane hypothesis" and,
    172
  cisternal, 169, 171
  exercise stimulus and, 47
  passive distribution of bicarbonate from
    blood to, 181–182
  pH of, 177–178
  plasma bicarbonate changes and, 182–185
  regulation of carbon dioxide pressure in,
    168–177
Cerebrospinal fluid-arterial P_{CO_2}
  arterial acidity and, 175–176
  cerebral blood flow and, 173–175
Cerebrospinal fluid bicarbonate concentration, regulation of, 177–187
Cerebrospinal fluid-blood potential difference, 179–181
Cerebrospinal fluid glutamine, hypercapnia
  and, 72–73
Cerebrospinal fluid intermediate metabolites, ammonia level and, 79–80
Cerebrospinal fluid-specific mechanism, lactic acid and, 184
Charged membrane hypothesis (Wien effect), 172, 186–187
Chelona mydas, 95, 103–104, 108

A
B
C 8
D 9
E 0
F 1
G 2
H 3
I 4
J 5